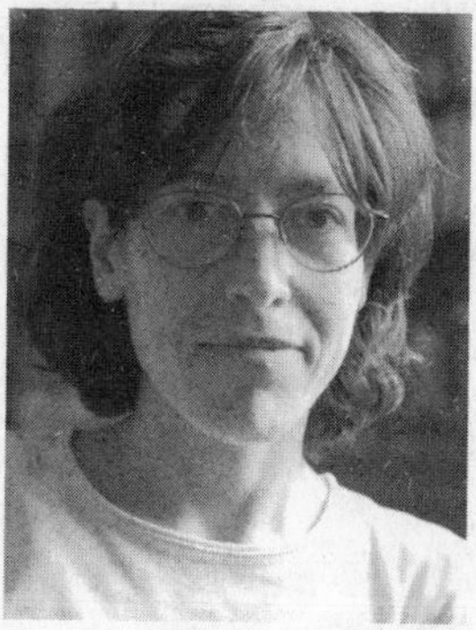

Peter Peter

Helen Epstein writes frequently on public health for various publications, including *The New York Review of Books* and *The New York Times Magazine*.

ADDITIONAL PRAISE FOR *THE INVISIBLE CURE*

Amazon.com #1 Science Book of 2007

"Intelligent and judicious . . . A reliable primer on the African epidemic."

—*Newsday*

"Courageous and thought provoking . . . Not only a book that should be required reading for people concerned in the least with AIDS or with Africa; it is also compulsively readable."

—*The New York Review of Books*

"Vivid descriptions of personalities, anecdotes, and organizations . . . [Epstein's] careful reporting and passionate stance make this book well worth reading."

—*Foreign Affairs*

"Epstein has done a great service to humanity by reminding us that complacency and knee-jerk assumptions do more harm than good."

—*National Catholic Reporter*

"An excellent primer on the complicated relationship between American medical science and philanthropy and the public health crisis in Africa . . . Reminds American readers that while good intentions are necessary, they're rarely enough."

—*Commonweal*

"Lucid, scientifically accurate, and well-referenced, *The Invisible Cure* is in many ways more informative than any multimillion-dollar international AIDS conference or collection of regression analyses in a peer-reviewed journal."

—*Population and Development Review*

"Provides vital insights into this ongoing tragedy . . . reminds us of our common humanity and our moral obligation to help people who share dreams and aspirations similar to our own lives of peace and mutual respect."

—*Chattanooga Times Free Press*

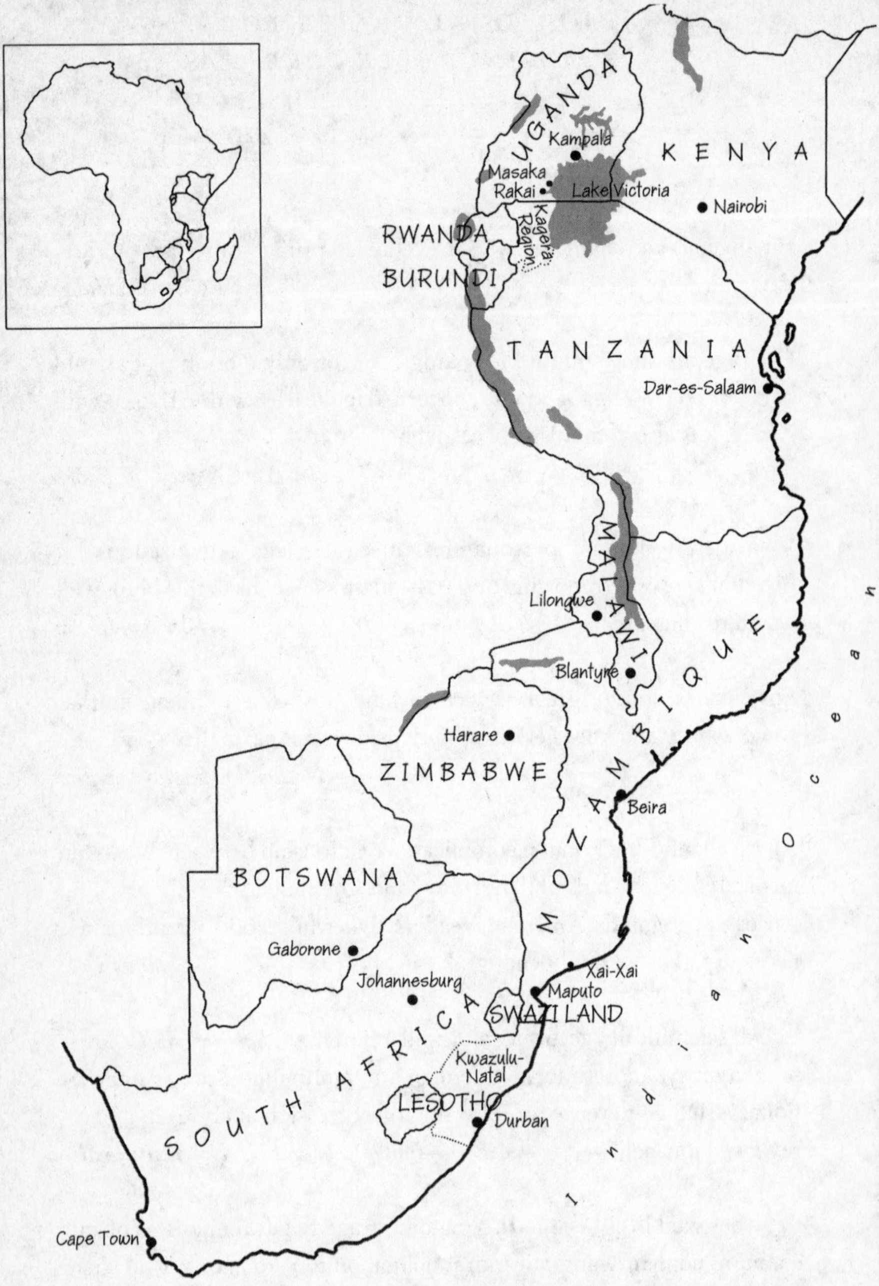

EAST AND SOUTHERN AFRICA

THE INVISIBLE CURE

Why We Are Losing the Fight Against AIDS in Africa

HELEN EPSTEIN

Picador
Farrar, Straus and Giroux
New York

To my mother, Barbara
In memory

www.picadorusa.com

Picador® is a U.S. registered trademark and is used by Farrar, Straus and Giroux under license from Pan Books Limited.

For information on Picador Reading Group Guides, please contact Picador.
E-mail: readinggroupguides@picadorusa.com

Designed by Robert C. Olsson

ISBN-13: 978-0-312-42772-6
ISBN-10: 0-312-42772-7

First published in the United States by Farrar, Straus and Giroux

10 9 8 7 6 5 4 3

AIDS has come to haunt a world that thought it was incomplete. Some wanted children, some wanted money, some wanted property, some wanted power, but all we have ended up with is AIDS.

—*Bernadette Nabatanzi, traditional healer*
Kampala, Uganda, 1994

CONTENTS

THE FRONT LINES

PREFACE

One morning in November 2001, two officials from a Kenyan AIDS organization picked me up from my hotel in Nairobi and took me on a drive. We drove and drove all day, over muddy tracks, through endless pineapple and coffee plantations, rural villages and slums, through all of Africa, it seemed, to arrive at a small field, perhaps half an acre, with some weeds growing in it and an old woman standing there with a hoe.

I had not expected this. I was reporting on AIDS programs for an American foundation, and most of the other projects I had visited were either medical programs, AIDS awareness campaigns using billboards, radio or television spots, or traveling roadshows designed to promote AIDS awareness or condoms or HIV testing. I was about to say something when one of my guides spoke first.

"We are very proud of this project."

So I said nothing. About twenty women had saved up for two years to buy this land. All of them were supporting orphans whose parents had died of AIDS, and they hoped the land would produce enough food for about fifty people in all. On a nearby hill, one of Kenya's vast corporate-owned coffee plantations loomed like the edge of the sea. The old woman kept glancing at it as though it might sweep her away. I was moved by what I saw, although I didn't understand at the time how this project was supposed to fight AIDS. This book explains how I came to do so.

The worldwide AIDS epidemic is ruining families, villages, businesses, and armies and leaving behind an immense sadness that will linger for generations. The situation in East and southern Africa is uniquely severe. In 2005, roughly 40 percent of all those infected with HIV lived in just eleven countries in this region—home to less than 3 percent of the world's population.[1] In Botswana, Lesotho, and Swaziland, roughly a quarter of adults were infected, a rate ten times higher than anywhere else in the world outside Africa. In other world regions, the AIDS epidemic is largely confined to gay men, intravenous drug users, commercial sex workers, and their sexual partners. But in East and southern Africa, the virus has spread widely in the general population, even among those who have never engaged in what health experts typically consider high-risk behavior and whose spouses have not done so either. Although there were predictions that HIV would soon spread widely in the general population in Asia and eastern Europe, this has yet to occur, even though the virus has been present in those regions for more than two decades. The UN AIDS Program now predicts it probably never will.[2]

Why is the epidemic in East and southern Africa so severe? And why has it been so difficult to control? I started thinking about this in 1993, when I quit a postdoctoral job in molecular biology at the University of California and went to Uganda to work on an AIDS vaccine project. My results, like those of many others, were disappointing.

For more than twenty years, scientists have been trying to make such a vaccine, and most experts predict it will take at least another decade.[3] The editor of Britain's prestigious medical journal *The Lancet* has even suggested that a truly effective AIDS vaccine may be a biological impossibility.[4]

I continued to work on AIDS as a writer and consultant for various development agencies after I left Uganda, and I continued to wonder about what might be done to arrest the epidemic, and whether some other device or program might substitute for a vaccine. In 1996, a combination of three antiretroviral drugs, taken for life, was found to dramatically relieve the symptoms and extend the lives of HIV-positive people. At the time, these drugs were patented and extremely expensive, and for years they were out of reach of the millions of poor African patients who needed them. Before long, a worldwide network of AIDS activists began to pressure pharmaceutical companies to cut the prices of these drugs and urged international donors to raise billions of dollars to fund AIDS treatment programs in developing countries. As a result, millions of Africans with HIV are now receiving treatment.

In this book, I do not deal at length with this extraordinary struggle, a story that has been ably covered by other writers, some of whom are activists themselves.[5] While the humanitarian urgency of AIDS treatment programs is inarguable, these drugs will not halt the epidemic on their own. They are not a cure, they don't work for everyone, and they can have severe side effects. In Africa, those most likely to spread the virus to others are often at an early stage of infection and are not in need of treatment. In many cases, their infections may not even be detectable by HIV tests.[6] Because Africa's health-care infrastructure is in such a dire state, treatment programs are expensive and difficult to administer, even when the drugs themselves are practically free. Those who do receive treatment can expect to gain, on average, only 6.6 years of life because the virus eventually develops resistance, necessitating second- and third-line treatment, presently all but unavailable in Africa.[7] It is impossible to put a price on six years of anyone's life, least of all that of an African mother whose children would otherwise be orphaned, so the international community must endeavor to expand the range of AIDS drugs available in Africa. However, it would be better by far if that mother had never become infected in the first place.[8]

To date, the closest thing to a vaccine to prevent HIV is male circumcision, which was shown in 2006 to reduce the risk of HIV transmission by roughly 70 percent.[9] The widespread practice of male circumcision in the predominantly Muslim countries of West Africa may largely explain why the virus is so much less common there than it is along the eastern and southern rim of the continent. It is urgent that as many men as are willing to undergo the procedure have access to cheap, safe circumcision services. But it may take years to develop such services and in the meantime, millions of people will become infected. In any case, HIV infection rates may be quite high, even in West African cities where nearly all men are circumcised.[10]

As international concern about the epidemic has grown, along with foreign-aid budgets for programs to fight it, a global archipelago of governmental and nongovernmental agencies has emerged to channel money, consultants, condoms, and other commodities to AIDS programs all over the world. During the past decade, I have visited dozens of these programs and spoken to hundreds of people. I never found a panacea, but I did learn a great deal. I learned, for example, that AIDS is a social problem as much as it is a medical one; that the virus is of recent origin, but that its spread has been worsened by an explosive combination of historically rooted patterns of sexual behavior, the vicissitudes of post-colonial development, and economic globalization that has left millions of African people adrift in an increasingly unequal world. Their poverty and social dislocation have generated an earthquake in gender relations that has created wide-open channels for the spread of HIV. Most important, I came to understand that when it comes to saving lives, intangible things—the solidarity of ordinary people facing up to a shared calamity; the anger of activists, especially women; and new scientific ideas—can be just as important as medicine and technology.

Like many newcomers to Africa, I learned early on that the most successful AIDS projects tended to be conceived and run by Africans themselves or by missionaries and aid workers with long experience in Africa—in other words, by people who really knew the culture. The key to their success resided in something for which the public health field currently has no name or program. It is best described as a sense of solidarity, compassion, and mutual aid that brings people together to solve a common problem that individuals can't solve on their own. The closest thing to it might be Harvard sociologist Felton Earls's concept of "collective efficacy," meaning the capacity of people to come together and help others they are not necessarily related to. Where missionaries and aid workers have, intentionally or not, suppressed this spirit, the results have been disappointing. Where they have built on these qualities, their efforts have often succeeded remarkably well.

It's easy to be pessimistic about Africa. Headlines from the continent chronicle apparently endless war, tyranny, corruption, famine, and natural disaster, along with a few isolated nature reserves and other beauty spots. Certainly there are many war-torn countries in Africa and many poor, sick people who need assistance. But sometimes helplessness is in the eye of the beholder. There is also another Africa, characterized by a striking degree of reciprocity, solidarity, and ingenuity. Time and again,

African people have relied on these qualities to save themselves—and at one time, the entire human family—from extinction. Now, faced with the scourge of AIDS, some of them, including the farmer I met in Kenya, are trying to do so again.

Most of the black Africans who now live in the region covered in this book are descended from Bantu farmers who began migrating from western Africa several thousand years ago, across the continent and then south.[11] On the way, some of them encountered other African population groups—the San and Khoi of southern Africa and the Nilotes of the Sahel, for example—with whom they exchanged aspects of language and culture and with whom they sometimes intermarried. Subgroups splintered off from each other and adapted to local circumstances.

Their story is, with some exceptions, not about the accumulation of great personal fortunes and the founding of cities with palaces, cathedrals, and libraries. It is a story of relatively small groups banding together to survive on a harsh and dangerous frontier, of natural disasters and political and economic crises.

Survival was not inevitable. The ancient, infertile soils of Africa could not sustain large permanent farming settlements, and the development of towns was further prevented by infectious diseases that spread rapidly as soon as populations reached a certain threshold. When farmers cleared large tracts of land to grow crops, malaria bloomed in the sunlit mud; as herds expanded, the animals succumbed to tuberculosis and sleeping sickness, which spread to their owners.

Faced with such a mutable, dangerous world, the people of East and southern Africa developed a genius for local improvisation, adapting to life in forests, deserts, or lakesides. Cut off by the Sahara from the developing technologies of Europe and Asia, they were forced to innovate and developed their own methods of agriculture, iron smelting, and mining. In a world without the apparent consolations of property and bureaucratic institutions, a powerful sense of spirituality provided moral order and solace to the suffering.[12] Few groups developed writing, but they relied on drumming, the patterns woven into cloth and beadwork, and their prodigious memories to transmit information and an ever-changing repertoire of stories and myths.

On the harsh African frontier, you were nowhere without other people, and this is still the case, even though the crises facing the continent are very different and constantly changing. It is almost impossible to be truly alone in Africa, and this has a profound effect on how people see the world and act in it. In remote villages, the poorest families will invite strangers into their houses and won't let them leave until they have eaten an enormous meal. Most Africans I know live in households that swarm with a vast and changing cast of inhabitants, including grown offspring, nieces, nephews, poor relations, aged aunts and uncles, and innumerable children. You would need a spreadsheet to establish who is related to whom and how.

These societies, wrote the historian Basil Davidson, "enclosed relations between people within a moral framework of intimately binding force. . . . an intense and daily interdependence that we in our day seldom recognize, except in moments of postprandial afflatus or national catastrophe. The good of the individual was a function of the good of the community, not the reverse."[13]

This sense of solidarity has a downside when it contributes to tribalism and social rigidity, but it can also be a source of power and creativity, and it has been at the heart of the region's most successful responses to AIDS.

What I didn't know when I was in Uganda in the early 1990s was that something remarkable was happening there. During the 1990s the HIV infection rate fell by some 60 percent in the arc of territory along the northern and western shores of Lake Victoria, an area comprising southern Uganda and the remote Kagera region of Tanzania. This success, unique on the continent at the time, saved perhaps a million lives. It was not attributable to a pill or a vaccine or any particular public health program, but to a social movement in which everyone—politicians, preachers, women's rights activists, local and international health officials, ordinary farmers, and slum dwellers—was extraordinarily pragmatic and candid about the disaster unfolding in their midst. This response was similar to the spontaneous, compassionate, and angry AIDS activism of gay men in Western countries during the 1980s, when HIV incidence in this group also fell steeply.[14] Why has such a response been so slow to emerge elsewhere? The complete answer may never be known, but in this book, I suggest that outside of Uganda and Kagera, health officials misunderstood the nature of the AIDS epidemic in this region, in particular why the virus was spreading so rapidly in the general population. As a result, the programs they introduced were less effective than they might have been and may have inadvertently reinforced the stigma, shame, and prejudice surrounding the disease.

Much of the stigma and confusion surrounding AIDS has to do with its common association with perceived "irresponsible" or "immoral" sexual behavior. However, what many people—from policy-makers, to public health experts, to ordinary African people at risk—did not realize is that most HIV transmission in this region results from normative sexual behavior, practiced by large numbers of people. It's not that African people have more sexual partners, over a lifetime, than people in Western countries do—in fact, they generally have fewer.[15] However, in many African communities, both men and women are more likely than people in other world regions to have more than one—perhaps two or three—overlapping or "concurrent" long-term partnerships at a time. A man may have two wives, or a wife and girlfriend, and one of those women may have another regular partner, who may in turn have one or more other partners and so on. This "long-term concurrency" differs from the "serial monogamy" more common in western countries, and the casual and commercial "one-off" sexual encounters that occur everywhere. But long-term overlapping relationships are far more dangerous than serial monogamy, because they link people into a giant network that creates a virtual superhighway for HIV.[16]

Concurrent sexual partnerships have strong cultural, social and economic roots in East and Southern Africa, and this has made fighting HIV very difficult. Fifteen years of vigorous condom promotion in many African towns and cities has had little effect on the epidemic, probably because most transmission occurs in long term relationships in which condoms are seldom used. As family planning experts have known for decades, people use condoms mainly in casual and commercial relationships, and inconsistent condom use offers poor protection against either pregnancy or STD transmission in long term relationships.

Urging African people to abstain or be faithful has its limitations too, because most people are faithful already, if not to one person, then to two or three. Many of those at highest risk of infection are the faithful partners of men or women with only one other trusted long-term partner; others are in mutually faithful relationships, in which one partner had concurrent partners in the past.

In this book, I argue that the key to the success of Uganda's early AIDS campaigns was that Ugandans, like the gay men of San Francisco and New York and like the Thai men of Bangkok, knew where their risks were coming from, and this made it easier for them to respond pragmatically. Although Ugandan public health officials didn't know the word "concurrency" they did know that the virus was spreading in relatively ordinary families and relatively ordinary relationships and that it wasn't just a problem for "promiscuous" people alone. This made it possible for everyone to speak more openly about how HIV had devastated their lives and to regard those affected by the disease with greater compassion. This openness in turn led people to take obvious steps to protect themselves.

Outside of Uganda, most AIDS prevention campaigns in Africa were for years aimed almost exclusively at so-called "high risk groups"—meaning prostitutes, truckers, soldiers, and other rootless, migrant men. Such an approach made sense in the rest of the world, where HIV remains largely concentrated in "high risk groups." But in East and Southern Africa, the concurrency "superhighway" puts virtually everyone at risk, from cabinet ministers to the women selling tomatoes on the street, even if they are not typically "promiscuous."

Much has been written about the lessons of Uganda's early success against AIDS, not all of it in agreement, either with the interpretation advanced here or with other interpretations. This is partly because the evidence for what happened in Uganda, and what it meant for billions of dollars in AIDS prevention funding, soon became the object of a tug-of-war between researchers and policy makers on the left and right of the political spectrum. Health officials on both sides interpreted the data in their own ways, and used their conclusions to support programs they favored. We will never know whether lives could have been saved had these policies been based on the evidence for what actually occurred in Uganda, but it is possible that this partly explains why fighting AIDS in Africa has been so difficult, and it may also suggest a way forward.

The AIDS epidemic is finally beginning to subside in many African countries, owing to increasing awareness and commonsense changes in sexual behavior. This is heartening, but it is possible that many lives might have been spared had policymakers better understood the nature of the epidemic early on.

Much of this book is concerned with donor-funded AIDS programs that failed in some way, beginning with my own vaccine project. I tell these stories not with a sense of satisfaction. I could not have done better myself at the time. But in science, failures are often as important as successes, because they tell us where the limits are. Only by looking honestly at our mistakes can we hope to overcome them. When it comes to fighting AIDS, our greatest mistake may have been to overlook the fact that, in spite of everything, African people often know best how to solve their own problems. They have been doing so throughout human history. Had they not succeeded, I would not be here to write these words, nor would you be here to read them.

A NOTE ON THE STATISTICS CITED IN THIS BOOK

Throughout this book, I refer to various statistical entities, including "HIV rate," "HIV prevalence," and "HIV incidence." "HIV rate" and "HIV prevalence" are synonyms meaning "the proportion of people in a given population who are HIV positive at a given time." In Africa, these figures usually refer only to adults aged fifteen to forty-nine, the group assumed to be most sexually active. Thus, to say that "the HIV rate in Uganda was 18 percent in 1992" means that 18 percent of adults aged fifteen to forty-nine were HIV positive in 1992. "In 1992, HIV prevalence in Uganda was 18 percent" means exactly the same thing.

HIV incidence is a measure of the speed at which HIV spreads. It refers to the proportion of people in a given population who contract HIV during a given time interval, usually one year. Thus, to say that "HIV incidence was 4 percent in 1987" means that 4 percent of the adult population contracted HIV that year. "HIV incidence in Kagera fell by 75 percent between 1987 and 1993" means that 75 percent fewer people contracted HIV in Kagera in 1993 than in 1987.

Most of the statistics cited in this book come from UN documents, the U.S. Demographic and Health Surveys, or the scientific literature. Most figures are derived from two different types of surveys, antenatal clinic surveys and population-based surveys. These two types of surveys sometimes give different results. Antenatal surveys tend to lead to higher overall prevalence estimates because pregnant women are by definition at higher risk because they have recently had unprotected sex. Also, HIV infection rates in Africa tend to be higher among women than men. Why this is the case is not entirely known. Women are not physically more vulnerable to infection than uncircumcised men are, and women also have fewer partners then men. One possible explanation is that when long term concurrent partnerships are common, an individual's risk of infection depends less upon her own behavior than on that of her partner.[1]

ANTENATAL SURVEYS

Antenatal surveys are based on tests of blood samples drawn from pregnant women in antenatal (or prenatal) clinics. As part of routine antenatal care, pregnant women are tested for syphilis and other conditions. In Africa, selected hospital labs are designated "HIV surveillance sites." At these labs, some of the women's blood samples are randomly selected to be tested for HIV, and the fraction found to be positive provides a rough measure of the HIV infection rate among sexually active women of childbearing age in the catchment area of the hospital. These surveys are usually conducted each year in selected African hospitals. They thus provide information not only about the HIV rate at a given time, but also about changes in the epidemic from year to year.

The dire condition of health services in many African countries means most women deliver their babies in their homes, not in hospitals. However, this does not significantly reduce the accuracy of antenatal HIV surveys because the vast majority of pregnant women attend a health clinic for antenatal care at some point during their pregnancies, even in the poorest African countries.[2]

Antenatal surveys are completely anonymous. The blood samples that arrive in the lab are labeled only with the women's ages and the hospital's name. There is no way of tracing a sample to a given woman, so neither the woman nor doctors and nurses nor lab technicians nor anyone else knows whether she is positive or not. Her confidentiality is thus entirely protected. A growing number of clinics in Africa now offer HIV counseling and testing for women who wish to know their HIV status.

The prevalence of HIV infection in pregnant teenagers aged fifteen to nineteen is sometimes used as a rough measure of the incidence of new infections in a population. This is because few children below age fifteen are HIV positive (see below), so most cases of infection in pregnant teens are assumed to have occurred recently.

POPULATION SURVEYS

Population surveys measure the HIV rate in the general population—including men, nonpregnant women, children, and the elderly, as well as pregnant women. These surveys are usually conducted by teams of researchers who go from house to house in a given area collecting blood or saliva samples that are then tested for HIV. In most cases, participants are offered the chance to learn their results or are referred to voluntary testing and counseling services.

Population surveys provide information about which population groups are most vulnerable to HIV. For example, they have shown that in East and southern Africa, HIV rates are higher among women than among men, while the opposite is the case in the rest of the world. Sub-Saharan Africa is also home to 90 percent HIV-positive children. Without antiretroviral drug treatment roughly 25 percent of babies born to HIV-positive women inherit the virus. Most of these children die of AIDS by age five, although a growing number are now being kept alive longer with AIDS treatment. HIV rates among children aged six to fifteen are extremely low, but then rise rapidly among sexually active teens.[3] Some population surveys are conducted annually, and this allows researchers to calculate the incidence of new infections in a given population.

HIV statistics are often regarded with skepticism. All statistics should be questioned, whether they refer to the chance of rain tomorrow, the proportion of dentists who recommend chewing gum, or the prevalence of HIV in Africa. However, HIV infection is one of the most accurately measured diseases in Africa. In many countries, we know far more about the HIV/AIDS situation than we do about malaria, measles, postpartum hemorrhage, or other serious public health problems.

But mistakes do happen. In 2004, demographers at UNAIDS discovered an error in the analysis of antenatal surveillance data that led to an overestimation of HIV in some rural areas in Africa. Since a large fraction of the population of sub-Saharan Africa resides in rural areas, this led to a downward revision of the UNAIDS HIV prevalence estimates in many countries by 25 to 40 percent. For example, in 1992, Uganda's HIV rate was estimated to be 30 percent, but the correction put the figure at roughly 20 percent. The error arose from the fact that the surveillance clinics used to estimate HIV prevalence in rural areas were actually located in towns and trading centers that had a distinctly urban character. Since HIV rates tend to be higher in urban areas, this led to an overestimation of HIV prevalence in rural Africa. The problem was corrected and now UNAIDS's estimates correspond well with those of population-based surveys, such as the U.S. Agency for International Development's demographic and health surveys.[4]

THE FUTURE OF THE GLOBAL AIDS EPIDEMIC

Estimates of the future course of the AIDS epidemic vary widely and are far less reliable than estimates of current prevalence. Predicting the future course of any event relies on numerous assumptions, and agencies generally present a range of possible scenarios. For years, UNAIDS; the World Health Organization; the Global Fund for AIDS, Tuberculosis and Malaria; and other agencies claimed that such countries as India, China, and Russia, which have generally had relatively low HIV rates, were "on the brink" of major epidemics on the scale of East and southern Africa.[5] For reasons described in this book, the spread of HIV in Asia and eastern Europe is almost entirely confined to clearly defined risk groups, including prostitutes, intravenous drug users, and their sexual partners, and it is very unlikely that HIV will spread widely in the general population in these regions.[6]

MEASURING SEXUAL BEHAVIOR

Declines in HIV infection rates are finally underway in various countries in Africa, Asia, the Caribbean, and Latin America. There is general agreement that these declines are due to behavior change and not simply to the deaths of high risk individuals.[7] However, there is considerable debate about what accounts for these welcome trends, particularly the most proximate behavioral changes—abstinence, faithfulness, or condom use—that must underlie them.

Sources of data on behavior change include the USAID-funded Demographic and Health Surveys, other national surveys and local research studies conducted by academic groups at Columbia University, Johns Hopkins University, Imperial College London, and others. The interpretation of these data should be straightforward. However, discrepancies sometimes arise in the measurement, analysis, and interpretation of the results. For example, indicators of condom use include "ever used," "used at last sex," "used at last higher risk sex," and "always use." Indicators of multiple partnerships include "multiple partners in last year," "multiple partners in past four weeks," and "sex with a non-spousal, non-cohabitating partner in past year." Affirmative answers to any of these questions could have very different implications for the interpretation of data and trends. For example, for years, the UNAIDS program used indicators that over-estimated both the fraction of people engaging in "risky sexual behavior" and the fraction of people using condoms effectively.

Measuring "risky sexual behavior" is especially complicated. For many years, it was assumed that "risky sex" meant sex outside of marriage or cohabitation. Thus, the many researchers measured "risky sex" with the indicator "number of people who had sex with a nonspousal, noncohabitating partner in past year" of "all those who had sex in the past year." We now know that in Africa, much HIV transmission takes place in ongoing relationships, including marriage, and therefore this indicator doesn't really capture all of the riskiest sexual encounters, especially for young people. For example, using the usual indicator, a very high rate of "risky" sex would result if 99 percent of all young people were abstinent, and 1 percent were faithful to a single partner whom they were neither married to nor living with. In that case, 100 percent of sexually active young people in such a society would be having "high risk sex"—even if they were all abstinent or faithful! More realistically, since men tend to marry late in Africa, most of the young men who have sex, have it out of wedlock, so even if they are faithful to their partners, they will show up in the "risky sex" category. In Rwanda, for example, the fraction of young men and women having so-called "high risk" sex in 2005 was 48 percent and 15 percent, respectively, (meaning with a "non-marital/non-cohabitating partner"—among all youth who had sex) but only 9 percent of ALL young men and 5 percent of ALL young women had premarital sex at all.

Since the late 1990s, the US-funded Demographic and Health Surveys have been reporting the much simpler and more informative indicator "fraction of people with multiple partners in past year," and as of 2008, UNAIDS will begin doing so as well.

When it comes to condom use, many researchers, report only the indicator "ever used," or "used at last higher risk sex" (meaning with a nonmarital, noncohabitating partner). But most HIV transmission in Africa takes place in longer term relationships and in such cases, condoms are only protective when used during every sexual act.[1] Some studies report such "consistent use," but the practice is rare. In 2007 a Ugandan newspaper ran a feature story about a couple that had managed to use condoms throughout their fourteen-year marriage. This was considered national news.

AUTHOR'S NOTE

This book is a work of nonfiction. To the best of my knowledge, everything in it is true, with the exception of some of the details of my work on insects, described in Chapter 1. Here, I have conflated aspects of my Ph.D. and postdoctoral experiments. In addition, throughout the book, the names of many people have been changed to protect their privacy, including most of those living with HIV and all of the doctors I worked with in Kampala during the early 1990s.

AIDS RESEARCH
FOR BEGINNERS

CHAPTER ONE

The Outsiders

APRIL 1993

About two weeks before I was supposed to leave for Uganda, I packed up the materials I would need for the experiment I planned to do there and called Dr. Arthur Murray, whom I would be working with, to confirm the shipping address.

"Maybe you shouldn't send the stuff just yet," he said.

"There's a problem?"

"There may be a problem."

"Is it a bad problem?"

"It could be."

"Is it a political problem?"

"Well, not the whole country."

"Just the project?"

"Yeah, just the project."

A few days later he called and said that everything was OK; the problem had had to do with a truck.

"A truck?"

"Yeah, a truck."

I knew there had to be more to it than this.

I arrived at Entebbe airport in a small propeller-driven plane from Nairobi and walked across the tarmac to a two-story building that had been almost completely gutted. The only light came through the doorway; fragments of electrical wiring and old plumbing fixtures, black with tar and dirt, dangled from the walls and ceiling. A man lounged on an elevated platform; a sign above his head said HEALTH. This was the man who checked your immunization papers. Before I left, I had been told that to be allowed past him you needed to show that you'd had injections for yellow fever, cholera, and typhoid. Malaria pills and injections for hepatitis A and B and rabies were recommended.

Arthur was there to meet me. During the drive to Kampala, we talked about my materials, which still hadn't arrived. I'd called the shippers before I left, and they'd told me they thought a project called CHIPS was closing and, thinking that my project was part of CHIPS, they hadn't sent anything out for me. I told the shippers to send my parcels anyway, but what was CHIPS?

When I asked Arthur, he became tense. "Just don't talk about that," he said. So I didn't. It was midday. I had been up all night on the airplane, and my first view of Africa out of the car window seemed like part of a waking dream. Soldiers in baggy green uniforms carrying heavy machine guns shambled by on the road. We drove along the shore of Lake Victoria, which sparkled in the sun. A bright yellow bird flew up out of a marsh, and vines cascaded from the crabbed and twisted branches of giant trees. I made myself a promise, which I would soon break, to learn the name of every plant and animal I saw.

Within a few miles of the airport, the road gave way to threadbare patches of tarmac and our progress slowed considerably. The air was heavy with diesel fumes, wood smoke, and fine ochre dust. We passed through towns: the road became an open-air market, with kiosks selling furniture, chicken coops, spare parts for cars, machine tools, jerry-built appliances of all kinds. Pale green trucks stood in the middle of the street wheezing black vapors. Their flimsy metal frames were piled high with bananas, foam-rubber mattresses, and chickens crammed in their cages, their feathers raining everywhere. Along the roadside, there were old men in baggy suits; dusty, barefoot workers; children dressed in rags; stray goats; and stout women in colorful wraps selling green bananas and charcoal from lean-tos constructed from stripped tree branches roped together with banana leaves. Everything seemed handmade, makeshift, rough-hewn.

Small, colonial-style cement bungalows, their roofs dented and askew, ranged untidily over the hillsides. Without a sterilizing winter, their foundations were riddled with cracks from the intrusions of tree roots, creeping molds, burning sun, and driving rain. Over the coming months and years, I too would have to contend with the forces of nature. There would be power cuts and water shortages and broken toilets and stuck doors and cars that started only when you kicked them. Most of the time, someone would find a way of rigging things to avert disaster.

ARTHUR DROPPED ME OFF at the house of his colleague, Dr. Celeste Quinn, on the campus of Makerere University, where I would be staying. Celeste was a gynecologist working with the urban poor in Kampala. She was also the director of CHIPS, the U.S. Agency for International Development–funded project that I was not supposed to talk about.

Like most expatriate residences in Kampala at the time, Celeste's house was a space pod of Western comfort. There were guards, servants, a telephone, a television. Celeste was a large, slightly intimidating woman, with a physician's scrubbed white hands. When we were introduced, she extended an ivory arm and gave me a brief smile. She was seeing off some friends at the door and seemed distracted, so I sat in a wicker chair on the back porch and played with her cat, which emerged from its cardboard box and slunk over to me.

I would be working in a lab at the Uganda Cancer Institute, a compound of weathered one-story concrete buildings on the grounds of Mulago Hospital, the only state-run hospital in Kampala at the time. The lab was next to the dental clinic, and the screams of the children being treated there could be heard all day long.

The Cancer Institute had two barn-like open wards that were so dark and overcrowded that most of the patients and their families lounged on the verandahs and gravel yards outside. They bathed their children under an outdoor spigot and prepared maize meal and mashed bananas on open wood fires. On the Cancer Institute grounds I saw people with growths on their necks the size of pineapples, and people without arms or legs. I saw a man without a nose.

My lab was a short distance uphill from the Cancer Institute. Arthur took me there the day after I arrived. We walked through the main lab, which was crowded with equipment and Ugandan technicians, and entered a much smaller room, which had no light and was full of empty cardboard boxes and rusty machine parts. When he pushed the door open, plumes of red African dust rose and swirled around us.

"We were thinking of putting you here," Arthur said. It was clear that some other place would have to be found for the boxes and machine parts. A plasterer and painter would have to be hired, and we would have to install a refrigerator, a light, and a table. Some time would pass before I could begin my experiment.

A few days later, a contractor was hired, but he quarreled with the institute's accountant over how much the job would cost. The two men negotiated within five dollars of each other before the contractor lost his temper and left. It took two days to get him to come back and accept his own terms.

I grew accustomed to such delays. The materials I had shipped from California were still missing in any case. The American shipping company assured me the boxes had been sent and should have arrived. The airline said the boxes were with customs, customs said they were with the clearing agent, and the clearing agent said they were at the Cancer Institute, where, according to Celeste, who kept track of the shipments that came in, they could not be found.

I had come to Kampala to carry out an experiment that I hoped would contribute to the development of a vaccine to protect Ugandans against HIV, the virus that causes AIDS. I became interested in the problem when I was doing postdoctoral work in California. I had been studying the sexual organs of a tiny insect the size of the letter *i* in ELIZABETH on an English penny, when I realized I was finding it increasingly difficult to concentrate. I had recently heard a lecture given by a scientist named Kathelyn Steimer about the HIV vaccine that her lab at Chiron, a biotechnology company near San Francisco, was working on. It had been injected into about two hundred volunteers so far, and the results were encouraging.

After the lecture, my mind never seriously returned to the insect world. My research had been bothering me for some time. In my university biology department, and others like it, "frontiers" were the thing. It was unfashionable to study anything for a practical reason. We thought of ourselves as the astronauts of the cell, exploring the logic left behind by evolution's intricate digressions. Our heroes were the men and women who described the structure of the gene, saw the first microtubule, and found out how ribosomes worked. We were not in the business of developing cures or vaccines.

My academic outpost near San Francisco was some distance from the frontier. In the 1920s, a German scientist discovered that if you stained the nucleus of certain insect cells and looked at them under a light microscope, you saw a black dot. He wrote a series of long, detailed articles on the subject suggesting that the black dot was a chromosome, and left it to posterity to figure out what it was for. My boss believed that the black dot was extremely important. He theorized that it determined sex, that it contained a genetic memory bank, that it was some sort of death clock. We spent hours discussing it.

The aphid-like bug I was studying was tiny and round and had six legs, each consisting of three segments. It had a pair of short antennae with seven segments and a tiny mandible. Its little body was covered with pores from which it secreted a white goo in which it hid.

I asked my boss whether we all shouldn't be out helping the poor and the sick, rather than studying the molecules inside the sex organs of a bug that was almost too small to see.

"The poor and the sick will always be with us," he said, "but we will change the way people think about the world." Although my boss didn't say it, I knew that he considered work like Steimer's pedestrian.

He had a point, I suppose, but when I looked around at all the people in the lab muttering recondite gene-speak, it all began to seem very strange. I longed for a biological problem that had meaning outside the world of academic conferences and biochemical journals. I had known several people who had died of AIDS. Most were young; all suffered horribly. Although scientists had spent billions of dollars trying to understand how the virus worked, they had as yet found no way to stop its spread. AIDS had devastated the gay enclaves of New York, San Francisco, and Los Angeles, and the news from the developing world was even worse. Millions of people in East Africa, Thailand, and India were already infected.

Steimer's vaccine consisted of a harmless suspension of molecules called gp120, and doctors had injected it into two hundred HIV-negative volunteers so far. Steimer hoped that the gp120 molecules would train their immune systems to fight off HIV if they were ever exposed to it. Many of the volunteers were homosexual men who had watched their friends die of AIDS. Some of these men were sexually active themselves, and thus they were also at risk of HIV infection. Although they had been advised to avoid risky sex and use condoms, not all of them complied with this advice. Soon Steimer would know whether her vaccine protected these men or not. She was hopeful because Chiron had developed a similar vaccine for hepatitis B that had saved many lives and earned the company billions of dollars. So far the results with the HIV vaccine looked promising too.

A few weeks after Steimer's lecture, I asked a doctor I knew who had worked on AIDS in East Africa if he thought a molecular biologist might be useful there. He suggested I write to a professor in San Francisco who was conducting a study of sexually transmitted diseases (STDs) in Uganda. Perhaps he would be able to give me some advice. I had read about the AIDS epidemic in Uganda. One-third of adults in the capital city, Kampala, were HIV positive, and the virus was spreading along trade routes into the countryside. Thousands of children had been orphaned by the disease, their farms left idle because their parents were dead or too sick to work. I wrote to the professor and phoned his secretary some time in August. She said he was very busy but had time to see me at eleven-thirty on October 23, 1992, for about fifteen minutes.

Professor Cornelius was about fifty, a small, round man with a tennis-ball fuzz of hair around his cheery face.

"So, you want to go to Africa!" he boomed. He talked about the poignant beauty of Kampala—the crowded, dirty city; the skeletal remains of the stone buildings, gutted by war; the surrounding hills and the vast slums in the folds of land between them—and about Makerere University and Mulago Hospital, once the most distinguished in East Africa, destroyed by Idi Amin, Milton Obote, and twenty-five years of murder, corruption, and neglect.

In the mid-1980s, when health officials first recognized the magnitude of the AIDS crisis in Africa, they feared that this great plague affecting heterosexual people would spread north, to Europe, the United States, and other developed regions. There were predictions that it was only a matter of time before large numbers of ordinary non-gay, non-drug-using Americans—college students, Wall Street executives, housewives—would find they were HIV positive. So the U.S. government, through the National Institutes of Health and the U.S. Agency for International Development, poured money into research. Professor Cornelius was one of those trying to find out why so many heterosexual people in Africa were infected with HIV. At the time, there were many theories about it, but Professor Cornelius and others believed that it had something to do with the prevalence of STDs there. HIV-infected cells and virus particles do not penetrate unbroken skin, and they don't survive long outside the body. In order to pass from one person to another, they must encounter mucous membranes, the slimy surfaces of the body's internal cavities, such as the vagina and rectum, and even then, it is not a certainty that infection will occur. STDs—syphilis, gonorrhea, herpes, and so on—cause genital sores and ulcers that Professor Cornelius and others thought created direct channels to the bloodstream through which HIV could pass very easily. STDs were common in Uganda. Although most cases could be cured with cheap antibiotics, two decades of civil war and economic demise had left half the population without any medical care at all, and the situation wasn't much better in other impoverished African countries.

Professor Cornelius was overseeing several projects related to AIDS in Uganda, one of which, CHIPS, the project I was discouraged from talking about, was being run in Kampala by his young colleagues Celeste Quinn and Arthur Murray. In the course of their work they had collected blood samples from thousands of patients at a public STD clinic in Kampala, which were now stored in a freezer. About half the patients were HIV positive. No one had yet studied these samples. Perhaps this was something I would like to work on? We discussed possible experiments. During the meeting, Professor Cornelius was interrupted by an urgent phone call, and his secretary appeared at the door making frantic gestures that I was not supposed to understand.

I HAD BEEN IN KAMPALA for three weeks. The plasterer had fixed up my little lab, which now had a light and a table, but I still needed a refrigerator.

The Cancer Institute's accountant authorized the money to pay for it, and Vicki, the large, beautiful Ugandan woman who ran the institute storeroom, said she would help me buy one. She warned that Ugandan dealers would double the price of anything a white person bought, and recommended we go to an Asian shop.

Traders from the Far and Middle East have been coming to East Africa for centuries. Until the 1970s, South Asians ran most of Uganda's businesses, factories, and sugar and cotton mills; they built many of the towns, taught in the university, and owned a great deal of property. Then, in 1972, Idi Amin threw them all out and gave their property to black Ugandans. Chaos ensued. The new African entrepreneurs were totally inexperienced and the economy fell into ruin. Amin spent what little foreign exchange remained in the country on whiskey and transistor radios to placate the army, and soldiers and other government henchmen looted at will.[1]

Yoweri Museveni, president since 1986, in a bid to both redress past injustice and restore the economy, offered the Asians the chance to return and reclaim their houses, shops, and factories, and many did.

The Asian shop Vicki took me to was small and crowded, but the man behind the counter seemed to know her, so we didn't have to wait long. He showed us a refrigerator called a Sno-Cap.

"How much?" Vicki asked.

"Twelve hundred thousand shillings."

"Eight."

"No."

Silence. "OK, eleven hundred and fifty."

"Nine."

"No."

"Come on, nine hundred."

"Eleven hundred and that's as low as I can go."

Vicki looked at me and I shrugged.

"OK," she said.

The refrigerator that arrived at the lab a few days later was half the size of the one we thought we had purchased.

My boxes were still missing. I consulted Celeste, but all she could do was sympathize. In the two years she had been working in Africa, she had seen this happen a thousand times. Sometimes things just vanished. Uganda was a developing country after all, and life here was chaotic.

Celeste had something to confide in me too. The project she was running was also in trouble. CHIPS—the Community Health Initiative to Prevent Sexually Transmitted Diseases—was a $1.5 million project funded by the U.S. Agency for International Development (USAID). Celeste was the director and had written the original request for funding and had hired the 132-person Ugandan staff. CHIPS had been running for about a year and was located in a Kampala slum called Kisenyi, which means "swamp" in Swahili. It lies between two hills, where two of Kampala's many cathedrals stand. Catholic and Protestant missionaries brought Christianity to Uganda in the 1870s, but within a decade the converts were at war. Thousands were killed and peace would not return for another twelve years. Religious tensions persist in Uganda to this day; Kampala's Catholic and Protestant cathedrals now face each other from adjacent hills, and Kisenyi lies in the depression between them. When it rains, garbage and silt run down the hills and collect in Kisenyi. The air smells of rotting banana peels, children gather food from garbage heaps, and rivulets of sludge course through the narrow passageways that serve as streets.

Kisenyi is where people displaced by war or poverty end up when they come to Kampala. Everyone is poor and unemployed, and yet everyone appears to be doing something. The men fix bicycles, make things out of wood, or steal. The women sell things: roasted bananas, cigarettes, sweets, themselves. The prevalence of both STDs and HIV infection was very high. CHIPS was established to see what effect a neighborhood STD clinic and HIV testing center would have on the spread of HIV. At the time of my visit, the only treatment available to people with STDs was the clinic at Mulago Hospital, which was overcrowded, far away from where most poor people lived, and frequently out of medicine.

Like many AIDS projects in Africa, CHIPS was an uneasy collaboration among three parties with different interests: USAID, which provided the money; Celeste, who was responsible for spending it; and the people of Kisenyi, on whom the money would be spent.

USAID's goal, determined by the US government, was to reduce the spread of HIV and other STDs and to promote family planning in developing countries. Its officials hoped that the CHIPS clinic would serve as a model for programs throughout Africa that would achieve both aims at the same time.

USAID had a lot of money to spend—some twenty million dollars in Uganda alone at the time—and therefore it also had considerable power. It gave jobs to scores of American experts in public health, waste management, education, and so on, who in turn hired hundreds of local people.

The interests of the people of Kisenyi were different. Free condoms and treatment for STDs were fine, but the CHIPS clinic was the largest, most modern building in the area. When they saw the walls going up, they must have wondered what it was all about. They must have hoped it would provide treatment to save the countless children in Kisenyi who die of malaria, diarrhea, and pneumonia every year, or the scores of women who die in childbirth. Perhaps it would even offer treatment for AIDS. Some people may have hoped to get jobs there.

Moreover, Celeste was a scientist. She wanted to know which STDs were most common in Kisenyi, and the best and cheapest ways of treating them. She also wanted to know exactly how many people living in the area contracted HIV each year, and how many cases of infection could be prevented by the services offered at the clinic. Such a project might seem simple, but she must have encountered many frustrations along the way. I can only imagine all the things that could have gone wrong.

AT MULAGO HOSPITAL, down the hill from the lab at the Cancer Institute, an American doctor was trying to determine how best to treat cryptococcal meningitis, which often affects people dying of AIDS. The doctor was ordinarily a mild man, but when I asked him if I could accompany him on his rounds, he agreed only reluctantly and seemed irritated. I asked if anything was wrong.

"You'll see," he said.

Cryptococcal meningitis is caused by a fungus that infects the fluid bathing the brain and spinal column. Everyone is exposed to the germ that causes the disease; its spores can be found on the leaves of certain trees or in the air. But the only people who get sick are those whose immune systems are in such disrepair, because of AIDS, cancer, or some other cause, that they can't fight it off. The symptoms are nausea, vomiting, disorientation, and headaches so severe that when a child dies of AIDS in Uganda, it is often said that he died of headache.

At the time, the powerful antiretroviral drug cocktails that can vastly improve the lives of AIDS patients had not been developed and would not become widely available in Uganda for another decade. The only treatment for cryptococcal meningitis available in Uganda at the time was amphotericin, a highly toxic medicine that, even in moderate doses, caused permanent kidney damage. The doctor was being paid to study a relatively new drug called fluconazole, which was not as toxic, but was very expensive. It was provided free to all AIDS patients willing to participate in the doctor's study, but without antiretroviral drug cocktails, most of these patients would die within a few months anyway.

Following the doctor on his rounds, I was not surprised by the chipped paint and grimy windows, the torn, dirty sheets, and the few items of rusty furniture. But I didn't expect to see someone lying in a pool of blood, or meet a man who had spent the previous night having a seizure. A nurse, had there been one, would have known how to stop it, but the man stopped it himself, by lapsing into a coma.

There were so few nurses at Mulago that patient care—feeding, washing, and alerting the doctors in emergencies—was virtually all done by family members. Mulago was a public hospital, and basic drugs and supplies should have been provided free, but they were rarely available. When a patient needed a drip line or an aspirin, a relative went to a market nearby. Some nurses and doctors also sold drugs and equipment—some of it stolen from the hospital stores—and they tended to overcharge. In the early 1990s, doctors at Mulago earned about $150 a month; nurses, fifty dollars. It was not surprising that some of them were so alienated that they made what extra money they could from their patients. Some, having taken other jobs, did not show up for work at all.

The doctor went from bed to bed. There was another man in a coma, and another so weak he seemed able to move only his eyes. One patient had a private room. The place was tidy and sunny and clean. He must have been rich. Someone had brought two straw shopping bags full of provisions: cups and saucers, a Thermos flask, books, a soap dish. The patient looked all right to my untrained eye, not thin, with no obvious rashes or sores, breathing quietly—although he was moaning and writhing and holding his head. The doctor said he would give the man codeine, but the only way to make him comfortable would be to knock him out completely. He died the next day anyway.

"Sometimes I don't know what I am doing here," the American doctor told me.

But I did, and so did this doctor's employers. Conducting this trial in the United States would have been far more expensive because the American patients would have required far better care. But ethical standards required that the pharmaceutical company needed only to ensure that the Ugandan patients received the standard of care in Uganda, which was very low indeed. At least the patients were getting something as a result of the trial, I thought. There was no placebo group, so everyone was treated. Nevertheless, the doctor knew that after the trial ended, he and the company would leave Uganda. No further patients at Mulago would receive free fluconazole until 2002, nine years later, when Pfizer, the company that makes it, under pressure from AIDS activists and manufacturers of generic drugs in Thailand and India, offered the drug free to African hospitals. Pfizer's donation program, though generous, has been slow to get off the ground, and even today, cryptoccocal meningitis remains a common cause of AIDS-related death throughout Africa.

Medical research in Uganda can be profoundly frustrating for the doctors involved. They are caught between the demands of their employers for convincing survival curves and those of their patients for help of any kind. A high proportion give up and leave. But for some, Mulago is a rewarding place, recalling a time when doctors were closer to their patients than they are now. Medicine in the West relies on expensive diagnostic techniques unavailable here, but some doctors I met in Uganda admitted that they had learned a great deal from being forced to rely only on a stethoscope. As one of them told me, "I never realized there was so much you could learn just from listening to someone's heart."

I withdrew after a while to sit on a bench beside a thin old man who was staring straight ahead and wheezing. Between patients, the doctor came over to me.

"Are you all right?" he asked. A funny question, I thought, to ask someone visiting such a place.

"I'm not sure I can take this," I said.

"I can understand that."

If only my materials would turn up so I could start my experiment, I might not feel so useless, I thought. I tried to think of ways around it, of what local substitutions I could make, of what I could borrow from other scientists around Kampala. But what I was trying to do—design an HIV vaccine for Uganda—was way out on the high-tech edge. Many of the materials I was expecting came from highly specialized labs in the United States, and existed in small quantities. They were made nowhere else. Some of the materials had been donated to me by scientists who cared about the AIDS epidemic in Africa and wanted to contribute in some way to my project. I had been in Uganda for only a month, and already, I was disappointing them.

WHEN HIV was first identified in 1983, many researchers thought it would be easy to develop a vaccine to protect people against it. But by the time I arrived in Uganda a decade later, this optimism was beginning to fade. To understand why it has been so difficult to make an AIDS vaccine, it helps to know what happens when a person first becomes infected with HIV.

HIV is a spherical virus whose surface is covered with tiny stalks. There is a ball at the end of each stalk that consists of a clump of molecules called gp120. The gp120 molecules function like a key, enabling HIV to break into particular white blood cells—called CD4 cells—that help protect the body from disease. Once inside the CD4 cells, the virus takes over the DNA copying machinery and forces the cells to churn out millions of new viruses, until the cells eventually burst open and disintegrate or clump together and die. In the bloodstream of HIV-positive people, a billion CD4 cells are hijacked and killed each day, and 100 billion new HIV viruses are produced.[2]

Right after infection with HIV, people feel nothing, but after a few weeks or months, some people become feverish, and the lymph nodes in their necks and armpits swell as the first immune response against HIV is being made. Lymphocytes and antibodies—Y-shaped molecules with mitten-like protrusions that latch onto and kill infected cells and microbes—clear most of the virus particles, but some viruses escape by mutating: they change slightly, infect new cells, and continue to reproduce. The body must make new lymphocytes and new antibodies to fight the mutants, but the mutants mutate again, necessitating a new immune response.

The human immune system is able to fight off most viruses and clear them from the body, but not HIV. By the time the immune system begins making cells and antibodies it is too late. The virus has embedded itself in so many CD4 cells that it is impossible for the immune system to clear it without destroying itself in the process. As the CD4 cells die off, the body loses its ability to respond to a range of other infections. The patient is slowly consumed by diseases that are harmless to other people and dies.

When I first heard Dr. Steimer's lecture, I learned that it might be possible for a vaccine to prevent the virus from taking hold in people who were exposed to it. This is what had encouraged me to abandon the tedious complexities of the insect gonads that I was studying. The vaccines that protect people against infections are usually made from harmless versions or fragments of the microbe that causes the infection itself. When the vaccine is injected into the body, the immune system reacts as though it were the real thing. The bone marrow and lymph nodes generate cells and antibodies that specifically kill that particular microbe. These cells and antibodies constitute what biologists call "immunological memory." They remain in the blood for years. If the real microbe enters the body, they are able to destroy it in hours rather than weeks or months, and clear it before it seizes control of vast numbers of CD4 cells.

Back in California, I had learned that there were about thirty HIV vaccines under development, but many researchers were already losing hope that any of them would work because of the vast number of mutants. By all accounts, the most promising vaccine at the time was the one designed in Steimer's lab at Chiron Corporation. Shortly after Professor Cornelius suggested that I might work with the bank of serum samples in Uganda, I contacted Dr. Steimer and she invited me to visit her lab.

Chiron was founded in 1981 by a group of molecular biologists from the University of California, San Francisco, who had been among the first to isolate a human gene and clone copies of it in a test tube. Cloning provided an entirely new mechanism for making drugs and vaccines, and it soon inspired visions of corporate empires in biology similar to the rapidly growing software empires that had been established a decade before. Biologists who had once scrounged through forests, swamps, and sewers to find natural molecules that might be effective in treating diseases could now engineer them in bright, clean laboratories, or so it was hoped. Chiron occupies a ten-acre lakeside compound near San Francisco, and employs two thousand people, largely paid for by its multibillion-dollar sales of a vaccine for hepatitis B, the first vaccine to be created by cloning.

I recognized Dr. Steimer immediately. She was tall, slim, and blond, and had the same efficient but melancholy and distracted manner I had noticed when she was giving her lecture. She showed me around the lab. We passed through the two main rooms, where work with uninfected specimens took place, and the isolation room, where technicians wearing blue bodysuits, booties, shower caps, rubber gloves, and face masks were working with live HIV virus. Was the virus really so dangerous to work with? I wondered.

Dr. Steimer explained that although HIV mutates, she and her colleagues had a strategy that might contain it. Her vaccine consisted of gp120 molecules that her technicians had cloned in her lab. Because gp120 was the "key" that allowed the virus to break into cells, part of it was "conserved"—meaning it could not mutate without destroying the function of the key. Steimer hoped her vaccine would stimulate the production of antibodies that would grab onto this special conserved part of gp120. Like a piece of gum on a door key, the antibodies would prevent the virus from unlocking the cells and infecting them. Steimer hoped that her vaccine would give the immune system a head start, so that it could make such antibodies early and kill HIV in hours, before it began flooding the body with mutants. Because the vaccine was made artificially by cloning, it contained none of the virus's genetic material and posed no risk of infection.

At the time, the DNA of the HIV mutants from about five hundred different patients around the world had been analyzed. No two of them were identical, but they seemed to fall into some ten distinct categories known as subtypes, which tended to circulate in different populations around the world. Most people in the United States were infected with the subtype known as B, and Dr. Steimer's vaccine was made from the gp120 of a subtype B virus that had been isolated from a patient in San Francisco. Dr. Steimer hoped that it would protect people from infection with subtype B, but she knew it would be unlikely to protect people from infection with other subtypes circulating in other parts of the world. Nevertheless, a vaccine for subtype B would be an enormous breakthrough.

A test of any vaccine involves three phases. First it is administered to a small number of volunteers to ensure that it does not make them sick. Next it is given to a larger group of volunteers, to see if it induces the production of the right kinds of antibodies and cells. Blood is drawn from these volunteers and added to the virus in a test tube. If the volunteers are making good antibodies, the blood will kill the virus. Phase III is a massive, fantastically expensive venture involving thousands of healthy volunteers, who receive either the vaccine or a placebo. After several years, the rates of infection in the vaccinated group and the placebo group are compared, and the statistics indicate whether the vaccine protects people or not. If the vaccine fails completely, equal numbers of people in the vaccinated group and the placebo group will become infected. If the vaccine is perfect, no one in the vaccinated group will become infected. If the vaccine is only partly effective, some members of the vaccinated group will become infected, but far fewer than in the placebo group.

While the volunteers in a Phase III trial are healthy, they are chosen because they have a high risk of becoming infected. In the case of HIV, they might be young gay men or intravenous drug users. They must be told that the vaccine is experimental and might not work and that in any case, they might receive only the placebo. They are warned to take every measure to protect themselves. The success of the trial depends on the fact that a significant number of these people—for whatever reason—will be exposed to the virus anyway, despite these warnings.

Dr. Steimer's vaccine was in the second stage of testing. It had been deemed safe, and the antibodies produced by healthy volunteers killed various laboratory mutants of subtype B. These lab strains contained pure stocks of virus that had been propagated in an incubator for years. Viruses taken from patients were far more diverse and complex, having adapted to survival in the body, in the presence of an active immune system, rather than in a plastic flask. Dr. Steimer and her colleagues were preparing to determine whether the antibodies her volunteers made would kill these "wild-type" HIV strains, taken from real people with real infections. If that worked, they would proceed to Phase III.

Chiron could not finance a Phase III trial of the vaccine itself, but the U.S. Congress, on the advice of the National Institutes of Health, was considering pitching in with $20 million. Their decision would depend on additional lab data, and was expected sometime the following year.

My thoughts were these: The World Health Organization (WHO), sensitive to the fact that the poorest nations might be overlooked in the high-tech scramble for an AIDS vaccine, had designated four developing countries as potential sites for AIDS vaccine trials—Thailand, Brazil, Uganda, and Rwanda. Dr. Steimer's vaccine was designed only to work against subtype B infections, prevalent in the United States. Nevertheless, if it worked, and if information could be obtained about the subtypes circulating in Uganda, the company might consider making a vaccine that could be tested there in the future. Although Ugandans would never be able to afford to buy such a vaccine, perhaps the United Nations or some other institution would pay for it.

My contribution would be to determine which subtypes of HIV were prevalent in Uganda. Some information about this was already available, but Chiron scientists had developed a new test that could identify HIV subtypes from blood samples very rapidly. Once the experiment was up and running, it would be possible to test hundreds of samples in a few weeks. This would enable me to find out just how common the different subtypes in Uganda were, and what kind of gp120 vaccine might work there. I could begin by testing some of the thousands of samples from the STD clinic that had been stored in the freezer at the Cancer Institute in Kampala.

Routine HIV tests, such as those offered in hospitals and clinics around the world, are designed to detect not the virus itself, but antibodies that react with HIV. Such tests, known as enzyme-linked immunosorbent assays, or ELISAs, were first developed in the 1970s. The ELISA forms the basis for home pregnancy tests, as well as tests carried out in doctors' offices for hormone deficiencies, infections, and other medical conditions. One of Dr. Steimer's colleagues had designed an ELISA that could distinguish antibodies against different HIV subtypes. It could tell if someone was infected with A, B, C, or some other subtype. Dr. Steimer suggested I use this technique to investigate the antibodies in the Kampala serum samples.

I worked in Dr. Steimer's lab on the vaccine project for a couple of months to earn money and learn the new ELISA technique. Meanwhile, I planned the trip to Uganda carefully. Not knowing what to expect, I packed as though I were setting up an ELISA on the moon. I packed scissors, pencils, tape, pipettes, chemicals, plastic ELISA dishes. These were among the materials that were lost on the way to Kampala.

Dr. Steimer was prepared to pay for the materials I would need to do the experiment, but not for me. In Uganda, I would have to support myself. The doctors in Kampala were prepared to let me use the stored blood samples in their freezers and give me space in a lab, but they would not pay me either. Nevertheless, I was happy about the arrangement. The project was very small, and although it would turn out that others were thinking along the same lines and would also publish surveys of HIV subtypes in Uganda, I felt like a pioneer.[3] Such feelings are rare in biology these days. The hour of the lone scientist following his or her imagination into the unlit corners of nature is passing. These were the days of the Human Genome Project, the biotech revolution, and the five-million-dollar grant. Whatever you might have wanted to do, others had thought of it already, and they had more money, more technicians, more pipettes, more frogs, more of whatever it takes than you did. So you joined their lab and you did what they said, or forget it. But here in Kampala, I was on my own.

I WAS STILL WAITING for my materials to arrive when Arthur offered to show me the blood samples stored in the freezer at the Cancer Institute. They had been collected over the preceding four years, subjected to a routine HIV test, and labeled with numbers but no names. Arthur carefully opened the upright freezer where they were stored. There must have been a hundred plastic sandwich bags filled with vials in there. He put out his hand to make sure they didn't fall on the floor.

"They're kind of a mess," he said. The vials were stored randomly, without regard to the age of the patients, or where they came from, or any detail of their medical history.

Arthur left me to sort through the bags. It took an hour to go through the first one, from which I retrieved four samples that I thought I could use. The next bag went more quickly, but it contained only three usable samples. By the end of the week, exhausted from boredom, I had 193. I decided to test these first and if my results were ambiguous, I would somehow find the strength to return to the freezer for more. But in order to proceed, I needed my materials from California, which still could not be found.

One day, while I was still waiting for my boxes to arrive, I took a taxi across town to visit a friend. The driver asked me what I was doing in Uganda. When I told him, he bristled. "How can you make a vaccine when the virus mutates so much? As soon as you make your vaccine, the virus turns into something else, and your old vaccine is useless." I explained that we hoped to get around that problem and told him about the neutralization experiments, the T-cell binding sites that we thought might make good targets for vaccine-generated antibodies, and so on. He seemed to accept this, but then he asked, "Why bother looking at this V3 loop?"

"Well, we think that's important too," I said.

I had similar conversations with a construction worker, a group of high school students, a hairdresser, and the man who mopped the floor of the lab. I had to confront questions about mutation rates, opportunistic infections, and why some people didn't get infected even though they seemed to be having a great many sexual relationships. Nowhere else had I found people so inquisitive and well informed about AIDS.

In Kampala, everyone talked about AIDS. There were AIDS clubs, meetings, conferences, marches, candlelight vigils, benefit breakfasts, lunches, and dinners; there were AIDS T-shirts, hats, banners, books, and cartoons; there were movies, plays, songs, poems, and dances about AIDS.

When I told the cab driver that I was impressed with how much people in Uganda seemed to know about HIV, he said, "Everyone is affected by it. Everyone has a friend, a sister, someone who is sick or dead because of AIDS."

During the following two years, I would hear over and over again that someone I knew had died or was burying a relative. Some of my colleagues in the lab seemed unusually thin, with shiny, feverish skin and eyes that seemed to grow larger every day. Twenty years of war and deepening poverty meant that Ugandans were used to seeing children die. For some, the death of a child was even considered natural. But fatal illness had always been rare among people in their twenties and thirties, even in Uganda. Now in some parts of the country, AIDS had increased the death rate among young adults fivefold.

In 1993, some two million Ugandans were living with HIV, and hundreds of thousands of people had already died. Around 18 percent of adults were HIV positive, the highest national HIV infection rate ever recorded at the time. Why was AIDS sweeping through Africa with such speed, and why had a similar epidemic in the West so far failed to emerge?

Some people attributed the African epidemic to extreme promiscuity, or to exotic rituals involving blood. But such explanations seemed unlikely. Surveys carried out in African cities suggested that Africans do not have more sexual partners, on average, than people in the West do. While bloody rituals involving the repeated use of sharp instruments—female genital mutilation and scarification, for example—are practiced by isolated groups in Uganda, these are not the groups with the highest levels of HIV infection. Anal sex and other forms of sodomy are rare here—or at least they are not admitted to.

At the time, most researchers pointed to the prevalence of STDs in Africa, as Professor Cornelius had explained to me back in San Francisco. Gonorrhea and syphilis were unknown in Africa before European contact, but once introduced, these diseases spread rapidly. During the first decades of the twentieth century, 20 percent of all patients at Mengo, Kampala's first missionary hospital, had STDs. The VD epidemic caused alarm among the colonial authorities, who blamed themselves for modernizing Uganda's tribes too quickly, causing moral breakdown. For some officials, Africa seemed like the Garden of Eden, and the Fall was taking place right before their eyes.

"Among the . . . unclothed Nilotic tribes, a notable degree of sexual morality is found to exist," wrote the British governor of Uganda in 1909. "Unfortunately, more clothes means less morals." The Baganda, "who have always been greatly addicted to wearing apparel, are of notoriously lax habits."[4]

Ugandans themselves also blamed the syphilis epidemic on the immoral influence of missionaries and colonial authorities. Tribal patriarchs claimed whites undermined their power to enforce traditional codes of behavior. To address this, "social purity" campaigns were launched, which promoted moral conduct with lectures and pamphlets; as in nineteenth-century England, single women suspected of prostitution were forced to submit to random pelvic examinations and sent back to their families. Well into the 1950s, all pregnant women attending mission hospitals were dosed with mercury solutions. Whether this harmed the unborn children of these women is unknown.[5]

When antibiotics became widely available in the 1960s, the VD hysteria subsided. Then during the 1970s, rates of syphilis and gonorrhea began to rise again.[6] At the time, President Amin was overseeing a campaign of terror that is legendary, even by African standards. Hundreds of thousands of people died and many of the country's institutions, including its health-care system, all but collapsed. Doctors were murdered or fled into exile, hospitals were looted of every movable item, the economy shrank by half, and imported medicines became a rare luxury. Amin was overthrown in 1979, and a series of civil wars followed, during which four successive leaders were toppled one after the other. When Yoweri Museveni took over in 1986, he brought peace and stability to the southern regions of the country, but reconstruction proceeded slowly and by the time I arrived in 1993 few Ugandan clinics were equipped to treat anything, let alone STDs. Most people had to walk for hours to reach a clinic of any kind. When they got there, they often found that antibiotics were out of stock, and few health workers knew the correct doses anyway. When Ugandans noticed genital lesions, they often ignored them and hoped they would go away, or they went to a traditional healer. Many continued to have sex until it became too painful.

CHIPS was a pilot project, a single clinic for STDs in a single urban slum. Similar clinics were planned for the rest of the country, but this was the first of its kind. We were on our way into town one day when Celeste told me she intended to close CHIPS. She said that she was preparing a flyer to distribute to everyone working on the project sometime in the next week. It would say that work had not been proceeding on schedule, and that USAID had decided to withdraw its grant. This meant that 132 Ugandans would lose their jobs, Kisenyi would lose its clinic, and people would continue to go without treatment for STDs.

She explained that it had taken nine months to set up the CHIPS clinic, to hire and train the doctors, nurses, counselors, drivers, accountants, statisticians, and data-entry clerks. During that time the building had been renovated in Kisenyi, and large amounts of equipment and supplies had been purchased from the United States, shipped to Uganda, and stored under lock and key at the Cancer Institute. Then Celeste left the country. She went to the Seychelles on a holiday, then to an AIDS conference, and then on a speaking tour of the United States. She applied for and was offered a prestigious job on the medical faculty of a midwestern university. She returned to Uganda three months later.

Back in Kampala, she found that the odometer on one of the CHIPS vehicles had advanced by hundreds of miles, that money had disappeared from CHIPS bank accounts, and that a Ugandan colleague had placed three of his sons on the payroll. Only thirty people had been treated at the CHIPS clinic.

Clearly the project had gotten off to a bad start. And yet, from what Celeste told me, it should have been possible to make it work. None of the crimes Celeste described seemed so terrible. Perhaps someone had used the vehicle to drive a sick person back to his home village or returned a dead body to its relatives for burial. Perhaps people in Kisenyi were not aware of the services at the clinic, or perhaps they were disappointed that the doctors there would treat only STDs, when they suffered from so many other afflictions. I wondered whether Celeste had not simply lost interest in the project, but it seemed unwise to ask, given her determination to shut CHIPS down.

The day CHIPS closed, I was out of town, visiting medical projects in western Uganda. At the time, AIDS was considered less of a problem there, because there were fewer cases and because other diseases overwhelmed it. I had gone with a doctor friend to the district of Kabarole, about two hundred miles west of Kampala, in the foothills of the Rwenzori Mountains, where tea is grown on large plantations. We stopped in a village where tea workers lived in a row of huts made of reeds and mud.

About twenty patients had assembled there. We met the children first. They wore ragged American T-shirts and peered at us from around trees. When I smiled back and tried to take a picture, the older ones scattered, laughing, and hid behind the huts; the little ones burst into tears.

A Ugandan doctor led us to a small building site that was under construction, "our new clinic," he joked, and the patients were asked to come in one by one. The first ones all had onchocerciasis, a parasitic disease affecting the skin and eyes, endemic in the tropics. Outside in the tea fields all day, the patients had been bitten by the blackfly that transmits the disease. They had lumps under their skin that contained coiled worms a foot long. Inside, the worms mated and reproduced, and their tiny offspring swam through the flesh, making it wrinkle and itch. I touched one of the lumps and could feel it move.

When the villagers learn that doctors are coming to town, they turn up with all kinds of complaints. There was a woman with an abscess, another with arthritis, and a child with a fever. A teenager came in, shy and giggling, and said something softly to the doctor. He turned her by her shoulders so that her back was facing us, and undid her dress from the front. Her back was covered with tiny sores, some of them bleeding. "This is not onchocerciasis," the doctor said. "I think she suspects what it is." This rash, I would learn, was an early symptom of AIDS.

Later, the American doctor and I drove farther north to visit the main hospital in the region. There was one doctor there—a German—and some nurses who seldom turned up. Water was supplied in jerry cans. The X-ray machine was powered by a generator for an hour a day, if there was enough fuel. The bathrooms had been completely gutted and did not function except as aviaries for the finches that made their nests in the porcelain scraps on the floor. Patients shared beds or slept on the floor. The doctor showed us a bed frame with half the springs missing. "We found a way to get this wire," he said, pointing to one of the remaining springs. "The people can bend it into springs themselves."

There are clinics and hospitals like this all over rural Uganda. Many have no buildings or drugs at all, and a nurse or doctor who rarely turns up. Some time later, a planner from the Ministry of Health would tell me that the problem was not that the buildings were falling apart: it is not impossible to work in a clinic with no beds or only one wall. What were needed most urgently were decent salaries for health workers and a system for ensuring drugs weren't stolen on the way to the patients. "With committed staff, you can set up a clinic under a mango tree," he said.

I thought of USAID and its grand aim to control AIDS with brand-new STD clinics and condoms. I thought of CHIPS: $1.5 million, a sizable fraction of Uganda's entire health budget at the time, spent on refurbishing just one such clinic. I wondered whether a more modest program to raise health workers' salaries throughout the country and improve the supply of cheap drugs for malaria and other infections, including STDs, might not have been a better strategy.

When I returned to Kampala, the CHIPS offices were desolate. A few people were hanging around the administration buildings. Some were told they could work until the end of the month, others a little longer. Perhaps because it was an AIDS project, CHIPS had been infused with enthusiasm. Its employees seemed to believe in what they were doing. Now the spirit had drained out of them. Because I was white, a few people asked me if I could help them find jobs, but what could I do?

That evening, Celeste was remote. She said she had detected veiled personal threats. She had been warned, menacingly, she thought, that it was dangerous to go out in Kampala at night. The following week, she went away on safari to Kenya. While she was away, her cat and dog were mysteriously poisoned.

Before Celeste left Kampala for good, her boss, Professor Cornelius, flew out to Uganda. He was overseeing various research projects in Kampala, in addition to CHIPS. He met with the Ugandan doctors at the Cancer Institute and learned how his work was going there. In addition to being in charge of a university department, he was the editor of a prestigious medical journal and he had recently been appointed the private physician of an Arab sheik. He lamented the closing of CHIPS but said very little about it. One evening, he accompanied some of us to a local expatriate hangout in Kampala, where a prostitute swanned up to him and put her hands in his pockets.

The professor was a little surprised to see me in Uganda. In fact, most of the doctors wondered what I was doing there. Unlike them, I was not employed by the University of California; nor was I currently employed by Chiron. I was in Uganda because I had managed to interest Dr. Steimer in the blood samples stored at the Cancer Institute and had managed to obtain approval from the doctors in Kampala to let me test them. So here I was, living in their rented houses, riding in their vehicles, working in their lab. They let me do this because of their hope that, if my project worked, and if Dr. Steimer's vaccine also worked, the World Health Organization might sponsor a vaccine trial in Uganda in the near future. In that case, there would be plenty of work for everyone, including me. But for the time being, I was just a hitchhiker, and as hitchhikers sometimes do, I became a little arrogant. Hitchhikers live cynical, parasitic existences, but sometimes they see the landscape more clearly than the drivers.

The professor threw a party during his visit and many people came, including a German doctor who had spent twelve years at an up-country hospital. He told us that during the civil wars in the 1980s, parties would last all night because it was too dangerous to go home. The shooting started at about four in the afternoon, and wherever you were then, there you would stay until morning. He and his Ugandan colleagues were on their own in those days. They had very few drugs and supplies; sometimes it was even impossible to find clean water to wash out gunshot wounds. As difficult as things were now, they were far worse then.

Our group of Americans looked up to this man, but I don't know how he felt about us. He told us, perhaps only partly in jest, that they talk about two kinds of AIDS in Uganda: slim AIDS and fat AIDS. People with slim AIDS get slimmer and slimmer and slimmer until they finally disappear. Fat AIDS afflicts doctors, bureaucrats, and foreign-aid consultants with enormous grants and salaries; they fly around the world to exotic places and get fatter and fatter and fatter. Fat AIDS had become so common in Uganda, he said, that if you said you were working on HIV, people thought you were a thief.

A CURIOUS THING happened a few days after CHIPS was canceled. My boxes turned up. They had been locked in a storeroom and had been there for more than a month. Celeste was the only one with the keys, but after the project closed, she handed them over to an official at USAID.

All the equipment and supplies there were due to be returned to their U.S. suppliers. I knew my boxes would be there. It was the only place I hadn't looked.

Celeste should have known the boxes were in there, since she was the only one with the key. But she had been distracted and upset and perhaps she overlooked or ignored them. The day I found the boxes, I told Celeste about it and she said, "Great!" and gave me a big smile.

Some of the Ugandans should have known about the boxes as well, because they would have put them there. The chief accountant kept track, or was supposed to, of everything that came and went from the institute. I remember describing the boxes to him in great detail, and presenting him with a list of their contents. He promised to search. I checked back with him every day. Every day he told me the boxes had not turned up, but he was sure they would do so soon.

And yet there they were. Whomever I chose to complain to would blame it on someone else, or just smile. By now, I was beginning to detect, in the way people phrased things, that there was a vague but consistent confusion between accident and responsibility. If something fell or broke, Ugandans said, "Sorry!" At first, I would reply, "Don't worry, it's not your fault," but I soon realized that they knew this already. When someone crashed his car, he said, "The car got an accident," as if it had caught a cold. Found stealing a cassette tape, the gardener said, "It just got in my pocket."

It reminded me of what physicists called Brownian motion, the random movement of particles, on a grand scale. The natural world obeys statistical laws. When you turn on the tap, the most likely outcome is that water will flow from the tank on the roof into the sink. But there is a very small probability, immeasurable, or nearly so, that all the molecules will drift the other way. In Uganda, the margins of probability were considerably wider. Water still flowed downhill most of the time, but sometimes the wily gardener turned off the supply. He blamed the old pipes the stingy landlord put in and requested "money to pay the plumber" to fix them. Disorder was driven by a tide so strong it pulled everything with it, and the careless, dishonest, and greedy coasted along in the current with ease.

I built and dismantled various paranoid scenarios. Maybe the Ugandans had something against vaccine projects. This would not be a trivial matter. In the early 1980s, a medical relief worker was vaccinating people against polio on the Ssese Islands in Lake Victoria when a rumor broke out that whites were using injections to sterilize or kill black children. The islanders rowed him out to a place where the water was deep, tied a rock to his neck, and threw him overboard.

Maybe the accountant didn't like me. Maybe the accountant didn't like Celeste, and didn't like me because I lived with Celeste. Maybe Celeste, angry about the outcome of her own project, didn't want my project to work either. Soon I became too busy to worry about it.

When I opened the boxes, everything was there: plastic jars containing powdered chemicals, three expensive micropipettes that were capable of measuring one millionth of a liter of fluid, aluminum foil, waterproof pens, a roll of pink tape. But in order to begin the experiment, I needed to find clean water. The water from the taps in the lab, when they worked, came from Lake Victoria and was sometimes a faint green color and had things floating in it. The experiment called for distilled water, but there was none at the Cancer Institute. The tests conducted there didn't need it because they came in prepackaged kits, shipped at great expense from the United States.

There was a medical research lab across town run by the government, which shrewdly recognized that Uganda's diseases might constitute a nontraditional export. The lab was associated with a military clinic, and it functioned on a for-hire basis. For a price, scientists from anywhere in the world could study sick volunteers who were being treated at the clinic. Many of these volunteers were Ugandan soldiers who were either HIV positive or, because they were young and sexually active, were at risk of becoming HIV positive. Arthur and Professor Cornelius were on friendly terms with the directors of this lab and often met them to discuss future research projects and other matters. There was a still at this lab, and I went there one afternoon to ask whether I could use it.

The lab was in a long white building with a well-kept lawn that was being meticulously cut with machetes by young men in green uniforms. Soldiers in camouflage stood at the entrance. The director was not in, but his deputy advised me that if I wanted to use water from the still, I should write a letter to the director, stating who I was, what my project was, and what I needed the water for.

I returned to the Cancer Institute and drafted a two-paragraph letter. There were no computers at the Cancer Institute, so I asked the secretary to type it. She did so, and I gave a copy to the Ugandan doctor who was the head of the Cancer Institute. He decided that it would be better if the letter came from him, since he was senior to me and in a better position to negotiate. Eventually, my letter, typed by the secretary and signed by the director, was delivered to the government lab. After a week, no answer arrived, so I went back to the lab to make inquiries. This time, the director was in. He had lost the letter. I explained everything again and he agreed to let me use the water in his lab.

The government lab was immaculate and vast. There were seven technicians working there, all wearing lab coats, ties, and clean white sneakers. Some were setting up cultures to diagnose tuberculosis; others were measuring out samples of an herbal mixture, which, it was claimed, relieved the nausea and diarrhea associated with AIDS. It had the color and consistency of alfalfa and was delivered weekly by a traditional healer, an enormous man with one front tooth and a puff of bushy gray hair.

I met one lab assistant whose only assignment seemed to be to watch water drip out of the still. He sat for hours on a white countertop and stared at the still with a cheerful, lazy smile. At lunchtime, he removed his lab coat and turned off the machine. As he headed out the door, I asked him to turn it back on.

"Don't worry," I said. "I'll watch it." I then went back to calculating how much sodium hydroxide I would need to adjust the pH of borate to nine.

When I looked up again, a gust of steam was pouring out of the still. Apparently the water supply had been cut off, and the machine's bare coil was about to ignite. A two-thousand-dollar piece of equipment, unavailable elsewhere in Uganda, had almost been ruined. The technicians were forgiving. They said it had happened before. The still could be fixed.

The demons of accident are a feature of scientific work, and the thoughts of most scientists, when they are not taken up with novel theories about nature, are mainly concerned with preventing things from screwing up. But I was used to problems on a smaller scale: a bad batch of some chemical, dirty pipettes, mislabeled test tubes, stray bits of fluff in the air falling in petri dishes, careless little mistakes. In Uganda, accidents were of an entirely different order.

At the end of the week, I was able to return to my own lab with a dozen bottles of freshly prepared solutions and begin the ELISA tests. After the refrigerator had been installed, there was no room for me, so I had to work in the main lab after all. The place was crowded; there were six of us in a very small room. Nurses came and went, delivering specimens from the hospital, vials of urine and blood and other things to be tested for pregnancy, diabetes, syphilis, HIV. Sometimes the nurses hung around, chatting. Once a person I didn't know sat down on the floor near my corner, blocking my only way out, and spread thousands of tiny pieces of paper everywhere. The other technicians were very big and we all tried to avoid sudden movements.

I ran through the experiment as I had learned it at Chiron, adapting it slightly for this African lab. It was a pleasure and a relief to see the readout of the first experiment. An array of green dots appeared on a plastic dish, each one corresponding to a single patient and a single HIV subtype. The greener the dot, the more antibodies the person had made to that particular subtype, and the more likely he was to have been infected with it.

On the first day, I processed four patients' samples. All were infected with HIV-1, but they carried different subtypes. One had antibodies against subtype A, and another had antibodies against subtype C. Two had antibodies against both subtypes A and D. The next day I processed four more samples. These patients had antibodies against C only, D only, both A and D, and nothing.

I was so relieved that the experiment was working that I didn't realize what I was seeing at first. I was intrigued by how different the patterns of these green dots looked from those generated by the blood samples from California. Almost everyone there had antibodies against subtype B, and only subtype B. But it was hard to identify any pattern in these Ugandan samples.

After three weeks, I had tested about fifty samples. I sent a page of data to Chiron to let them know the work was under way. I said I thought the results were interesting and wondered if they did too. I spoke by telephone to a postdoc in Steimer's lab, and he said he was pleased that the experiment was working. He told me to keep going.

One morning I arrived to find the lab dark. The chief technician sat by a window, reading a newspaper. Two other technicians, one a skeptic, the other a Catholic, were arguing about the Ten Commandments. The Cancer Institute had a backup generator, but it had burned out from overuse. The hospital engineer had stopped by, looked at the generator, and shaken his head. The administrator went to call the electricity company, but the phone was out of order. We drove to the electricity company, found the manager, and told him that we were doing AIDS research at Mulago, that our work was being ruined, that lives were at stake, that he had to do something.

The problem was with the transformer, he said. There was nothing he could do. He wouldn't even accept a bribe.

Was anyone working on it?

No. The engineers were busy elsewhere. We went back to the lab and the lights were, miraculously, on, but it was too late to start an experiment.

That night the transformer at the hospital exploded in a flash that lit up the sky over half the city. A friend watched it burn from a balcony café in town. Then the hill where the hospital was went dark. My friend called me. "Don't bother coming to work," she said, "for a week at least." She was being pessimistic. After a few days, the lights were on again.

As the weeks wore on, more problems occurred; although always unpredicted, the novelty soon faded. Sometimes I wondered if I should have stayed in the United States, where boxes don't disappear, refrigerators don't shrink, water flows on demand, and labs rarely blow up. But AIDS research in the United States would have meant a contract and a salary and a boss. The boss would have told me that what I was trying to do wasn't worth it. The vaccine would fail, and condoms and STD treatment services would control the epidemic on their own. But mine was a romantic, naïve, ill-conceived mission that just might work, and for that reason the struggles and disasters were never too hard to endure.

Perhaps, I thought, CHIPS collapsed because it belonged to no one. When it got into trouble, USAID didn't care because it was only one of many projects—including STD projects—they were supporting throughout Africa. Taxpayers were unlikely to find out about the failure of one of them, and if they did, they were unlikely to be up in arms about it. The Africans didn't care because they wanted doctors and medicine more than they wanted buildings and condoms. And Celeste had other plans.

While I was working on the ELISAs, the phlebotomist at the Cancer Institute died. Toward the end, I was told, he was so sick that he frightened the patients. He wore a scarf to hide his swollen neck. I asked the American technologist in charge of the lab if she thought many people who worked at the institute were HIV positive. "You know that cute little pregnant nurse who hangs around the ward?" she asked. I did. She was beautiful—small, with perfect features like a child's—and enormously pregnant. She was married to the phlebotomist.

After I had been in the lab for some time, I began helping a technician who was growing cells from HIV-infected patients in dishes in the incubator. There were indications that something was wrong. Some of the cells were dying some of the time, but we couldn't predict when or figure out why. Most of the cells were fine and producing lots of virus particles, perhaps as many as a hundred per second. I suggested to the technician that he test his cultures to see if they were too acidic or too alkaline. He put a drop of one culture on a piece of litmus paper. Impatient to know the answer, I grabbed the wet piece of paper with a bare hand. The pH was within acceptable limits. Then I realized what I had done: the solution was far more infectious than any bodily fluid, including blood. I washed my hands four times.

I did some research and discovered that quite a few lab workers around the world had been infected on the job. Most cases involved an accident with a needle or scalpel. But one technician had been infected when blood splashed on his chapped hand. Another technician was infected when plasma splashed in her eye. Since 1978, there had been thirty-two cases of infection among lab workers where no other risk factor was present. In four cases the technician could recall no incident but percutaneous exposure. That is, HIV got through the skin somehow, through a small cut or rash or maybe the edge of a fingernail.

I thought of all the careless mistakes I had made over the years. Once I found I had spilled acid in a wastepaper basket, and another time I contaminated a test tube with radioactivity. On both occasions I was the only one who could have done it, but I had no memory of it; I must have done it unconsciously. How many times had I done this kind of thing? And how many times had it involved the AIDS virus?

Over the next couple of weeks, a mild headache came and went. I felt tired, I had a fever, diarrhea, an ear infection. I became aware of my neck and armpits. Everyone in the health field worries about accidental HIV transmission. The American technologist told me that she tests herself every six months or so by ELISA—a test similar to the one I was using for the subtyping experiments. The readout from the test is also an array of dots, each corresponding to a different person. The dots tell you who is infected. If the dot is clear, the person is uninfected. If the dot is green, the person is infected. Once she looked at the test plate and in the place where her own sample should have been, there was a green dot. She was infected. One of the other technicians noticed that she had been staring at the plate for a long time. He looked over her shoulder and told her she was holding the plate upside down. She was not infected.

For months I thought I felt mildly ill. I knew I should have a test. The doctor I went to see told me she had been a surgeon in Africa for six years. She had done operations, deliveries, cesareans. Forty percent of the women attending the hospital were HIV positive. The doctor said she had cut herself, stabbed herself with needles, been forced to work without gloves because the hospital was too poor to supply them. She had not become infected. While I waited for the results, I went for a walk, I went shopping. The world seemed surreally beautiful.

I was not infected.

At the end of three months I had data on almost two hundred patients, enough to convince myself that Ugandan HIV subtypes were a very mixed bag. Most patients had antibodies against subtypes A, C, or D, but there were many people who had antibodies against more than one subtype, such as both A and D, both A and C, or A, C, and D. I saw almost every conceivable combination. Perhaps these people were infected with more than one virus in the first place. On the other hand, they may have been infected with different, novel subtypes that simply shared characteristics with some of the known ones. Whatever the case, the diversity of viruses there appeared to be very great.

I was not surprised. Scientists theorize that HIV originated somewhere in West or central Africa. If true, this would mean it had existed in this region longer than anywhere else, so you would expect a greater diversity of subtypes. Perhaps HIV had been propagating for decades through African populations. During that time, it mutated and evolved into an array of different subtypes. Subtypes A, C, and D spread east to Uganda. Then, perhaps in the 1970s, one or a small number of HIV-positive people brought subtype B to the Western Hemisphere. After the first clusters of HIV infection occurred in gay men in the United States, subtype B fanned out all over the Americas and Europe.

This was interesting, but the practical implications were disturbing. My results showed that Chiron's HIV vaccine, which was based on subtype B, would have to be redesigned if it was to be tested in Uganda. It would have to include a cocktail of HIV strains, including A, C, D, and perhaps others. It is not clear whether the immune system would even be capable of making protective lymphocytes and antibodies against such a complicated mixture of viruses.

I sent my results to Chiron by fax. I looked forward to discussing the implications of what I had found, and learning how the subtype B vaccine trial was going. There was no reply for several days. Then there was a weekend, and then no reply for a few more days.

"You have to accept that what happens in Africa doesn't matter that much back home," said Arthur, when I asked him if he had any idea what might be going on.

Finally, I got a letter from one of the postdocs at Chiron. He said that in order to draw any conclusions from my results, more work would have to be done on the Ugandan serum samples. Would it be possible, he asked, for me to send some of the samples back to Chiron? If Chiron confirmed my results using more technically refined methods, then perhaps we could write a paper about HIV antibodies in Uganda and their implications for vaccine design.

It happened that Arthur was preparing to go back to San Francisco to take up a medical fellowship. We spoke to the director of the Cancer Institute, who agreed to allow him to take twenty-five vials of serum back to San Francisco.

When Arthur and I said goodbye, he promised to send the vials across the bay to Chiron, a forty-minute trip by car, as soon as he arrived. I was grateful for this and for all the other help he had given me. It was thanks to him that this venture had worked at all. He had convinced the doctors at the Cancer Institute to let me work in their lab, and he had driven me around town in search of boxes and water. He had been working in Uganda for two years, counting people as they got sick and died; he had become depressed by Uganda's dilapidated hospitals and its public health campaigns, which, though vigorous, had yet to show signs of success. He and I shared the hope that the answer to AIDS in Uganda would emerge from an incubator in the West someday.

We were to be disappointed. Further experiments showed that Chiron's subtype-B vaccine might protect people from lab strains of the virus, but not from the "wild-type" viruses circulating in infected people in the United States. It turned out that the surface of each gp120 molecule is covered with sugar molecules that form a barricade around the "conserved" part of the molecule that Steimer hoped would be the Achilles heel of HIV. As the virus proliferates and mutates in the body, this "sugar barricade" shifts, generating a battalion of decoys that are impossible for the immune system to keep up with.

In 2004, the editor of the prestigious British medical journal *The Lancet* looked back on twenty years of failed vaccine research and warned that we might never catch up. This virus can run faster than the human immune system, and much faster than our technical capabilities in vaccine research.[7] This is just what everyone had warned me about: the HIV researchers I spoke to in the United States before I left for Uganda, and even the cab driver in Kampala.

In May 1994, a multimillion-dollar trial of Chiron's subtype-B vaccine was looking pretty unlikely. That June, a committee of experts at the U.S. National Institutes of Health decided they felt the same way. They unanimously recommended that Congress reject a proposal to finance a trial of the Chiron vaccine in the United States. In November 1996, Kathelyn Steimer, my boss at Chiron, died of cancer, and the company, along with other labs around the world, scaled back its HIV vaccine research.

At that time, many AIDS researchers pinned their hopes instead on STD treatment services and condoms. Shortly after CHIPS closed, researchers from Columbia University launched a study of "mass STD treatment" in southern Uganda. Thousands of people were dosed with antibiotics in the hope that this would heal their genital sores and slow the spread of HIV. Unfortunately, this program had no effect whatsoever on HIV incidence. To date, five other studies of STD treatment have been undertaken in Africa, but only one modestly reduced the incidence of HIV.[8] It is likely that STDs accelerate the spread of HIV only when the epidemic is at a very early stage.[9] By the time the virus has spread widely in the general population, as it has throughout East and southern Africa by now, it is too late; treating STDs makes little difference.

What I didn't know when I was in Uganda was that the HIV rate was falling anyway, even though the programs for people with sexually transmitted diseases had failed and there was no vaccine.

Years later, I returned to the country to try to discover how this had happened. But by then much had changed, and I felt like a pilgrim exploring a place where a miracle was said to have occurred long ago. Everyone had a different story about it and half the evidence was missing. I eventually drew my own conclusions, but we are getting ahead of the story.

As Arthur was leaving, our parting words were these: "So, you're going to send those samples to Chiron?"

"I promise."

"I'm counting on you. All you have to do is ship them across the bay."

"I know. I will."

The samples never made it.

Everyone seems to know what Africa needs, but sometimes I think our minds are not really on it. Most of us see only Africa's contours, and we use them to map out problems of our own. Africa is a career move, an adventure, an experiment. It fades into an idea.

We aren't really looking. I think of the dot in the cells of the bug under the microscope in the lab back in California. Although the fine machinery of insect cells means less to me now, I did draw at least one lesson from that work: inanimate objects obey the laws of physics, but there are no corresponding laws for living things, and in biology grand theories are nearly always wrong. Nevertheless, if you look hard enough at a problem, you may find surprising truths that no one could have predicted. But you have to look very hard. You must enter a different world, follow its logic, and forget your own.

From the moment you are exposed to the HIV virus to when the infection can be detected with a test takes about three months. For three months I had lived with the possibility that I had HIV. Sometimes it seemed a certainty. Every morning on the way to the lab, I passed a clinic where HIV-positive patients lined up on benches on a porch, waiting to see the doctor. He weighed them, took a blood sample, and sent them home. Sometimes a man or woman had to be carried up the steps from the road, thin and weak, with arms swinging like a marionette's. I wondered how the others who were not yet sick dealt with this. They said nothing and looked away. AIDS can be a lonely disease. You die slowly, in great pain, and many people are frightened of you. I realized now that as I passed them, I could almost see across the distance of continents and race. Very briefly, I thought I saw AIDS their way.

CHAPTER TWO

The Mysterious Origins of HIV

After Celeste left Uganda, I moved to a house on Makindye Hill, a Kampala suburb that was at that time still very rural. On the way to my new house, I would walk up a red-dirt road, dispersing clouds of butterflies. Small plots of cassava and banana had been cut out of the bush, and goats and chickens grazed on the verges. A troop of green monkeys swung in the trees outside my window, and one morning I woke up early and saw a wild gray parrot take off from his perch on a bush. I shared a room with an assortment of insects: ants, grasshoppers, millipedes, and a shoehorn-sized flying beetle in need of pilot lessons. It tripped over things on the floor, bumped into walls, and made a sound like a small helicopter with its wings. I watched it one night during a case of insomnia brought on by the antimalaria pills I was taking. The problem seemed to be that when it landed, it fell over on its side and then had to buzz its wings to right itself. How could such a species endure? It seems as though almost anything can survive in the green equatorial girth of the Rift Valley, as though there were only variation and no selection. Life pours out of here as from a volcano. It is the only place on earth where a feeble, unsteady, slow-moving, hairless species like man could have evolved.

These fragile species constantly feed off each other, as parasites within parasites and predators upon predators drive the bitter process of evolution. Where did HIV—our fiercest predator yet—come from? How did it enter human populations and spread all over the world? In thousands of years of human history, not a single person is known to have been infected with HIV until 1959.[1] It is possible that there were cases before that year, but no colonial medical officer, African doctor, or traditional healer ever noticed them and they are absent from all known historical records.

Some scientists have claimed that we don't need to know where HIV came from. In 1992, a WHO official told *Rolling Stone* magazine that "the origin of the AIDS virus is of no importance to scientists today." Another irate AIDS researcher told the same reporter, "Who cares what the origin of the virus is? . . . It's distracting, it's non-productive, it's confusing to the public."[2]

Is there any value in knowing where HIV came from? I think there is. HIV viruses crossed into human populations from primates at least twice and perhaps more often, probably around 1930.[3] The only way to prevent other chimp or monkey viruses from doing so again is to know how these transfers occurred in the first place.

Also, the mystery of AIDS—why it emerged when it did, why it is spreading so rapidly among certain populations—is one of the most frightening things about it. Twenty-five years into the epidemic, rumors about the virus's origins swirl through every community where the virus is common, derailing research, treatment, and prevention programs.

In 1986, an item in various African newspapers alleged that HIV had been developed at a U.S. military lab and was then introduced into Africa by American and British doctors. The authors, assumed to be Soviet propagandists, would insert the names of local white physicians wherever the story appeared. The Ugandan version implicated Wilson Carswell, a British surgeon who had been working at Mulago Hospital since the 1960s. Carswell had conducted some of the earliest studies of HIV in Uganda, and had sent several shipments of blood samples to Porton Down, a germ-warfare lab in England and one of the few places in the world capable of conducting HIV tests at the time.

Shortly after the articles appeared, a series of mysterious incidents occurred at Carswell's house in Kampala. He arrived home early from work one day and found an intruder rummaging through his computer files. A few weeks later, his two-way radio disappeared, and then two of his servants were bludgeoned with digging hoes. When he made a casual remark about Uganda's staggering AIDS epidemic to a visiting journalist, Carswell was thrown out of the country.[4]

Rumors about AIDS betray a painful sense of confusion and shame. People want to know, What happened? Why us? Why now? Is the virus new? Then where did it come from? Was it always there? Then why didn't it spread before? Has the virus changed? Or have we? Knowing the answers might foster a more pragmatic response to the disease. In any case, if a group of African spies came to the United States and, however improbably, unleashed the most hideous plague in living memory, I think we'd want to know.

SOMETIME IN the early decades of the twentieth century—probably before 1930—five deadly retroviruses emerged from the African bush. Two of them were strains of HIV-2, and three of them were strains of HIV-1, one of which—known as HIV-1M—gave rise to the global AIDS pandemic. Many researchers theorize that there is a perfectly simple explanation for how this happened—that it resulted from what they call "natural transfer." Some thirty-six species of African monkeys and apes carry viruses—known as SIVs, for simian immunodeficiency viruses—that closely resemble HIV, and researchers speculate that the HIV viruses are really primate viruses that somehow jumped into human beings. HIV-1, the virus responsible for most cases of AIDS to date, came from a chimpanzee, and HIV-2, a less aggressive virus more common among West Africans, came from a monkey called the sooty mangabey.

According to the natural-transfer theory, AIDS is really an old disease, and viruses similar to HIV were always fairly common in a small number of forest-dwelling communities that hunted monkeys and apes for food. These viruses were passed to hunters when they cut their hands subduing or butchering prey, and chimp or monkey blood seeped into the wounds. In the past, most African people lived in isolated tribes, and this kept these viruses from spreading beyond the remote villages where the hunters lived. Then twentieth-century upheavals in African society changed everything. The far-flung regions of the continent were suddenly drawn together as never before by highways, labor migrations, and refugee movements. It is plausible that these highways for people were also highways for germs. At the same time, the trade in "bush meat" from wild animals caught in the forests of West and central Africa boomed.[5] Today, some five million tons of antelope, snakes, gorillas, and elephants are eaten every year in this region. The roasted hands, skulls, and limbs of gorillas, chimps, and other primates are gruesomely displayed at food markets throughout West Africa. Many of these species carry SIV viruses, any one of which could mutate in the bloodstream of a careless hunter or butcher into a new strain of HIV.

During the past century, African wars of independence, the growth of African cities, new highways and truck routes, and the expansion of African mining industries drew unprecedented numbers of men out of the countryside. They left their families behind in the villages, and prostitution flourished wherever they went. Now the HIV viruses had many opportunities to escape from the bush, and every urban community, every truck stop and military barracks, was a breeding ground for HIV. All that was necessary for the virus to break out of the jungle was for a hunter or meat seller to cut his hand while butchering an infected chimp, and then for that hunter to migrate to a city or join an army and have sexual relations, perhaps in a brothel. The virus might then spread from the prostitute who had sex with the hunter to other customers, and then perhaps to other brothels visited by those customers, and then to yet more customers, and eventually to the wives of customers.

This is a plausible theory, even if there is something Victorian about it. During colonial times, Europeans fretted about the impact of urbanization on fragile native souls, and the transition to modernity was sometimes invoked to explain why Africans were so susceptible to tuberculosis, syphilis, and a range of other diseases.[6] The natural-transfer theory implies that AIDS is the price Africans have paid for modern development, independence, war, urban drift, sexual license, and being cruel to chimps and monkeys.

But there are other reasons to question whether the natural-transfer theory provides a complete explanation for the origin of HIV. In 1999, the British journalist Edward Hooper alleged that HIV leapt from apes to human beings during a laboratory accident in the Congo jungle during the 1950s, where American researchers were conducting polio experiments on chimps and monkeys. Very little evidence has been produced to support Hooper's theory, but his book—*The River: A Journey to the Source of HIV and AIDS*[7]—is interesting less for its pursuit of the polio-HIV connection than for its skeptical treatment of the natural-transfer hypothesis.

As Hooper points out, early colonial and precolonial Africa was not all quiet villages and stable families. Since the sixteenth century, African wars have grown increasingly widespread and complicated, involving diverse tribes and European invaders. In the early nineteenth century, land disputes among rival chiefs in southern Africa ignited the "Wars of Wandering," named for the extensive migrations that followed. Prostitution flourished in the growing colonial cities of nineteenth-century Africa, but no one died of AIDS.

The slave trade, which reached deep into the interior, existed in Africa long before colonial times, and accelerated after the arrival of the Portuguese in the fifteenth century. Between 1700 and 1850 some twenty-one million Africans were enslaved, and at least nine million were marched to the coasts and shipped all over the world. During the two World Wars, African men were recruited as soldiers to fight in North Africa and the Middle East. These migrations did spread HTLV-1—a virus similar to HIV—that also seems to have come from chimpanzees, as well as malaria and yellow fever. So why not HIV?

Hooper also maintains that the AIDS epidemic must have been set off by something more than a hunter's wound. Africans have been killing and eating monkeys for at least fifty thousand years, and yet African and colonial doctors never saw anything like AIDS until the 1960s. HIV-1 is largely absent from the pygmy communities that still live in the forests of central Africa and hunt chimpanzees that carry viruses closely related to HIV-1. Pygmy hunters use rough tools to butcher their prey, so if the natural-transfer theory is correct, pygmies, if anyone, should be infected with HIV. However, the only HIV-positive pygmies identified to date are those who have had significant contact with larger towns and almost certainly picked up the virus through sexual intercourse. Pygmies do carry HTLV-l, which also spreads through blood and comes from chimpanzees, but not HIV.

It's possible that the monkey and chimp versions of HIV—or SIVs—are not harmful to human beings unless they undergo a genetic "shift" that transforms them into killers. In 2004, researchers from Johns Hopkins University analyzed blood samples from a thousand people living in the bush-meat-consuming areas of West Africa, where HIV is thought to have emerged. They found several people with benign HIV-like viruses that closely resembled viruses from mandrills, mangabeys, and other exotic species that are commonly hunted or kept as pets. But these viruses did not cause disease in those people, and did not spread to others.[8]

In 1990, a laboratory worker became infected with a monkey SIV virus related to the one thought to have given rise to HIV-2 in West Africa. He* was working with the blood of a macaque monkey that had been infected with an HIV-like virus from a sooty mangabey. The lab worker had been suffering from a case of poison ivy and the rubber lab gloves hurt his hands, so he didn't wear them. It is likely that he spilled something—blood or some other fluid with virus in it—on his hands and that the virus seeped in through the sores. The lab worker's immune system made antibodies against the virus, but the virus itself grew very slowly, and the lab worker never got sick. Similarly, several Africans, including two Liberian rubber-plantation workers and a woman who sold monkey meat at a market in Sierra Leone, were infected with the sooty mangabey virus thought to have given rise to HIV-2; but again the infections neither progressed to AIDS nor spread to others.[9] This is virtually unheard of with real HIV infection, which never clears and almost always causes AIDS.

Perhaps Hooper is right. Perhaps something did happen in central Africa in the early twentieth century—and perhaps simultaneously in West Africa—to cause a very small number of previously harmless monkey and ape viruses to become deadly to human beings. Somehow they developed the ability to creep into semen and other secretions, and spread from person to person, and grow so rapidly in human blood that they were able to overwhelm the immune system and destroy it.

NONE OF THE AIDS researchers I have spoken to share Hooper's belief that HIV came from a polio vaccine.[10] Most assume that a small number

*Or she: the sex of the lab worker was not reported.

of SIVs mutated by chance into human viruses and then spread widely across twentieth-century Africa, blown by the winds of change sweeping the continent, including urbanization, migration, and war. While I agreed that a single virus might mutate by chance into a killer and then be swept up by those winds, it still seemed odd that five viruses would do so in such a narrow space of time. After all, despite accelerated urbanization, the growth of prostitution and the bush-meat trade, and an endless series of civil wars and refugee crises, no new HIV viruses have emerged since the 1950s. Why not?

The reason may remain forever a mystery, but one hypothesis that Hooper pursues only briefly in *The River* intrigued me. A small number of scientists have suggested that the introduction of vaccination campaigns or possibly blood transfusions into Africa during the early twentieth century could have facilitated the evolution of HIV.[11] While I was talking to Patricia Fultz, who studies HIV-like viruses in monkeys at the University of Alabama, she mentioned the work of Opendra Narayan, a virologist at the University of Kansas. I discovered that Narayan had actually succeeded in turning an apparently harmless monkey virus into a deadly killer in his own laboratory.

Narayan was working with a genetically engineered version of HIV known as SHIV—simian human immunodeficiency virus—which is used to infect lab monkeys. SHIV is a weak virus. It grows in monkeys but does not cause disease in those monkeys, and it is not passed to other monkeys through sex, biting, or other natural means. However, SHIV can be passed from one monkey to another in laboratories through blood transfusions or bone-marrow transplantation. If SHIV is transmitted artificially from one monkey to another and then another rapidly enough, through a process known as passaging, it can turn into a virus that spreads easily and causes a monkey version of AIDS.

"This has been known since Pasteur's time," Narayan told me. "If you take any virus and 'passage' it through a new species often enough, eventually you get a more pathogenic virus." To prove that this would work with SHIV, Narayan and his colleagues injected it into a monkey and waited for it to grow.[12] Usually the monkey's immune system controls the virus and clears it, but this takes a month or so. During this time, the virus makes millions of copies of itself. As it does so, it mutates, so that not all the copies are identical to the original virus. After a few weeks, Narayan took a small sample of virus from the monkey's bone marrow, where it was still reproducing, and injected it into another monkey. The viruses used to infect monkey number two would have been the most robust of all the mutants, having withstood attack by the immune system of monkey number one for the longest period of time. Thus Narayan was using natural selection to give the virus a head start in its battle with the second monkey's immune system. A few weeks later, Narayan took virus from the second monkey's bone marrow and injected it into a third monkey. The virus caused no disease in the first two monkeys, but it caused mild disease in the third monkey. But when, after a few more weeks, the third monkey's virus was passed to a fourth monkey, the virus caused AIDS in almost every subsequent monkey Narayan injected it into.

Something similar may have happened with HIV. If a hunter or monkey-meat butcher became infected with a harmless monkey virus and then shortly afterward passed it on to someone else, who then passed it on to someone else a few weeks later, it is possible that the monkey virus might have turned into HIV. Like Narayan's SHIV, the monkey virus might not have been able to cross from the hunter to other people by sex, but it just might have been able to cross to others through blood. This might have happened in the clinics and hospitals of early twentieth-century Africa.

Many medical campaigns conducted around the time HIV first emerged involved what now seem like highly unsafe practices. During World War I, for example, six syringes were used to treat some ninety thousand people with sleeping sickness in the Belgian Congo. In 2000, the University of California anthropologist Jim Moore suggested that HIV might have undergone serial passaging during the smallpox campaigns carried out in West Africa during the early twentieth century, when thousands of people were inoculated with material from pox vesicles—blisters filled with weakened smallpox virus and with white blood cells, the primary home of HIV in the blood.[13] These pox vesicles had been scraped from the arms of other people who had recently been inoculated themselves. Such arm-to-arm inoculation was common in Africa until World War I.[14]

Another possibility is blood transfusion. Hypodermic needles were introduced in Africa in the early twentieth century, and blood banks were introduced later, probably after World War II. Perhaps a hunter or butcher carrying a benign monkey virus gave blood at a hospital. In Africa, people who receive transfusions sometimes donate blood themselves once they have recovered from their illness. Perhaps the person who received the hunter's blood became a donor himself a few weeks later and the virus was then transferred to a third person through another transfusion. This might have been enough to kick-start the virus. It might have evolved through such passaging so that it could grow vigorously in human cells and infect new people through means other than inoculation or blood transfusion. It might have become sexually transmissible, and deadly. I asked Dr. Narayan whether primate HIVs might have first adapted to human beings after being passaged through blood transfusions or inoculation, just as his SHIV adapted to monkeys through successive bone-marrow transfers. "Yes," he said, "that might have happened."

Such passaging events might be very rare. "We used to talk in terms of lightning rods," the AIDS researcher Preston Marx told Hooper. "You know—lightning can't strike twice unless there's a lightning rod. The lightning rod's the needle. That's why it struck twice in the same place—HIV-1 in central Africa and HIV-2 in West Africa."[15]

Hooper dismisses Marx's hypothesis, and many scientists, although intrigued by it, remain skeptical. Although the theory is hard to prove, it is worth considering the possibility that new medical technologies introduced into Africa in the early twentieth century sparked the global AIDS pandemic. New diseases tend to emerge when our relationship to nature changes. If HIV entered human populations through such new medical technologies as needles, blood transfusions, or inoculation campaigns, it would not be the first time that a new microbe flourished in the wake of human development. Epidemics of polio emerged only in the nineteenth century with improvements in sanitation. Smallpox, brucellosis, tuberculosis, and anthrax probably jumped from cattle to people during the process of domestication. Likewise, influenza evolved from chicken and pig diseases; the common cold from a horse disease; and measles, rabies, and hydatid cysts from dog diseases. The prions that cause BSE and its human cognate, new-variant Creutzfeldt-Jakob disease, or nv-CJD, emerged when producers began using the carcasses of sheep—some of which carried scrapie, a disease similar to BSE and CJD—to make feed for cattle, ordinarily a noncarnivorous species. More recent developments in intensive farming may have made possible the evolution and spread of yet more diseases, including West Nile virus and perhaps avian flu.[16] Vaccinations, blood transfusions, animal farming, and sanitation have saved generations of human beings from malnutrition and disease, only for new plagues to emerge in their places.

CHAPTER THREE

Why Are HIV Rates So High in Africa?

After I left Uganda, I moved to England to study public health at the London School of Hygiene and Tropical Medicine. I lived among the greenswards and gray, rain-slicked tile roofs of Clapham Common, far from the dust and noise and glaring equatorial sun of East Africa. But my mind kept returning to AIDS. From its early niche in the northwest corner of Lake Victoria, deep in the folds of the Rift Valley, HIV was now spreading throughout the entire eastern and southern arc of the continent. The maps and bar graphs in the UN reports and public health journals that came into the London School of Hygiene library looked like the field drawings of a conquering army. In 1985, virtually no one in Botswana was HIV positive. By 1992, 10 percent of pregnant women carried the virus, and by 2005, nearly 40 percent did. In South Africa, the HIV infection rate rose from 5 percent in 1993 to 20 percent in 2005.[1] By 2004, 42 percent of all pregnant women in Swaziland were HIV positive.

These rates were astronomical compared with most of the rest of the world. The HIV rate in the United States never exceeded 1 percent; in Russia and India, the figure also hovered around 1 percent. Even in Thailand, with its thriving sex and drug trades, the national infection rate peaked at only around 2 percent in the early 1990s.[2] At first, some UN officials predicted that HIV would spread rapidly in the general population of Asia and eastern Europe, but the virus has been present in these regions for decades and such extensive spread has never occurred. Instead, the virus remains confined to those with well-known risk factors, such as prostitutes, intravenous drug users, and gay men who might have scores or even hundreds of partners a year. In East and southern Africa, virtually everyone is at high risk of HIV infection, even though intravenous drug use is rare and few people have large numbers of sexual partners.[3]

Why has HIV spread so rapidly in East and southern Africa? Because HIV prevalence in Africa is highest among heterosexual men and women, most people suspected it must have something to do with sex. But what were Africans doing differently?

In 1995, this was a question few people wanted to discuss. Everyone knew that certain groups—gay men, prostitutes, intravenous drug users, and Africans—were much more likely to be infected with HIV than other people. These groups already faced discrimination, now exacerbated by the terrible stigma associated with AIDS.[4] During the 1980s, journalists from Europe and the United States had flocked to the heavily AIDS-afflicted villages of southern Uganda, now all but abandoned. In fact, this had less to do with the ravages of AIDS than with President Museveni's crackdown on smuggling, which had been the main livelihood in these border villages in the Amin and Obote years.[5] Nevertheless, the "abandoned AIDS villages of Uganda" left a vivid impression on the public. So did such statements from American and European experts as this: "There is profound promiscuity in Uganda. The average Ugandan has sex with great frequency, with a great number of partners."[6] Such claims, under tactless headlines like "Doomsday Reports Shock Whitehall: African AIDS 'Deadly Threat to Britain'"[7] angered African leaders and intellectuals across the continent. One Ugandan diplomat accused the West of launching "a smear campaign against us." After all, HIV had first been identified in the United States, one letter writer pointed out in a Nigerian newspaper, where "society had gone berserk with its sexual habits during the 1960s."[8]

Most African leaders reacted to the furor over AIDS in Africa by downplaying the significance of the epidemic in their countries. The governments of Zambia and Nigeria discouraged local newspapers from reporting on the AIDS crisis. When community-based AIDS organizations in Kenya tried to register with the government so they could begin operating, they faced endless bureaucratic obstacles.[9]

Diplomatic public health officials feared that drawing attention to the unique severity of AIDS in Africa would only drive African leaders further into denial, so they tactfully emphasized the global nature of the AIDS epidemic. Even though the statistics suggested otherwise, most public health officials insisted it was only a matter of time before the AIDS situation would be similarly severe in other poor world regions.[10]

But the question did not go away. After all, it was hard to know what to do about Africa's staggering AIDS epidemic without knowing what was causing it. In the pages of academic journals, theories about the mysterious concentration of AIDS in Africa sprang up and faded year after year.

At first, the answer seemed quite simple. In 1989, the Australian demographer John Caldwell and his colleagues argued that the virus was spreading rapidly in Africa because people there had a unique "sexual system" characterized by higher rates of casual and premarital sex.[11] He pointed to the cultural desire for many children, the tradition of polygamy, and the relative freedom of African women—at least compared to Asian women, many of whom were forbidden even to speak to unrelated men and were sometimes confined entirely to the home.

Caldwell's theory sparked controversy, not only because it seemed to revive tired stereotypes about African sexuality, but also because studies suggested that Africans were not more promiscuous than heterosexual people in other world regions.[12] In Africa, sexual debut tends to occur in the late teens, as it does in Europe and the United States. African men and women report roughly similar, if not fewer, numbers of lifetime partners than do heterosexuals in many Western countries.[13] According to the World Health Organization, men in Thailand and Rio de Janeiro are more likely to report five or more casual sexual partners in the previous year than men in Tanzania, Kenya, Lesotho, or Lusaka, Zambia. And very few women in any of these countries report five or more partners a year. Certainly Africans aren't nearly as promiscuous as American gay men of the 1970s and '80s, who routinely reported one hundred or more partners a year. And yet the HIV rate in some African cities was just as high as it had been in the gay enclaves of New York and San Francisco.

Some people wondered whether it was not the amount of sexual activity in Africa that mattered, but its exotic nature. They pointed to African sexual customs, such as "widow cleansing"—in which a designated village elder is expected to sleep with all newly widowed women—or "dry sex," in which African women clean their vaginas with plants and other substances. Perhaps the drying made women more susceptible to HIV by creating vaginal sores.[14] But this didn't make sense either, because widow cleansing is quite rare in the urban communities where HIV rates are highest, and many AIDS-afflicted communities prefer "wet sex."[15] In any case, the evidence that women who practice dry sex are at higher risk of HIV is equivocal.[16]

Others wondered whether Africa's high HIV rates had anything to do with sex at all. A Harvard molecular biologist proposed that Africa was home to "killer" strains of HIV that spread especially rapidly.[17] But he has produced little evidence to support this claim. African HIV strains have been found in European and U.S. patients but have not given rise to large epidemics in either place.

Another theory held that Africans were vulnerable to HIV because their immune defenses had been weakened by malnutrition and parasite infections common among the poor.[18]* But this didn't explain why the HIV rate was thirty times higher in Botswana than in India or Bolivia, much poorer countries.[19] Nor did it explain why Africa's most impoverished, parasite-infested, and war-torn countries, such as Liberia, Congo, Sierra Leone, Ethiopia, and Somalia, had low HIV rates, while rich, peaceful countries, such as South Africa and Botswana, had high HIV rates.[20] Even within these countries, the poorest people, the farmers and refugees, were less likely to be infected than traders, small businessmen, and other relatively rich, otherwise healthy people.[21]

Most of my professors in London believed that the African epidemic was caused by sexual behavior, but they maintained that what mattered most was not the number of sexual partners people had, but who those partners were. In 1991, the epidemiologist Roy Anderson of Oxford University theorized that Africans were susceptible to AIDS because of "sexual mixing" between "high-risk groups"—prostitutes and their male

*In 2006, researchers discovered that malaria enhances the transmission of HIV (see Laith J. Abu-Raddad et al., "Dual infection with HIV and malaria fuels the spread of both diseases in sub-Saharan Africa," *Science* 314:5805 (December 8, 2006), 1603–1606. Malaria infection increases the concentration of HIV in the blood, making HIV-positive malaria sufferers more likely to transmit the virus to others if they engage in unprotected sex. The researchers estimated that in Kenya, where malaria is common, the HIV infection rate was 8 percent higher than it would have been without malaria. This is a serious problem and further motivation—if it is needed—for malaria control in developing countries, but it cannot explain the HIV epidemic. The HIV rate in Kenya would still be very high even if there were no malaria in the country, and HIV rates are astronomical in Lesotho, Botswana, and South Africa, where malaria is uncommon.

clients—and everybody else.[22] In the West, AIDS mainly affected gay men, who tended to have sex with other gay men, and intravenous drug users and their sexual partners, who also tended to spread the virus among themselves. But in Africa, Anderson claimed, sex crosses social boundaries more frequently than in the West. It occurs between rich and poor, urban and rural, old and young, and this sexual mixing gave rise to an "epidemiological pump" that drove the virus through the population.

Anderson claimed this "pump" had been created partly by the legacy of colonial rule. Beginning in the late nineteenth century, the economy of southern Africa as far north as Tanzania was tied to the newly opened gold and diamond mines of South Africa. In order to attract labor for the mines, the British colonial authorities imposed a tax on every hut or dwelling, effectively forcing millions of African men to leave their villages behind for months or years at a time in search of wages to pay their taxes. The effect on the African family was devastating.[23] Beginning in the 1920s, rates of STDs such as syphilis and gonorrhea soared in the anomic slums and mining camps of South Africa, with their bawdy, lowlife culture of prostitutes, migrant workers, and drifters.[24] As migrants shuttled back and forth between rural and urban areas, they brought their sexually transmitted diseases with them, and when HIV began spreading in the 1980s, it followed the same migrant routes.

At first, Anderson's "mixing" hypothesis seemed to explain everything. In the mid-1980s, nearly half of the AIDS patients in East African hospitals were either prostitutes or migrant workers such as miners, itinerant businessmen, or truckers.[25] In 1985, Wilson Carswell conducted a survey of Ugandan "bar girls"—impoverished prostitutes who worked in the towns and trading centers near Lake Victoria. He noticed that many of the towns where the bar girls worked were truck stops, with wide turnouts for the giant vehicles that heaved along the Trans-African Highway from Mombasa on the Kenyan coast to Nairobi, Kampala, Kigali, and other cities in the interior. When Carswell tested the truck drivers, one in three turned out to be HIV positive.[26] He saw then how these men could spread the virus throughout East Africa and then south to Zimbabwe, South Africa, and beyond.

Throughout the 1990s, most experts reasoned that the best way to stop HIV from spreading was to stem the epidemic at what they thought was its source—prostitutes and their male clients, especially mine workers, truckers, soldiers, and other migrants. Lecturing such people about abstinence and faithfulness was assumed to be futile, so their main prescription was for condom programs and treatment services for STDs such as syphilis and gonorrhea.[27] Programs to warn the general population about the dangers of AIDS were considered a lesser priority.[28]

But as the 1990s wore on, and the virus tore through the general population in East and southern Africa, some people began to worry. The epidemic that had begun among prostitutes and migrants was now killing ordinary men and women in huge numbers. Teachers, shopkeepers, policemen, and cabinet ministers were almost as likely, and sometimes more likely, to be HIV positive than prostitutes and migrant workers were.[29] Meanwhile, prevention programs were failing disastrously. As condom use soared, the HIV rate soared as well.[30] Improving STD treatment services also made little difference.[31] Some people were beginning to wonder whether the "high-risk/low-risk mixing" theory entirely explained the African AIDS epidemic after all.

IN 1993, Martina Morris, now a professor of sociology and statistics at the University of Washington in Seattle, set out for Uganda. Morris had followed Anderson's research closely, and she wanted to test his mixing theory using data on sexual behavior from an African population severely affected by AIDS. Like Anderson, she assumed that African HIV rates were high because typical high-risk groups were spreading HIV to everyone else.

Morris had helped devise a computer program that would predict how HIV would spread through a population, based on such factors as the number of sexual partners people had and the length of each relationship. She planned to collect sexual histories from thousands of Ugandan people, plug the data into her computer model, and see whether the computer generated the HIV infection rate measured in Uganda at the time. If the model worked, she planned to use it to forecast the spread of HIV in other countries.

"Just after I arrived in Uganda, I had to give a lecture to a group of doctors at the medical school in Kampala, telling them what I planned to do," Morris told me in 2003. "At the time there was talk in Uganda about helicopter scientists—whites from the United States and Europe who just parachuted in, took data, and didn't work with local African experts. I was the only American woman in the room, and it was a tough audience. The HIV rate was estimated to be 18 percent at the time, and here I was trying to explain how mathematical models were going to help people. In the middle of my talk, one man raised his hand and asked, 'Can your computer handle situations where people have more than one partner at a time?' I said, 'No, that's too difficult to model.' The man walked out of the room. Afterward, the others sat down with me and said I had to include concurrent partnerships in my model. Otherwise it would be irrelevant."

Morris's lecture in Uganda was a turning point. Until then, she and other experts had been trying to understand the spread of AIDS in Africa in terms of behavior typical of AIDS-affected communities in the West. In the gay community and among prostitutes the world over, "risky sexual behavior" meant having dozens or even hundreds of different sexual partners a year. In Africa, relatively few people were anywhere near as promiscuous as that—even migrant workers seldom had more than ten or twenty partners in a lifetime, and most people had far fewer.[32] However, as Morris and others soon discovered, a relatively high proportion of African men and women had ongoing relationships with a small number of people—perhaps two or three—at a time. These "concurrent" relationships might overlap for months or years, or even, in the case of polygamous marriages, a lifetime.

Such behavior is normative in many African societies, especially for men, and is practiced by large numbers of people who are neither prostitutes nor especially promiscuous. This pattern differs from the serial monogamy more common in Western cultures, or the onetime casual and commercial encounters that occur everywhere. But as Morris discovered, concurrent or simultaneous sexual partnerships are far more dangerous than serial monogamy, because they link people up in a giant web of sexual relationships that serves as a superhighway for the rapid spread of HIV.

The idea that long-term simultaneous partnerships might increase the spread of HIV was first proposed by the British epidemiologists Robert May and Charlotte Watts in 1992.[33] But Morris had not seen their article when she set out for Uganda in 1993, and the mathematical tools she had at the time were not up to the complicated task of modeling multiple long-term partnerships anyway.

But with the Ugandan doctors' advice in mind,* Morris began collecting detailed information about sexual behavior in Uganda. This meant asking more than a thousand people to answer some very intimate questions about their lives. Sex surveys are fascinating, but they sometimes give misleading results.[34] Women tend to underreport the number of partners they have had, while men tend to exaggerate. To help mitigate this problem, Morris replaced the impersonal language of standard questionnaires with a structured conversation. She trained a team of interviewers to collect detailed sexual histories by first asking each person whom he or she last had sex with, how the couple met, how long they had been together, and whether they were still together. Then the interviewers asked about the respondent's previous sexual partner, and the one before that, and so on. "Respondents love it, because it's really like gossip," Morris explained. "In a way, people are telling the story of their lives."

*It is not clear where the Ugandans at Morris's lecture first learned about the concurrency hypothesis. However, some months earlier, some of them had received a visit from a young British doctor named Christopher Hudson. In a 1992 scientific article, the Ugandan researchers had noted that Ugandan women with very few partners were at extremely high risk of infection. They attributed this mainly to high rates on untreated sexually transmitted diseases, but Hudson suspected that it might have more to do with the fact that the women's few partnerships were concurrent, and that they were thus on the HIV "superhighway." The Ugandans were intrigued by Hudson's idea and this may be why they urged Morris to pursue it.

Hudson had become interested in concurrency during a stint at a London sexually transmitted diseases clinic, when he noticed that some diseases, such as genital warts, seemed to be more common in his white patients, whereas others, including gonorrhea, were more common in blacks, many of them recent immigrants from the Caribbean. When Hudson took sexual histories, he discovered that the black and white patients, broadly speaking, behaved differently. Both groups had the same average number of lifetime sexual partners, but his white patients tended to engage in "serial monogamy"—one partnership at a time—whereas the blacks were more likely to have steady, long-term "concurrent" relationships with perhaps two or three people at a time.

Hudson had a hunch that these different patterns of behavior might help explain the spread of the different diseases. People with warts are infectious for years, but those with gonorrhea are infectious only for about six months. So if a "serial monogamist" who switched partners every year or two contracted gonorrhea, the disease probably would have run its course before he could pass it on to a new partner. But if a man with two long-term "concurrent" girlfriends contracted gonorrhea, he would spread it to both of them immediately—and if either of those women had another long-term partner, she would spread it to him right away, too. In this way, gonorrhea could spread rapidly to large numbers of people.

If his "gonorrhea theory" was correct, Hudson realized, it would have profound implications for the spread of HIV—a far more serious problem because like gonorrhea, HIV also has a brief—roughly month-long—period of especially high infectiousness.

(See DS Serwadda et al. "HIV risk factors in three geographic strata of rural Rakai district." AIDS 1992: vol 6 pp 983–9; CP Hudson "Concurrent partners and the results of the Uganda Rakai project." AIDS 1993; vol 7 pp 286–7 and the reply by DS Serwadda et al on pp 287–8).

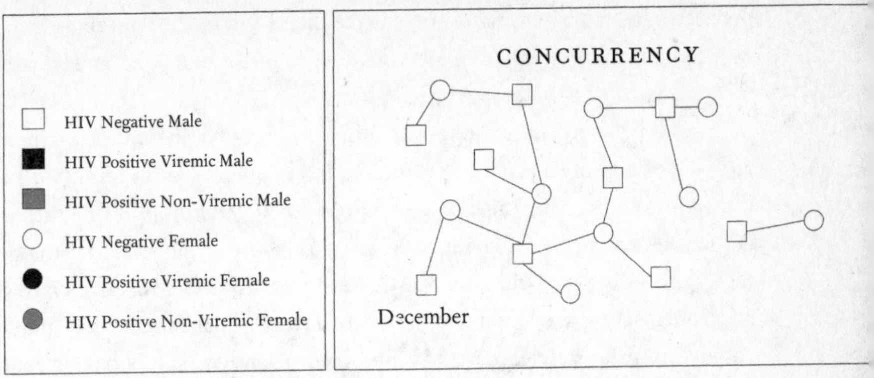

THE EFFECT OF SEXUAL NETWORKING ON HIV TRANSMISSION. This chart begins a series of diagrams illustrating the spread of HIV through two hypothetical populations, one in which long-term concurrency is common and one in which serial monogomy is the norm. They are arranged so that readers may thumb through them, as with a "flip-book." It is clear that HIV transmission is much more rapid in the former case. Diagrams by Stewart Parkinson, Population Services International.

The technique allowed Morris to calculate not only how many partners people had had in their lives, but how many were ongoing at the same time and the length of time that concurrent relationships overlapped. Similar surveys were being carried out by other researchers in Thailand and the United States at the same time, and when Morris compared the findings from the three countries, the results were fascinating. The average Ugandan had fewer sexual partners over a lifetime than the average American, but America's higher rates of promiscuity did not result in a higher rate of infection. The HIV rate in Uganda peaked at 18 percent in the early 1990s, but it never exceeded 1 percent in the United States.

A key difference between Uganda and the United States, Morris found, is that although heterosexual Americans tend to have several long-term relationships over a lifetime, they usually have them sequentially, not concurrently. If an American contracts HIV from a boyfriend, she probably won't pass it on to anyone else until the couple breaks up and she finds a new partner. She might well infect that new partner, but then the virus will be trapped in this new relationship for months or years, as long as the couple stays together. If one member of the couple has a one-night stand, the casual partner has a good chance of escaping infection because HIV transmission is what mathematicians call a "stochastic process." It occurs as a matter of chance, like the flip of a coin or a game of Russian roulette. Also, casual and commercial sexual encounters are very likely to be protected with condoms.

Sexual behavior in Uganda was different. Around 40 percent of men and 30 percent of women told Morris's interviewers that at least two of their most recent relationships overlapped for several months or years.[35] About 20 percent of Ugandan men are formally polygamous, but many men with only one wife have mistresses or girlfriends with whom they sleep at closely spaced intervals, on a "rota basis," as one former Ugandan cabinet minister described it.[36] While women tend to be less open about their extramarital affairs, some of them also carry on what President Yoweri Museveni of Uganda has referred to as "surreptitious side relations."[37]

Similar patterns of behavior have been reported from other African countries. WHO surveys from the late 1980s found that in Tanzania 18 percent of men and 10 percent of women said they had more than one long-term partner; in Lusaka, Zambia, 22 percent of men and 10 percent of women said so; and in Lesotho, 55 percent of men and 40 percent of women did. In Thailand, Sri Lanka, and Manila, only 2 percent of men said they had concurrent long-term partners, and virtually no women did.[38]

Other studies have challenged the concurrency theory—but these studies are themselves open to challenge. In a commentary on Martina Morris and Mirjam Kretzschmar's 1997 article "Coining a new term in epidemiology," the epidemiologists Geoff Garnett and Anne Johnson of the Imperial College of Science and Technology claimed that the authors failed to control for the number of partnerships in their model, and that the increased transmission in the "concurrency" scenario was due to a greater number of partnerships therein. However, Garnett and Johnson made an error: the number of partnerships was, in fact, controlled for in Morris and Kretzschmar's model.[39]

During the 1990s, researchers working under the auspices of the World Health Organization found that the proportion of people practicing concurrency did not correlate with HIV infection rates in five African cities.[40] This study probably understimated the effect of concurrency for at least three reasons. First, rates of male circumcision, which is highly protective against HIV, differed markedly among the cities and would have made the effect of concurrency harder to detect (see chapter

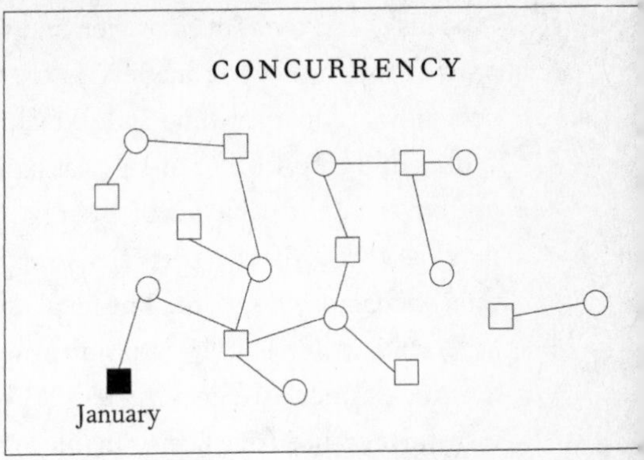

11). The study also failed to account for the fact that the important factor may be not one's own concurrency, but one's partner's concurrency. A 2004 study conducted in the United States found no correlation between concurrency and an individual's risk of sexually transmitted infection. However, people whose partners had concurrent partners were three and a half times more likely to be infected than those whose partners did not have concurrent partners. This would explain the common observation in Africa that many faithful women are infected with HIV even though they themselves are not practicing concurrency. It's their husbands' behavior that puts them at risk.[41]

The WHO researchers also failed to distinguish short term from long term concurrency. The duration of the overlap of concurrent partnerships may vary from a single day (if a man with one wife has a fling with a prostitute) or for years (if he has another long term partner). As discussed above, short term flings are generally safer because they involve less exposure and are also more likely to be protected with condoms. But in the WHO authors' analysis, all concurrent partnerships would have been treated equally.

Even though the Ugandans Morris studied had few partners over a lifetime, the relationships they did have gave rise to a stable interlocking sexual network that served as a "superhighway" for HIV as the series of illustrations beginning on page 57 show. If a man with two long-term partners contracts HIV—perhaps from a fling with a prostitute—he will very likely pass the virus on to both of his partners in a very short time. If either of his partners has another partner, these "partners of his partners" will very soon become infected too, along with any other partners they might have, and so on. In this way, concurrent sexual relationships link people up into a web of sexual relationships that can extend across huge regions. If one member contracts HIV, then everyone in the web is immediately placed at very high risk as well.

This risk extends even to men and women who are faithful to a single partner, because what matters is the nature of the network, not the behavior of any particular individual. Faithful men and women—stray spokes in the network—are also at high risk, not from their own behavior, but from the behavior of their partners. Even monogamous couples may be at risk, if one partner had a previous partner who was part of the concurrency network. This explains why so many African people—especially women—who are not promiscuous and have had very few lifetime partners are nevertheless HIV positive. Because so much HIV transmission in Africa occurs in long-term relationships in which there is a degree of intimacy and trust, condoms are seldom used, and this makes the epidemic even more difficult to control.

In Thailand, Morris found yet another pattern of sexual behavior, which differed from both the long-term concurrency of Uganda and the serial monogamy of the United States. Most Thai men had only one long-term sexual relationship in a lifetime—with their wives. However, half the Thai men in Morris's survey said that they had sex with prostitutes on a fairly regular basis, on average five times a year. Many Thai prostitutes are HIV positive, and one would think that this would place the men—and their wives—at high risk of HIV. However, it turned out that the men's risk of infection was relatively low—less than 2 percent of Thai men were HIV positive at the time of Morris's study, and the rate has declined since then. The reason so many of the men escaped infection is that they usually slept with a given prostitute only once and very often used a condom when they did.

In 1993, Morris teamed up with the mathematician Mirjam Kretzschmar of the National Institute of Public Health in Holland to develop a new computer program that could compare the spread of HIV through two populations: one in which concurrent partnerships were common and one in which serial monogamy was the norm. The computer program allowed the researchers to see what would happen if they introduced a hypothetical virus into these populations, and the people in them then formed and dissolved relationships over a five-year period. The two populations were exactly the same size, and over five years they formed the same number of sexual relationships, but the virus spread ten times faster in the population practicing concurrency than it did in the popula-

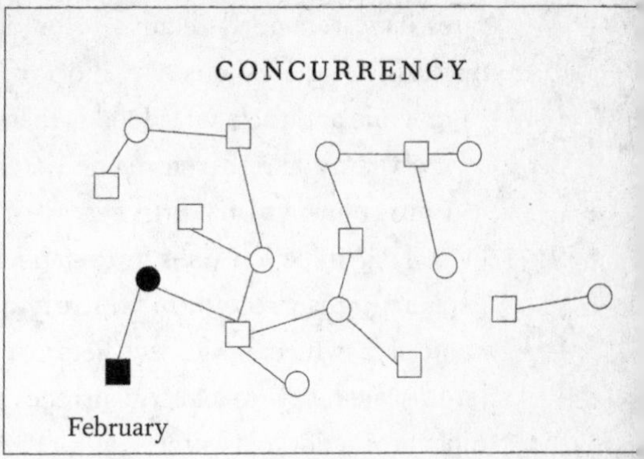

tion practicing serial monogamy. Even in populations in which people had, on average, only two partners over a five-year period, a huge epidemic resulted if a significant fraction of those partnerships were long-term and concurrent.[42] The researchers then ran the computer program with actual data on sexual behavior from Uganda, Thailand, and the United States, and the simulations reproduced the same prevalence of HIV observed in those countries in the early 1990s, when the data were collected.

What Morris and Kretzschmar did not know when they developed this computer program was that HIV has evolved a genetic "trick" that allows it to spread even faster through long-term concurrency networks. It turns out that HIV-positive people are much more likely to pass the virus on to others in the first few weeks or months after they have been infected themselves. The infectiousness of HIV varies with the concentration of virus in the blood—the more virus there is, the more likely it will get into genital fluids and be passed on during sex.[43] During the first few weeks or months after infection, a person's blood teems with virus. But then the immune system produces antibodies and cells that attack HIV. Virus levels fall and may remain low for years, rising again only when the person's immune system eventually fails and AIDS symptoms appear. A recently infected person may be a hundred or even a thousand times more likely to transmit the virus than someone who has been infected for a few months or years.[44] This means that sexual networks in which some people sleep with two or three partners at intervals of days or weeks are probably even more dangerous than Morris's computer program predicted they were.

The existence of a "viremic window" early in infection, when transmission is especially likely, also sheds light on why HIV spreads so slowly in populations practicing serial monogamy. By the time our serial monogamist has moved on to a new partner, his viral load will have fallen, so he is unlikely to infect her. The viremic window also explains why HIV rates have remained relatively low in Thailand. Although many Thai prostitutes are HIV positive, most of them have been infected with HIV for a while and their viral load is therefore low.

Polygamy, and therefore concurrency, is fairly common in the largely Muslim countries of North and West Africa and the Middle East. However, HIV infection rates are relatively low in these regious. The likely explanation is twofold: first, nearly all men in Muslim societies are circumcised, which limits the heterosexual spread of HIV; and second, large-scale heterosexual concurrency networks can only emerge if a significant fraction of women, as well as men, engage in concurrent long-term relationships. But in many Muslim societies, women's sexual behavior is under strict surveillance by male relatives, and the penalties for female infidelity are severe.

MAXINE ANKRAH was not present at the meeting where Martina Morris first learned about long-term concurrency but, like most of her colleagues in Uganda, she had a pretty good idea of why the virus was spreading so rapidly there. Ankrah, an African-American sociologist who has lived in Uganda since the early 1970s, participated in Uganda's early AIDS campaigns and, like the Ugandan doctors who attended Martina Morris's lecture, she knew that Anderson's high-risk/low-risk mixing theory of the HIV epidemic did not make sense in East Africa. She had never heard the word "concurrency," but she knew that typical sexual promiscuity and prostitution could not explain why so many people were dying of AIDS in Uganda. "Our focus was on the ordinary woman," she told me years later. "We did not focus just on the sex workers."

In 1992, Uganda became the first African country to begin to see a sustained decline in its national HIV infection rate. Elsewhere, the epidemic would not begin to subside for almost another decade. The reasons for Uganda's success are controversial and will be explored in later chapters, but the crucial insight that every sexually active person—not just prostitutes, promiscuous people, and their partners—was at risk of HIV formed the centerpiece of Uganda's AIDS campaigns in the early years of the epidemic. In 1989, Philly Lutaaya, a famous Ugandan musician, took the stage at Makerere University. Beside him stood Dr. Sam Okware, then head of Uganda's AIDS Control Program.[45] Before a packed audience of students, Lutaaya, emaciated and clearly dying, declared, "If there is any one message I would like to leave with you tonight, it is that AIDS is not a disease that only affects the other person or a particular class of person. Anyone can get it."

CONCURRENCY

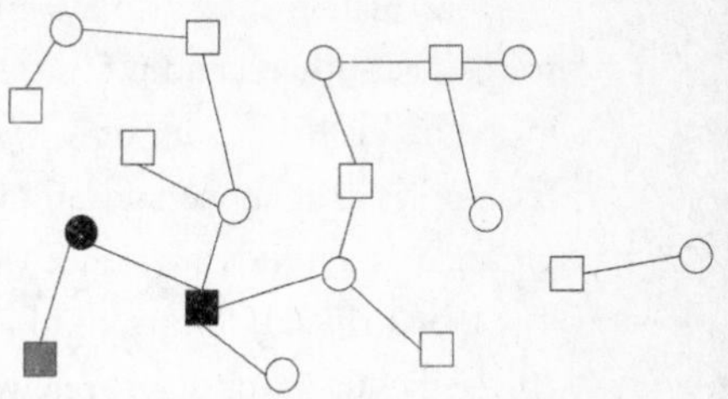

In other African countries, most prevention programs were "segmented" and "targeted"—in the language of public health—to high-risk populations. Ordinary African people had to learn the hard way that the virus was everywhere, all around them, and they too were at risk, even if they did not engage in typical "high-risk" behavior.

Once, at an AIDS meeting in Washington, D.C., Ankrah told Roy Anderson that she disagreed with his high-risk/low-risk mixing theory. "I didn't know much about computer modeling," she told me, "but I made my statement anyway. I did have the courage to say what I thought was true."

Today, few health officials working in Africa would argue with her. "We were poorly informed," Johannes van Dam, director of reproductive health programs for the Population Council, admitted to me in 2005. "There was a theory that intervening with high-risk groups would have a substantial effect on the epidemic, but we should have focused more broadly on the sexual networks in the general population."

"It took a while for everyone to catch up with Maxine," says Joseph Amon, director of HIV/AIDS programs for Human Rights Watch, who knew Ankrah in the early 1990s. "She was a bit of a voice in the wilderness back then, but I think everyone understands what she was saying now."

Why didn't African medical experts in other countries besides Uganda see this too? It is possible that when it came to fighting AIDS, Uganda had an advantage over other countries in Africa: a cadre of talented medical doctors and academics—including Ankrah and the Ugandan doctors at Morris's lecture—who had a foot in both Western science and African culture. They rapidly demystified the disease, understood how it was spreading, set their own policies, and didn't wait for Western experts to tell them what to do.

The British made many mistakes in Uganda. They favored some tribes over others, and when they departed in 1962, they left the country in the hands of a cadre of schemers and hooligans, setting the stage for the political violence and ethnic tensions that persist to this day.[46] But Uganda's colonial experience was relatively benign compared with those of other British possessions in Africa. After the American Civil War, the British began searching for new sources of cotton for the Lancashire textile mills, and Uganda, with its mild, rainy climate and fertile soil, was ideal. Local administrators encouraged Ugandan farmers to grow cotton on their own plots of land and sell it for profit to Indian traders. White settlement was discouraged, and at the height of the colonial period there were fewer than six hundred British people in the entire Ugandan protectorate. Most land remained in African hands, and some tribes maintained their traditional forms of government.[47]

A moderately prosperous Ugandan middle class emerged, whose children were eager for education and advancement in such modern professions as medicine, law, and administration. For them the British built a university and medical school—Makerere—that was once known as "the Harvard of Africa." Makerere soon became a magnet for intellectuals from all over the world. The writer Paul Theroux, who taught there in the 1960s, called Kampala a "small green city," and Uganda "prosperous and full of distinguished people."[48]

In the 1970s, Idi Amin's henchmen killed some Makerere professors and hounded others into exile, but the university still produced a cohort of doctors and scientists with the sophistication, confidence, and insight to grasp something about the AIDS epidemic that outsiders would miss.

In Europe's other African possessions—South Africa, Mozambique, Rhodesia, and Kenya—white settlers threw blacks off their land, corralled them into the migrant labor system, and barred them from higher education. In some cases, native Africans were banned altogether from certain fields, including medicine.[49] Talented Africans who would have joined these professions were thwarted, or driven from the continent by war, poverty, or discrimination.

Many of those who remained were instilled with a sense of inferiority,

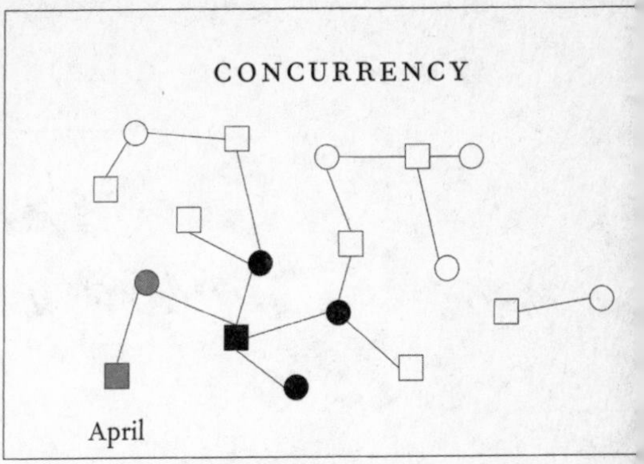

shame, and powerlessness that would later inhibit discussion of sexuality and paralyze the response to AIDS on much of the continent. The British have much to answer for in Uganda, but the people they left behind when they departed may have been in a better position than other Africans to address the AIDS crisis pragmatically, and not simply adopt whatever programs foreign advisors prescribed.

On visits to other countries in Africa, I often find myself having casual discussions about AIDS with all sorts of people. When I explain the difference between Anderson's high-risk/low-risk group mixing theory and Morris's long-term concurrency network theory, I am always amazed to see how people's expressions change. Young people, especially those not yet sexually active, are eager to know more. Even poor, illiterate adolescents have told me—through an interpreter—that the explanation makes sense to them. They understand perfectly how long-term concurrency can spread HIV, because they see such relationships all around them. But older people often go silent when I explain it. Some of these older people have been officials working for large nongovernmental organizations that specialize in programs for high-risk groups. Others were bureaucrats working for governments that have been far less proactive about AIDS than Uganda's was. The indifference of some of these governments to the AIDS crisis suggests a heartlessness that is hard to fathom. How could government officials look the other way when faced with such a threat to their own people? Their indifference recalled the heartlessness of the Reagan administration, which turned its back on the crisis in America and scorned its mainly gay and drug-injecting victims. How could African leaders, faced with a far more widespread catastrophe, do the same? Perhaps these bureaucrats went silent when I told them about Morris's long-term concurrency theory because they were thinking about their own behavior and wondering if they themselves might have been infected by a concurrency network. Perhaps for the first time they were seeing the AIDS crisis for the tragedy it is.

CHAPTER FOUR

The African Earthquake

After I learned of Martina Morris's long-term concurrency theory, I set myself a task. The concurrency hypothesis made sense on paper, but it didn't tell you much about how people experienced such relationships, or why they might behave this way. In my own culture of middle-class Europeans and Americans, relatively few men and women conduct simultaneous affairs, except during the brief period of experimentation with sex, emotions, and peer competition in high school and college, and perhaps in the few years after. One-night stands are common in every culture, but long-term concurrency—sleeping with more than one partner at closely spaced intervals for months or years—is relatively rare in mine. Married men have mistresses, of course, but many such men are sexually estranged from their wives.*

Most of the men and women I know who have engaged in long-term concurrent affairs agonized over them. They expressed despair over their guilty feelings, as though they themselves were the bereaved party, and sought psychological counseling as though they were somehow ill. To be "normal" was to settle down into a pattern of serial monogamy, in which two people proclaimed exclusive love for one another, if only temporarily. An affair might last decades, years, months, or weeks; it might be passionate or warm or boring or abusive; but the exclusive, transient love affair is the essential narrative of our culture. It is the subject of much Western

*French politicians may be another exception. See Christophe Deloire and Christophe Dubois, *Sexus Politicus* (Paris: Albin Michel, 2006).

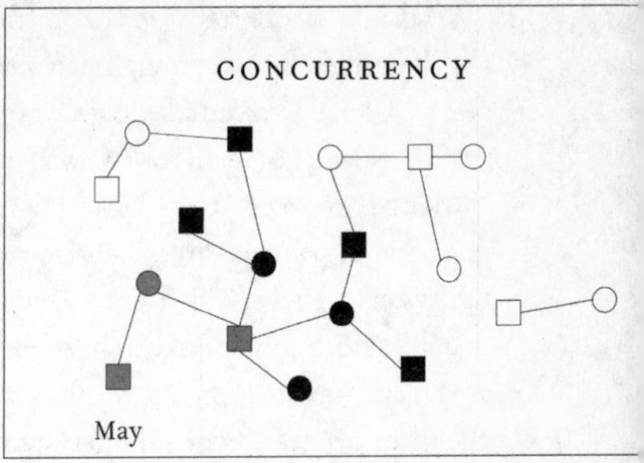

literature and art, and love's grand finale—the breakup—is the climax or nadir of many people's lives. It's also a one-way street. Once abandoned, few affairs are rekindled.

Not so in East and southern Africa. "You mean you just split? For good?" a Ugandan friend of mine, roughly my age, asked me in astonishment when I explained this to him. It was hard for him to imagine abandoning a relationship with a woman, especially if he had children with her. He would feel obliged to support her, and regular sexual relations would be expected by both parties, even if one or the other had other partners. The duration of such relationships, and the complications they entailed, tended to limit the number of affairs both men and women had in a lifetime, and this might explain why many surveys find that Africans have fewer partners over a lifetime than Westerners do.

In an effort to learn more about gender relations in Africa, I collected sexual histories from roughly one hundred people—Kenyans, Ugandans, South Africans, Tanzanians, Batswana, Mozambicans, Zimbabweans—many of them HIV positive. They told me about their lives, their sexual relationships, and about living with HIV. Some I contacted through AIDS organizations, and others I met in taxis or on the street. I was surprised at how open people were with a stranger and how willing they were to share their experiences. From their stories, I came to see how the AIDS epidemic in Africa has been triggered by one of the most rapid social and economic transitions in world history, from an agrarian past to a semi-urbanized present. For millions of African people, an entire way of life, with all its roots and certainties, has been lost in a few generations. The resulting upheavals in social life have generated an earthquake in gender relations that has opened wide channels for the spread of HIV.

IN SEPTEMBER 2002, I was hired as a consultant for Human Rights Watch to report on the upcoming presidential election in Kenya. When I arrived in Nairobi, tension was in the air. Daniel arap Moi, the tyrant who had ruled Kenya for eighteen years, was retiring. His preferred successor, Uhuru Kenyatta, a drowsy bon vivant and the son of the nation's first president, Jomo Kenyatta, was unpopular. Local monitors had been working hard to ensure a fair election, but Moi was a powerful, wily old man, and everyone feared the vote would be rigged. There were rumors that violent gangs, allied with Kenyatta and Moi, were training in the countryside. People spoke in hushed tones, fearful of spies.

One of my informants, a young man named David, told me that the people of his tribe were not interested in the elections. "We just graze our cows and follow our traditions," he told me. "We live close to nature, like the people you call 'hippies' in your country." I knew this was not true. David was a member of the Masai, a proudly traditional pastoralist tribe whose ancestors once grazed their herds across the vast beige pan of the Rift Valley. Masai leaders claim that the entire region once belonged to them, before members of other tribes, working for the British, cheated them out of their land in the early twentieth century. In protest, some Masai still herd their goats down city streets and set up homesteads in empty lots and on other people's fields. They wear traditional tribal costumes, walk with long strides, and even in crowded slums they seem to be gazing far into the distance. In recent years, Masai, armed with traditional weapons and sometimes guns, had clashed with other tribes over land and water rights, and several people had been killed.

As the conversation began to flag, I asked David whether the Masai were worried about AIDS. Suddenly he was eager to talk to me. For years, the Kenyan government had downplayed the presence of HIV in the country. Statistical reports were shelved and donor money for AIDS programs went unspent. But lately the newspapers and radio were reporting on the epidemic daily and people were frightened and confused. David's village was in a remote area of the country. There were no functioning health centers nearby and few AIDS information campaigns. David asked me whether I would come to his village and talk to people about AIDS. It was an irresistible offer. Here was a chance to visit one of Africa's most famous indigenous tribes, the protagonists of explorers' tales and the keepers of ancient African myths and culture. It was also a chance to learn

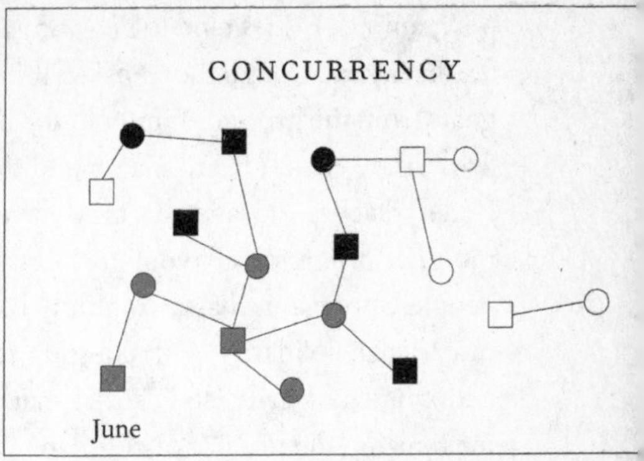

more about their sexual customs and try to help them by telling them what I knew about AIDS.

David's village was three hours outside of Nairobi. On the way, we passed through a game park. At the approach of our car, herds of zebra galloped away in clouds of dust as scavenger birds soared in the sky above them. An enormous giraffe hovered in the bush, then turned and disappeared without a sound. At a lake, we stopped to watch a pod of hippos. Eight pairs of eyes and ears bobbed out of the water in unison with eight snorting snouts and descended again. I learned that an adult hippo can eat 160 pounds of grass a day. Their dung is picked over by giant herons as tall as I am. The herons' eggs are eaten by alligators, and herons, in turn, sometimes eat baby alligators. At one time, before we deluded ourselves that we had broken free of nature, we knew our place in this world too. Epidemics like AIDS are not arbitrary natural disasters like earthquakes and tornadoes. They are embedded in the social ecology of the populations through which they spread. We may not like to think so, but we are still part of nature, and our fate is entwined in a constantly evolving system of relationships to each other, our predators, and our prey.

It was early afternoon when David and I reached the Masai village. It consisted of a circle of small huts made from woven reeds and fenced around with brambles, surrounded by a sea of windswept dry grass and soft brown hills. Some twenty men were waiting for us, all wearing the brightly colored garments and beaded hair and ear ornaments characteristic of their tribe.

I soon found that I had as much to learn about AIDS from these Masai men as they did from me. I had only recently learned about long-term concurrency, but from that day, I came to understand it as never before. It was as though these Masai had just leapt out of Martina Morris's computer program.

Like most tribes in East and southern Africa, the Masai are traditionally polygamous. Brides tend to be young, many still in their teens. Marriages are arranged through the transfer of bride price, usually a gift of cattle or goats from the groom's family to the bride's. As men age and their herds grow, they can afford to marry additional wives, and by the time a clan leader reaches old age, he may have accumulated five wives or even more, of progressively younger ages. For the Masai, as for many African peoples, polygamy has a traditional social and economic basis. It promoted clan solidarity by linking up families through the trade in cattle and women, and it also ensured that all women were married off, thus maximizing the fertility of the clan.

But polygamy created obvious tensions. Young women had little say about whom they were married off to, and the inevitable shortage of young, marriageable women meant young men hankered after old men's wives. The Masai had a customary way of defusing this tension. Young Masai men, known as morans, or warriors, are organized into age regiments, and together they undergo a long period of exile from the clan in the surrounding bush. During this time, they are circumcised and learn the techniques of warfare, hunting, and other manly duties. They are also kept away from older men's wives. However, during their exile, some morans sneak back into the village and appear at the door of one of the young wives of a tribal elder. Often the pair have a prior understanding and she invites him into her hut. Sometimes she is coerced. But she never complains about it. "The morans wander in the wilderness," an expert on Masai customs explained to me later, "and if one comes to the village at night and wants to sleep with a certain girl, no one will disagree. Even if she is someone else's wife. You have to give them special privileges. Women are well aware."[1] The resulting children belong officially to her husband—not to the moran—and nothing is said about the affair.

When the Masai men explained this to me, I immediately saw how HIV could spread rapidly through this village, from a young moran to his secret girlfriend, to her husband, and then to her co-wives, and then to their secret moran boyfriends, and so on. If only one person in this network contracted HIV, the virus would soon spread to many others. Even faithful wives who slept only with their husbands were at risk, and so were young morans with only one girlfriend. The risks of having two partners—which hardly qualifies as promiscuity in this day

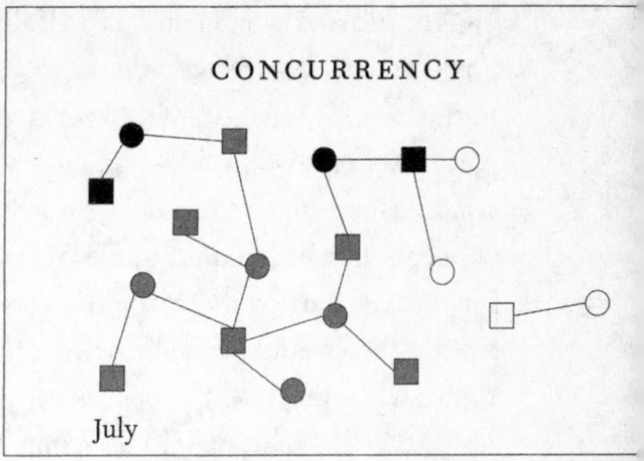

and age—would likely have been astronomical.*

When I explained to the group that their sexual customs put them at risk of HIV, they said they understood but could do nothing about it. "You see, we go out in the forest and eat meat and grow very strong," a young moran wearing white sneakers and a tartan shawl explained. "You feel you have to have sex." When I suggested the idea of abstinence, or sticking to one sexual partner, hysterical laughter broke out all around me, and the moran in sneakers respectfully told me that was not possible. Indeed, it did seem unlikely that these young men might be persuaded to abstain until marriage—which might not occur until their families had accumulated enough bride-price cattle, by which time they might well be in their thirties.

As it happened, I had obtained from the U.S. Embassy a large carton of condoms, and I asked the group if they would like to see how to use them. The HIV epidemic in Kenya had been raging for nearly two decades by then, but because government prevention programs had been so desultory these men had never seen such a demonstration. The crowd grew rowdy, especially the elders, who had earlier been enjoying their chiefly prerogative of getting drunk on a Sunday afternoon. "We want a live demonstration!" said one, who was wearing a traditional Masai beaded necklace and a small gold hoop earring.

I borrowed a wooden walking stick from one of the young morans. The old man with the earring had a fly whisk, made from the hair of the tail of a bull. After removing the condom from its wrapper, I explained that the penis had to be like the walking stick before the condom went on, and not floppy like the fly whisk. Everyone laughed except the man with the fly whisk. "Everyone must listen! This is serious!" he shouted, and gravely contemplated the fly whisk.

*The HIV rate in Masai communities is actually relatively low, probably because the Masai practice male circumcision, which is highly protective against HIV. Local experts estimated that some 5 percent of Masai are HIV positive.

Afterward, the men enthusiastically grabbed the condoms out of the box. I realized then that it would soon be empty and no one would come to this remote village again to replace it. In any case, the men and their partners would soon find—as men and women everywhere find—that condoms are uncomfortable and awkward to put on, and they prevent conception, which many couples want. If women wished to use condoms but the men did not, there would be little the women could do. I only hoped that the men would continue to use condoms if they were ever to visit prostitutes when they went to sell their livestock in town. At least that might keep HIV from getting into this complex sexual network in the first place.

LATER ON, David took me to meet a group of Masai women. We found them in a tiny hillside church, listening to a preacher in a canary-yellow suit. Since the mid-twentieth century, Masai women have flocked to evangelical churches like these, many seeking relief from what they call "spirit possession." Spells of weird body pains, nightmares, uncontrollable fits, and long periods of listlessness had afflicted Masai women since early colonial times. Victims attributed the symptoms to supernatural forces, but Dorothy Hodgson, an anthropologist who witnessed an epidemic of spirit possession when she lived with the Masai in the 1980s and '90s, interpreted them as women's rebellion against their loss of status in an increasingly male-dominated world.[2]

In precolonial East Africa, the Masai economy was controlled largely by women, who bartered livestock for cloth, tobacco, and other goods. Then, in the early twentieth century, the British replaced this messy, informal system with a male-controlled cash economy that could be more easily monitored and taxed. With the shift, women lost a degree of autonomy and power over the distribution of household resources. When Hodgson interviewed them, many expressed bitterness about their loss of status. "Now men treat us like donkeys," a young woman told her. Abuse and beatings became more frequent, and men became less willing to share domestic tasks. Unable to confront men directly, women sublimated their anger into an "illness" caused by evil spirits, and turned to the church for community and relief. But the church's prudishness about sexual matters threatened to further disempower these women and put them at even greater risk of HIV.

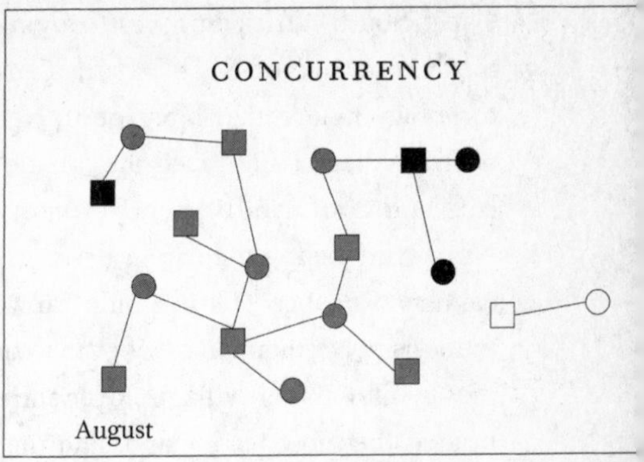

When the preacher concluded his sermon, I was introduced to the group as a special guest. But when I said I had come to talk about AIDS, half of my small audience fled. When I mentioned condoms, more women rushed out, and by the time I had finished, only three women remained. They sat politely in silence and asked no questions.

FEW PEOPLE in East and southern Africa live according to the old tribal ways anymore. Most young Africans these days strive not to own cows or slay lions as the Masai do, but to obtain an education and a job in an office. They wear Western clothes and attend Christian churches. They learn English and listen to pop tunes on their radios and watch soap operas on TV. Formal polygamous marriages are rare and the exchange of bride-price cattle is increasingly viewed as a quaint tradition, practiced mainly by the rich and sentimental.

Nevertheless, HIV infection is even more common in the rapidly developing, semi-industrialized countries of the southern cone of the continent than it is in Kenya, where the Masai live. Generalizing about sexual culture is always difficult; social life everywhere is complicated and constantly changing. But just a few generations ago, most people in southern Africa lived in polygamous tribes, just as the Masai do now, and I wondered how patterns of sexual behavior—especially concurrent partnerships—had been affected by modernization and development, and what was putting so many people in southern Africa at risk today.

IN 2004, I visited Ngcingane, a village that lies on a green plain amid misty hills about fifteen miles from Umtata, a large town in the Eastern

Cape, South Africa's poorest province. The Eastern Cape is home to the Xhosa, one of South Africa's largest tribes, who settled here centuries ago in large kinship groups. Nelson Mandela's forebears lived in a nearby village and grazed their cattle and grew sorghum and millet on large plots of land. Then, throughout southern Africa, villages like Ngcingane began their long descent into destitution. In the nineteenth century, European settlers built railways, mines, and cities and coerced millions of young men to work in them, forcing them to leave their families behind in their villages for months or years at a time. Whites appropriated the most fertile land, and the black population was resettled in independent "homelands" run by leaders appointed by the apartheid government. Many of these leaders were cynical and corrupt, and some still are. In 2002, 80 percent of the provincial budget of the Eastern Cape was unaccounted for.[3] Many people I met had been robbed or carjacked at least once. While I was waiting at a stoplight in the middle of town, I spotted a man in the lunchtime crowd casually loading an automatic pistol.

Corruption, along with persistent drought and barriers to agricultural trade imposed by Western nations, have all contributed to the economic crisis that has gripped much of sub-Saharan Africa since the 1970s. Today, the small-scale agricultural economy that sustained people for centuries, enabling them to maintain a livelihood on the land as the Masai still struggle to do, has been all but demolished. Because there are few unskilled jobs in South Africa's blighted rural areas, unemployment rates exceed 70 percent in places like Ngcingane. Most people rely financially on government pensions and remittances from migrant workers living hundreds of miles away.

Rachel Jewkes, an epidemiologist with South Africa's Medical Research Council, has been conducting research on the sexuality of young people living in the villages around Umtata for many years. She's an expert on HIV, teenage pregnancy, and violence against women, and she had found, as she told me, that gender relations in South Africa "are in a very bad state."

On a Saturday morning in January, Jewkes's research assistant, Lindiwe Farlane, introduced me to some of the young women participating in one of Jewkes's research projects. Seven of them were waiting for us under a tree in the yard outside a clinic in Ngcingane. The first thing that struck me was how stylish they were. Just looking at them, with their elaborately braided and colored hair, their fashionable clothing, and the way they yakked and giggled into their cell phones, they seemed to me a world away from the shy, disempowered Masai women I had met in Kenya.

SERIAL MONOGAMY

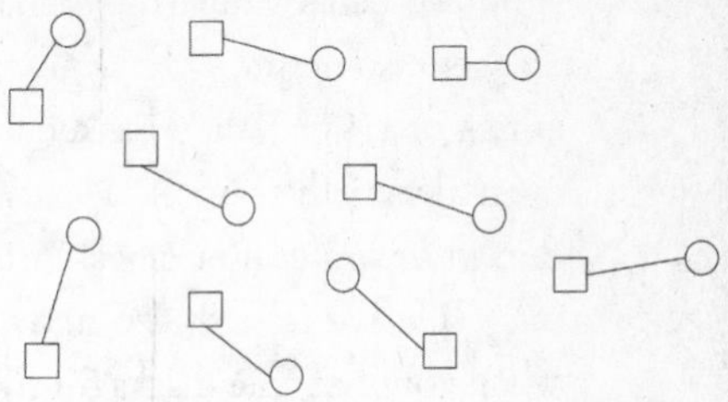

But their stories seemed strangely familiar. "He beats me once every two months or so," said Mcha, a cheerful eighteen-year-old high-school student, of her boyfriend, a twenty-two-year-old mechanic. "He beat me the day before yesterday." She showed me the bruises on her head. "Someone called me on my cell phone, and I was on my way to the bathroom and I answered. When I came back, my boyfriend said, 'You have a boyfriend!' I decided to say yes, since he'd beat me anyway. Sometimes he forces me to have sex when I don't want to."

South Africa has the highest recorded rate of rape in the world, but as Jewkes has shown, women like Mcha are at far less risk of HIV from the rapist who climbs in through the window than they are from the men they know best—their husbands and long-term boyfriends.

All of the young women I spoke to that day said they had only one boyfriend, but most were aware that their boyfriends were not faithful to them. "He does have other girlfriends," said Mcha, who had never been tested for HIV but had been treated for a sexually transmitted disease a few months earlier. "He even told me." So does the boyfriend of Mcha's friend, twenty-one-year-old Thokozile. He works in Cape Town, and Thokozile sees him once every few months. She's unhappy about his other girlfriend. "I don't know how much care he gives her compared to me. He might be loving her more." Thokozile hadn't been tested for HIV either.

Throughout my travels in South Africa, I would hear such stories again and again. The pattern of relationships—men with multiple partners, women acquiescing to the sexual demands of abusive men—resembled the polygamous ways of the Masai. But these women should have had choices. They were all in high school or had recently graduated; they had all been drilled about AIDS in school; they were exposed to modern ideas about women's rights. Why did they put up with men who openly cheated on them, sometimes physically and sexually abused them, and put them at risk of HIV? When I asked the girls in Ngcingane, the answer was almost always the same. "Because I love him," both Mcha and Thokozile said in separate interviews. "But why?" I asked. "I like that he's working," Thokozile said, "so he won't ask for money from me. It's boring when your boyfriend asks for fifty cents for a cigarette. This one can help me out with financial problems when I have them, not like the others. Sometimes he loads airtime on my cell phone."

"He gives me support, even if I owe fees at school," echoed Mcha. "Sometimes I use the money to buy clothes or do my hair."

Sexual relationships everywhere are motivated by a combination of physical attraction, emotional rapport, and financial calculation. But the last of these seems to have particular weight in southern Africa, where "transactional" sexual relationships, in which women expect gifts of cash or consumer goods from boyfriends, are by many accounts extremely common.[4]

"It's totally different from prostitution," said Mzikazi Nduna, a research psychologist who worked with Rachel Jewkes. "Prostitution is seen as a business. You go into the street and set a price. With transactional sex, the nature of the relationship is different. There are feelings involved. It's more committed."

Although transactional sex, like prostitution, involves the exchange of cash and other goods, the gifts themselves are often of less importance than the social connections and relationships they signify. Two University of California sociologists, Susan Watkins and Ann Swidler, have argued that transactional relationships are an extension of the kinship system, the network of dense interdependence and patronage that forms the basis of social life in many developing countries where bureaucratic and social-welfare institutions are weak. Like a kinship system, networks of transactional relationships provide a social security system for women and a source of power and self-esteem for men.[5]

Even though transactional sex differs from prostitution, it may be even more risky when it comes to HIV. Jewkes and colleagues have

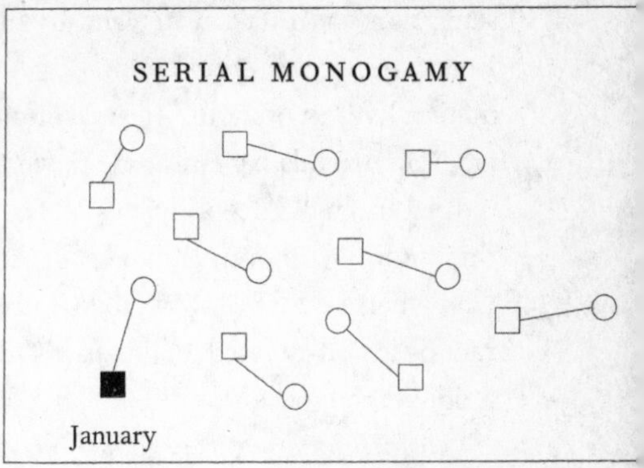

shown that women who enter transactional relationships are more likely to be HIV positive than other women, even if they—like Mcha and Thokozile—have had very few sexual partners in their lives.[6] Women in transactional relationships may be more vulnerable to HIV because they are more likely than other women to tolerate an unfaithful partner and also to seek out additional concurrent sexual relationships themselves.

Transactional sex in its current form has probably become much more common since the economic crisis of the 1970s, says Mark Hunter, an AIDS researcher at the University of California, Berkeley. As oil prices around the world rose, and banks began calling in their debts, African governments found themselves with a shortage of foreign exchange. As a condition for receiving further loans, the World Bank and other donors forced African governments to cut spending and remove barriers to free trade, such as import tariffs and subsidies to farmers. Then the growth of large commercial farms, many owned by multinational companies, all but destroyed, in a few generations, the system of small-scale, family-based agriculture that once sustained millions of people. At the same time, millions of African factory workers and civil servants would lose their jobs to budget cuts and the removal of trade barriers. Many of the factory workers were women, who increasingly came to rely on informal liaisons for survival.[7]

The tendency to form transactional sexual relationships has probably also been heightened by the penetration of the global market in consumer goods—makeup, clothing, cell phones, cars, and so on—into impoverished communities throughout southern Africa. Income inequality in South Africa and Botswana is higher than nearly anywhere else on earth. On the main roads in large cities, BMWs and Mercedes-Benzes swish by, their occupants shuttling between chic shopping malls and lush suburbs. But about 60 percent of black South Africans live beneath the poverty line, and 50 percent are unemployed.[8] Millions of people lack sanitation and piped water and live in shacks with dirt floors. Even in Botswana, a prosperous country by African standards, a third of the population lives in poverty.[9] In such circumstances, the gifts women receive from boyfriends have become powerful symbols of maturity and glamour. Even small gifts of lipstick and packets of cookies are prized, because they signify commitment and suggest that further gifts are forthcoming. And when a poor young woman is invited to a shopping mall or a restaurant by a well-dressed man with his own car, it must be like being offered a ride on the space shuttle.

Unfortunately, these glamorous men are also the most likely to be unfaithful, and thus HIV positive.[10] This is a lesson Lulu, a twenty-five-year-old HIV-positive South African woman, learned the hard way. "I was telling myself, 'He's my husband-to-be,'" she said of the twenty-six-year-old man who infected her with HIV when she was eighteen. "He was the director of a newspaper. He was a family friend and knew my parents from a long time back. He took me out, to lunch, dinner, to the zoo, the ocean. Maybe we went out eight or nine times. He was very good-looking, very well dressed, with a car and lots of money. Everything was easy. When we went to a mall and I asked for something, it was coming. I was feeling so happy, so excited. Then one day he invited me to a party, but he took me to a hotel instead. I didn't want to go, but I didn't know that he had already booked a room." At first, Lulu said no, but the man begged her. This was Lulu's first sexual experience. I asked her if she reported it to the police, but this never occurred to her. "It wasn't rape. I took my clothes off myself. I didn't scream." After that, the newspaper director didn't come back for six months. During that time, Lulu was tested for HIV and discovered that she had become infected through her single sexual encounter. "For me it was terrible," she said. She tried to contact her boyfriend by phone, but he was always away or about to leave town. "He'd say, 'I'm in Canada,' 'I'm in Cape Town.' I was hurt that he didn't come back. Then I found out he was married at the time. He already had a son."

"When a girl gets something in a transactional relationship, she sees it as a sign of love, not as an exchange for sex," explained Muriel Kubeka, a research assistant with South Africa's Medical Research Council. Unfortunately, men don't always see it the same way. Transactional relationships are more likely to be coercive and violent, Jewkes has found, probably because the exchange of money and gifts gives men a sense of ownership over a girlfriend's sexuality. Even nonviolent transactional relationships like Lulu's often involve pleading, nagging, and coercive pressure—the man's way of enforcing what he sees as an implicit sexual contract. If a woman is suspected of flirting with other men, a boyfriend may feel that, because he is giving her gifts, he has the right to beat her.

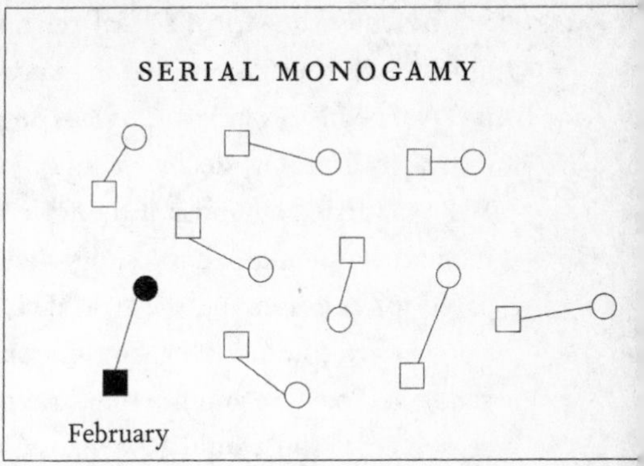

"He used to look at my footprints in the sand outside the house," a young HIV-positive teacher I met in Botswana told me of her abusive former boyfriend. "I told him I had been at work, but he wanted to check which direction I had come from." She knew that he was the unfaithful one—she even knew his other girlfriend.

In some cases the fighting escalates to tragic heights. During the past few years, a spate of "passion" murders has occurred in Botswana and South Africa, in which men have killed their girlfriends and then themselves. Dipheko Motube of the Botswana Police Service told me virtually all the passion killings occurred in long-term transactional relationships. "In a typical case, someone, usually the female, wants to end the affair, or else the man suspects she's been cheating. The man will say, 'But I have been supporting you!' Then he will kill her, and kill himself immediately afterwards."[11]

Domestic violence affects one in three women worldwide. Abusive partners are responsible for half of all female homicides, and their victims are also more prone to HIV, STDs, miscarriage, depression, and other mental-health problems. Although abuse occurs everywhere, it is far more common in developing countries, according to the World Health Organization, perhaps because gender relations are particularly vulnerable to the upheavals of social and economic change.[12]

In southern Africa, sexual relationships are haunted by traditional norms and expectations that in many cases can no longer realistically be met.[13] The historian Jeff Guy has described how in precolonial southern Africa, everything depended upon a man's ability to control women. Women carried out most of the agricultural labor—the hoeing and weeding and planting and harvesting—and gathered firewood and water and cared for children and the sick. This was arduous work. Droughts and floods were common; the soils of southern Africa are, for the most part, sandy and barren, and the thin, fragile topsoil erodes easily. After a few seasons, the soil would be exhausted and, as kin groups watched their harvest dwindle, they gathered their meager possessions and moved on. Men's responsibilities amounted to negotiating with other clan leaders—and sometimes fighting with them—to acquire better land, and then clearing it for the women to farm. There was very little of material value in this harsh world, no plantations or grand houses filled with coveted possessions, so men measured their wealth in people: wives who could work the land and produce children who would help them form alliances through marriage to other clans. Control over women and their children was thus a vital measure of a man's worth, and women's loyalty and obedience to men was a defining social feature of these societies.[14]

Much has changed in southern Africa during the past century. Gone, for the most part, are the rural polygamous homesteads dominated by powerful patriarchs; disappearing too are the unskilled occupations—such as mining and manufacturing—that enabled some men to earn enough money to maintain a traditional polygamous household, even in early industrial times. Soaring unemployment rates mean everyone must now struggle to earn a living. Success is based on education and skills, and women are trying to succeed at the same game as men.

Nevertheless, "traditional patriarchal ideas still linger," observed the anthropologist Iona Mayer in the 1970s, "but since the property base has practically vanished, they linger rather unconvincingly, like the smile on the Cheshire Cat."[15] Many men still aspire to have multiple partners, and to exert control over those partners. In *African Renaissance*, a 1999 essay collection with a prologue by South Africa's current president, Thabo Mbeki, the South African philosopher Lesiba Teffo writes, "The more

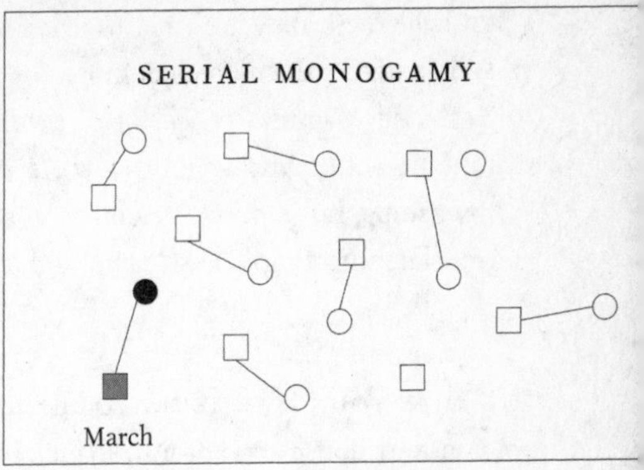

women a man has, the greater his stature in society."[16] "Respect" is a crucial dimension of African social life, he continues, and he approvingly cites the example of the ideal African woman, "who would not look her husband in the face when making an offer of any kind. She would rather crawl toward him whilst facing downward or sideward until she offers what is at hand."

Many South African women see the "ideal" relationship differently. During the 1970s, the South African anthropologist Virginia Van der Vliet asked scores of South African men and women about their expectations of marriage.[17] Most women wanted a "modern" type of family, in which husbands and wives shared household duties, friends, and recreational activities, and both partners aspired to a monogamous ideal. Most men, on the other hand, idealized a more "traditional" arrangement, in which they made all the decisions, and where husbands and wives lived largely separate lives. Women were to be occupied with rearing children, cooking, cleaning, and gardening, while men engaged in their own separate pursuits, which included drinking and having affairs. In the old days, their concubines might have become additional wives, but by the 1970s, few men could afford to support more than one wife and her children. Instead, men often behaved as if these women were semi-wives, whom they helped with gifts and money from time to time.[18] They expected their true wives to behave with "respect," which meant that they did not confront their husbands about these affairs.

Women, Van der Vliet found, were becoming increasingly repelled by these "traditional" male attitudes and mores. But few men were willing to change, because they feared being looked down on by their peers as "henpecked" or as following the ways of whites. As the divide between men and women widened, marriage rates plummeted.[19] Many single women now support themselves with jobs or else rely on occasional support from men with whom they sleep. But because they are not married to these men, they are freer to leave them or take up with someone else, which angers the men even more.

"It's low-intensity warfare," a young man at a conference on gender told the South African journalist Kerry Cullinan in 2001. He saw it in the townships, he said, where common slang words for "to have sex with" translate into English as "to hit with a pipe" or "to stab."[20]

WHILE YOUNG WOMEN in southern Africa complained to me of coercion and abuse by unfaithful men, young men without much money lamented that women always left them for richer men. "A man's beauty is considered by his wealth," said Siya, a university student in Umtata who lost two girlfriends in a row to wealthier men who, he heard, were abusive. "The boys I know think love is impossible," he said. "They've been disappointed so many times."

Unlike the Masai, modern southern African societies have no way of defusing the sexual tensions created by young women's preference for older, wealthier men. So some poor young men devise their own cold-blooded tactics.

"It's easy to get a beautiful girl," said Junior, a twenty-seven-year-old HIV-positive man I met in Gaborone, Botswana. "But you have to lie to them and tell them you have things you don't really have." Junior recounted for me a decade of philandering. You could see that girls must have loved him. He was athletic and witty and extremely good-looking, although he was now very thin and his voice was raspy with pneumonia. "When you go out, you're competing for girls. I can't remember their faces or names. Most of our targets were girls who acted snobbish, untouchable. It's not like you want to be a Casanova, you're on the defensive side—let me play her before she plays me." If a woman works in a shop or a bank, he told me, "she'll even look through the accounts. My father once gave me a check. When I went to cash it, the girls at the bank were smiling at me in a way I wasn't used to. The whole problem is love. It's a failure of love. I never had anyone I could pour out my soul to."

Patrick Mokhele, an HIV-positive South African man whose long-term girlfriend left him as soon as he lost his job, told me something similar. "The women of this country have no true love, that's why this thing"—meaning AIDS—"is hitting here more than other countries. Here money buys love. If you don't have it, you can't have love."

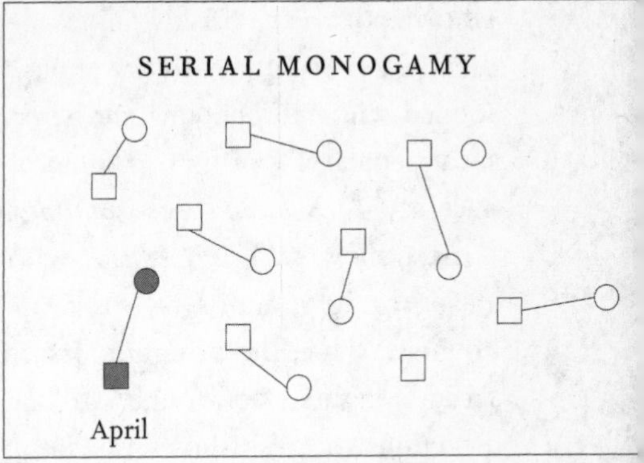

A day after speaking with Junior, I met Natasha, a twenty-eight-year-old HIV-positive woman who also lived in Gaborone. "Botswana men aren't very loving and caring," she told me. "They're just users." She ruefully described her schoolgirl romances. She wasn't interested in other students. "I liked guys from outside, the ones who were having money. You know, when you are in school, and someone shows up in a car to get you, you are a star." When someone told Natasha that one of her longer-term boyfriends was HIV positive, she replied, "Are you jealous because he has a BMW?"

Natasha was never beaten or raped by boyfriends, but she felt the sting of their infidelity. "When someone doesn't tell you the truth, you've been abused mentally. All the guys had other relationships, some were married. I never met a guy who was just by himself. . . . I want a kind, loving person, an honest person, with a very open mind, who'll tell me what he wants," she said.

"What if he doesn't have a lot of money?" I asked. I was thinking of Junior, also HIV positive, also wishing to turn over a new leaf.

"What?" she replied. "Why would I want that? How are you going to survive if he doesn't have money?"

After the fall of apartheid in the early 1990s, it was assumed that South Africans would be preoccupied with issues of race for at least another decade. Instead, notes Deborah Posel, a sociologist at the University of the Witwatersrand, gender relations, not race relations, have taken center stage in political and cultural debates.[21] When I was in Botswana and South Africa, the battle of the sexes raged on radio call-in programs and in gossip and advice columns. "Wishing cards" containing sentimental love poems sell briskly all year long, and on Valentine's Day, which seemed to be taken nearly as seriously as Christmas, the streets were festooned with red balloons and streamers. Throughout the region, the most popular TV programs are local soap operas and American imports such as *The Bold and the Beautiful* and *All My Children*. On the South African show *All You Need Is Love*, couples—black, white, Asian, multiracial, straight, and gay—declare their mutual love before the entire country. When the program airs on Tuesday evenings, this nation of freedom fighters and tough Afrikaner pioneers nearly grinds to a halt. Reactions to these shows can be profoundly personal. In 2003, Don Mlangeni, an actor who plays an unfaithful husband on the South African soap opera *Isidingo*, was slapped by a stranger in a shopping mall. He and the actress who plays his mistress have received a flood of hate mail and have found themselves ostracized at parties.

In her book *Talk of Love: How Culture Matters*,[22] Ann Swidler, a sociologist at the University of California, Berkeley, argues that culture—meaning discussions as well as artistic and other expressions of our humanity—flourishes in the unsettled corners of our lives, where the rules are uncertain or changing.[23] Perhaps the preoccupation with sex and love in southern Africa has something to do with the fact that the AIDS epidemic and sexual violence are forcing people to search urgently, and painfully, for greater understanding of the vicissitudes of love and personal relationships in a rapidly changing world.

These discussions may already be having a positive effect on gender norms. When Rachel Jewkes first began her research ten years ago, between 20 and 30 percent of young women in surveys claimed that their first sexual experience was the result of either rape by a stranger or an acquaintance or, more commonly, forced sex by a boyfriend.[24] Today, she and other researchers find the frequency of forced first sexual intercourse is far lower, reported by some 10 percent of young women in repeated surveys, a rate only slightly higher than that in the United States.[25]

"I think the level of forcing has genuinely fallen," Jewkes said. She also has noticed that young South Africans are much more likely to talk about sex and are developing "a vocabulary for discussing feelings and desires."

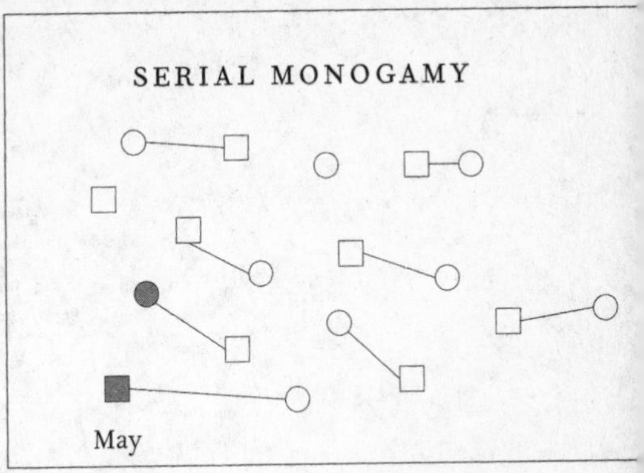

WHAT MAY HAVE helped spare the West a heterosexual AIDS epidemic on the scale of Africa's is the romantic belief that there is a "perfect partner," a "soul mate," to be cherished "for richer or poorer"—if not for life, then for a long time. This convention, inculcated in us from earliest childhood by fairy tales, novels, and movies, forms the cultural underpinning of monogamy, or at least its aspiration. It is also responsible for many Western ills, including divorce and the neurotic pursuit, through painful serial relationships, of an ideal conjugal love that may not exist.

In some African communities, this romantic ideal may take some getting used to. Back home in New York, I came across a study of sex and marriage among the Bemba of present-day Zimbabwe conducted by the anthropologist Audrey Richards in the 1930s.[26] Richards was amazed at the emotional distance between men and women. "Intimacy between a husband and wife is laughed at," Richards wrote. "I have heard a man laughed at because 'he sits on the verandah at night talking to his wife' . . . and another condemned less explicitly in the simple statement 'That man is a fool, the way he loves his wife.'"

"The two sexes eat and play apart throughout adult life," she observed. They share a house, but "this is the limit of their intimacy." Richards once asked a young man, "'Is X very fond of his bride?' He looked surprised and answered, 'How can he be fond of her? How can he know what her heart is like until they have grown old together? He has asked the other women of the village if she is a good wife for him. They are the only people who can tell him.'

"I once amazed a group of elderly Bemba," Richards continued, "by telling them an English folk-tale about the difficulties experienced by a Prince in winning the hand of his bride—glassy mountains, chasms, dragons, giants, and the like. An old chief present was genuinely astonished. 'Why not take another girl?'" he asked.

WHAT HAPPENED IN SOUTHERN AFRICA

CHAPTER FIVE

Gold Rush

IN THE LATE 1990S, the government of Mozambique first became suspicious, and then suspicion turned to alarm, about rising rates of HIV infection in the southern provinces of the country. Nuns at a Catholic mission hospital in a small railway town in Gaza province had begun noticing that the number of patients coming to them with AIDS was rising sharply. Meanwhile, Ministry of Health surveys were showing that the proportion of adults infected with HIV in Maputo, the capital city, was also rising, from an estimated 1 percent in 1992 to over 10 percent by the end of the decade. In Gaza province, the infection rate among pregnant women would rise to 27 percent by 2007.[1]

The HIV infection rate in Gaza was striking, particularly since this is a largely rural area. Most people in southern Mozambique are farmers who live on the land in quiet, sultry villages. Time here is measured by the sun and rain, and during good years, mangoes droop from the trees and the gardens are cluttered with pineapple plants and fat stalks of maize. The men wear battered old suits, and the women long colorful wraps printed with pictures of fruits or birds or African presidents. They are, in general, a polite and formal people. When friends meet, they engage in long, elaborate greetings, with handshakes, bowing, and curtsying. In Gaza, attendance at Christian churches is quite high, and adultery, though not uncommon, is publicly frowned upon.

This drowsy world is not where you would expect a terrible AIDS epidemic. At the time, most experts associated HIV with truckers and prostitutes, drug abuse and rootless city life. But the virus was now more common in the largely rural Gaza than it was in Maputo, where there were far more prostitutes and more customers who could afford them. I asked one of the epidemiologists who analyzed Mozambique's HIV statistics about the situation there. She admitted it was terrible, but it wasn't so unusual. It was typical of many rural areas throughout southern Africa, including KwaZulu-Natal in South Africa, Botswana, and Lesotho, where rates of HIV had soared in the past decade.

What all these regions had in common was that they sent large numbers of migrant workers to South Africa. Some of the migrants picked up jobs on plantations and construction sites, and others became involved in prostitution and petty crime. However, the most fortunate migrant workers were miners with jobs in the Witwatersrand gold mines in South Africa. During the past century, the rural provinces of Mozambique, Botswana, South Africa, Lesotho, and Swaziland have sent millions of mine workers to South Africa. In 2001, about 300,000 were working there, some 40,000 from southern Mozambique alone. The miners signed yearly contracts and might spend twenty years or more as migrant laborers, traveling back and forth between the mines and their rural farms, hundreds of miles away.

The migrant labor system in southern Africa has been blamed for many of the region's ills, including the disruption of family life and rural underdevelopment. Now it was also being blamed for the spread of HIV.[2] The long absences from home; the tedious, dangerous work; the drab anomie of life in all-male miners' hostels; the gangs of prostitutes clinging to the chain-link fences around the mines—all were assumed to contribute to miners' higher risk of HIV infection.

The Chamber of Mines of South Africa, which represents such mining companies as Gold Fields and AngloGold, denies that the migrant labor system has exacerbated the spread of HIV in southern Africa.[3] But the findings of the nuns in Mozambique seemed to contradict this. When I visited them in September 2001, they told me that nearly all the male AIDS patients who began turning up at their hospital six years before had been migrant workers in South Africa. Of those who were migrants, most had been Witwatersrand gold miners. More recent studies had found that the virus was now widespread in the general population of Mozambique—and the HIV rate was just as high among migrants as among nonmigrants.[4] But the doctors' findings provided pretty strong evidence that returning gold miners played an important role in bringing HIV to this region in the early 1990s.[5]

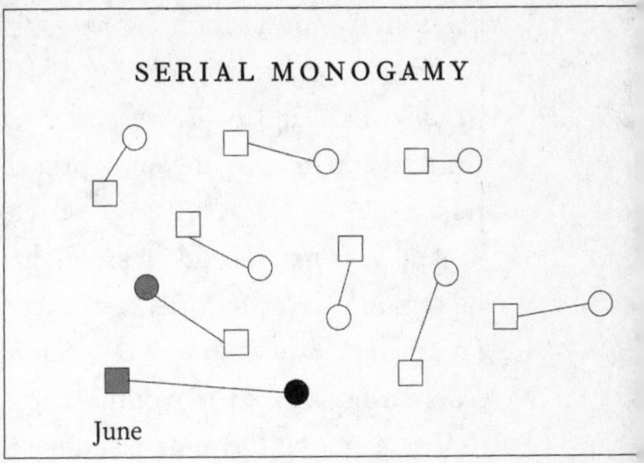

In an effort to understand the relationship between gold mining and HIV, I visited a South African gold mine one Saturday afternoon in September 2001. I was brought there by a couple of acquaintances who were gold miners themselves. We headed for the bar, where a few hundred glassy-eyed African men sat around a courtyard drinking. Some of them were passing around old paint tins containing homebrew, a foaming beverage made from molasses, millet, and other ingredients. The men sat in groups more or less according to nationality—the tall Basotho wrapped in gray blankets, and the South Africans in wool caps and parkas. Deafening African music issued from a pair of loudspeakers, virtually everyone was drunk, and the atmosphere was one of total oblivion. A few men danced by themselves and one fell gracefully over a chair, as if in slow motion, and then lay on the ground.

There were about twenty women in the courtyard; some of them sat joking with the men and others circulated through the crowd in pairs. These bar girls were local prostitutes, who might have sex with twenty different men every week, either in a shack somewhere or in the wooded areas around the mines, under makeshift tents made from plastic bags and twigs.[6] The mines provided condoms to the miners, and the miners used them, or so they told me, although they were so drunk, I seriously wondered whether they were really capable of doing so.

Migrant miners and prostitutes were what AIDS experts refer to as "high-risk groups."[7] During the 1990s, these experts maintained that it was particularly important to encourage members of these groups to use condoms and take other HIV prevention measures because their risky behavior endangered everyone else. Working with these groups was for years the foundation of most AIDS prevention programs in southern Africa. Mpholo Moema, who worked for the Mothusimpilo project, an

AIDS-prevention group in one of the mining towns, explained it to me this way: "This is what we know. This has been shown by the World Health Organization and by USAID, by everyone. You have to target high-transmission groups in your approach to prevent HIV in the community in general."

And yet I had recently learned that evidence from the very same mining region where Mr. Moema worked suggested that high-risk groups did not entirely explain how HIV was spreading in southern Africa. Two years earlier, a group of South African epidemiologists had measured the HIV rate among the miners and the prostitutes who solicit in the bushes around the mines. Almost as an afterthought, the researchers also measured rates of HIV infection among ordinary women living in a township about fifteen miles away from the mines. The researchers were not surprised to find that 80 percent of the prostitutes were HIV positive, or that 30 percent of the miners carried the virus as well.[8] But what really surprised them was that nearly 60 percent of the women in the township between the ages of twenty and thirty were also HIV positive. The women in the township were not prostitutes, and they were not particularly promiscuous. About half said they had had sex with fewer than three different men in their entire lives, hardly high-risk behavior. And yet they were almost as likely to be HIV positive as the prostitutes were, and they were twice as likely to be HIV positive as the miners themselves.[9]

"So, am I to understand that the 'low-risk' people are at higher risk than the 'high-risk' people?" I asked a South African nurse who worked with AIDS patients living near the mines.

"Yes," she replied.

"We were stunned," said Brian Williams, one of the epidemiologists who conducted the study. It turns out that miners, not surprisingly, prefer long-term girlfriends in the townships to hasty tussles in the wet grass with prostitutes. Only about 5 percent of the miners said they had visited a prostitute in the past year, whereas nearly half had had a girlfriend or mistress. When they did have sex with prostitutes, they knew it was risky, so they usually used condoms. But they trusted their longer-term township girlfriends, who trusted them in return, and condoms were used far less often in these relationships.[10] Nevertheless, because many of the miners had more than one long-term partner—perhaps a wife or girlfriend back home as well as one or more in the township—they were unwittingly caught up in a concurrency network and were thus at very high risk of infection themselves and of passing the virus to others.

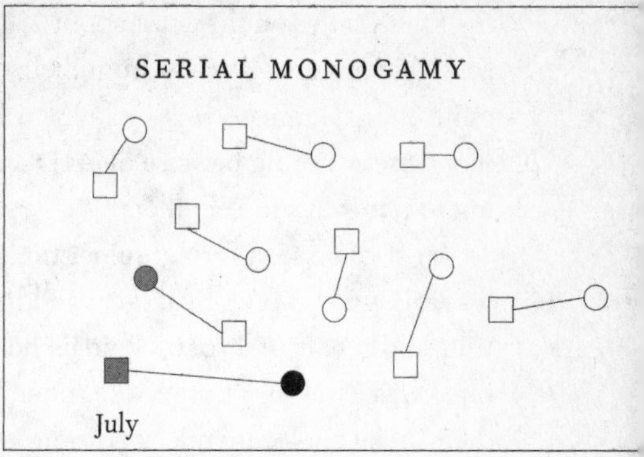

I WONDERED WHETHER HIV was spreading in a similar way in southern Mozambique, where many of the miners came from. I wanted to follow the epidemic back to Mozambique and speak to rural women from the villages that sent miners to South Africa, villages where HIV rates were now very high. I thought they might be able to tell me why the virus had spread so quickly, not just among miners and their wives, but to everyone else as well. Were condoms even available in these remote villages? Did people use them? If they didn't use them, why not?

The best way to find Mozambican women who might be willing to discuss HIV was through local nongovernmental, community-based organizations that were helping rural communities cope with AIDS, poverty, and other calamities. Certainly there were hospitals in this region, but the powerful antiretroviral drugs that can extend the lives of people with AIDS were all but unavailable in Mozambique at the time, and doctors could do little to help AIDS patients except give them relatively inexpensive antibiotics and send them home to die. But I knew from my experience in Uganda that small community-based organizations could do a great deal to help patients and their families cope. If only I could find such organizations in Mozambique, I thought, they would be able to help me find women to talk to about HIV.

But finding such organizations in southern Mozambique was not easy.[11] Eventually a journalist from one of the local newspapers suggested I contact the Mozambican miners' union, which is called AMIMO, and speak to its director, Moises Uamusse. I telephoned Mr. Uamusse at his headquarters in Maputo, and he told me he was just about to leave for a town called Xai-Xai. Would I like to go with him? I said I would. In that case, could I by any chance give him a lift?

Xai-Xai lies on the coast about 150 miles east of Maputo on the main road that miners travel on from their home villages to the South African mines. Mr. Uamusse said he knew a lot of mining families in Xai-Xai that were suffering because of AIDS, and through his union he was trying to find ways to help them.

Mr. Uamusse, a former miner himself, was about forty years old. He was tall, with a long, oval face, and he wore the frayed pieces of an old suit, and a pair of broken sandals held on with string. His mission, he said, was "the vindication of miners' rights, and the improvement of their social and economic condition." In practice, this meant writing letters of inquiry to the United Mine Workers Union, the AFL-CIO, the International Labor Organization, and other institutions to request funds. To these letters, Mr. Uamusse received few replies, although he had managed to raise a few thousand dollars from the World Bank, which he said he was using to conduct lectures on the dangers of AIDS to new recruits at the mine induction center near the border. He was also making a list of all the families that had been affected by AIDS in Xai-Xai, and he had a consignment of sewing machines that he was distributing to the widows of miners who had died of AIDS so they could earn some money making and repairing clothes.

The drive to Xai-Xai took three hours, and Mr. Uamusse talked nearly the entire time. The AIDS problem in the rural communities around here was caused by immoral behavior, he said, but not so much on the part of migrant miners. It was the women who were the problem. Because the men were always away, they were not able to impose discipline on their families. "Say you get a wife," he said hypothetically, "and then you go to South Africa to work. You come back twelve months later, and you find that wife pregnant. You find you have to fire that wife. Then you get another one, and that one is also unfaithful. This is what is happening."

Mr. Uamusse's words were harsh, but he had a point. International public health officials frequently attribute African women's vulnerability to HIV to sexual coercion and poverty that drives them into unwanted relationships, but studies of poor African women themselves suggest there is more to it than that. In 30 to 40 percent of "discordant couples," in which one partner is positive and the other negative, it's the woman who's positive, not the man.[12] Some women are sexually coerced, but many probably contract the virus in consensual premarital or extramarital relationships.[13] When the University of Pennsylvania sociologists Linda Tawfik and Susan Watkins asked poor Malawian women why they had extramarital affairs, they cited many reasons, including sexual pleasure, desire for attractive commodities, and revenge on an unfaithful spouse, as well as poverty.[14]

SERIAL MONOGAMY

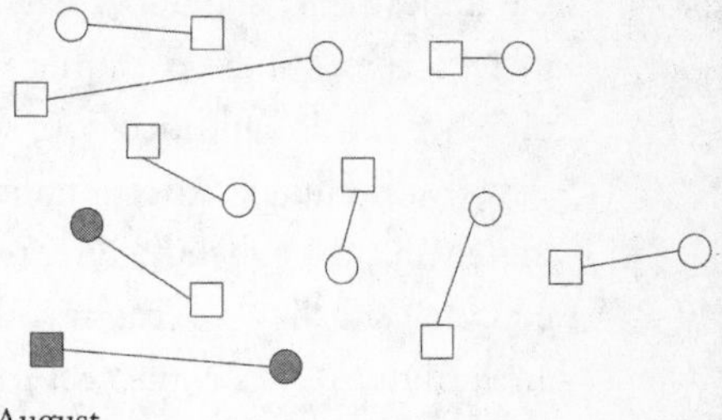

Mr. Uamusse approved of the fact that the mining companies in South Africa distributed condoms to their workers, but he did not believe they should be given to women, because it encouraged disrespect and promiscuous behavior. Mr. Uamusse's views seemed to be widely held in Mozambique. Condoms were cheap and generally available, but only nine million were sold in 2001, two for every male adult in the country.

It was late afternoon, and the countryside glowed in the shallow sunlight. Xai-Xai lies in a floodplain near the Limpopo River and the Indian Ocean. In recent years, oceanic cyclones had pelted this region with terrible floods, but now it was the dry season and plumes of dust blew off the fields into the clear sky, warning of drought. The road was smooth and fast and there was little traffic except for the buses, of which there were two kinds, Mozambican and South African. The Mozambican buses were great wheezing wrecks, belching smoke, traveling at thirty miles an hour and stopping everywhere. Teetering on the roof were huge bundles of pineapples, charcoal, and maize meal, which occasionally fell off. I had ridden on one of these buses a few days before, and as it drew nearer to the city, it became so crowded that passengers near the door could fit inside only if they all turned their heads in the same direction and pressed them up against the ceiling. Sleek new South African buses sped past us. These buses are almost exclusively used by returning mine workers, and they all tow small trailers loaded with goods—televisions and stereos still in their cartons, bicycles and mattresses wrapped in plastic—that are luxury items in this part of the world.

Miners earn relatively high salaries compared to other Mozambicans, and they are among the richest people in these communities. But mining is also dangerous work. About one in thirty miners doesn't make it out of the mines alive, and about half are permanently disabled by the end of their careers. Miners in southern Africa have the highest rates in the world of tuberculosis and silicosis (a severe immune reaction to silica dust that destroys the lungs). But a miner's greatest fear is that the walls of the mine will cave in behind him, trapping or crushing him. When this happens, the shock waves can travel for hundreds of kilometers. "It was like an earthquake; we could feel it in the hostels and then we knew people were being killed," Mr. Uamusse said. There were other dangers too. The miners came from all over southern Africa, and workers on the same mine might speak ten or more languages. Sometimes tensions arose in the cramped, all-male hostels. Sometimes there were fights, and sometimes the men killed each other.

However, in southern Mozambique, men cherished a job in the South African mines because the local economy was a shambles. In the early 2000s, Mozambique was often cited as a development success story, and according to the World Bank, its economy was growing strongly. But most of this growth was confined to Maputo, the capital city.[15] Rural incomes had been rising far more slowly, if at all. Agriculture, which supports most Mozambicans, grew by only 1 percent in 2000. The construction industry and a single aluminum smelting plant in the southern region accounted for most of the nation's recent growth, although money earned illegally may also have contributed. In 2001, Joseph Hanlon, a writer and expert on southern Africa, estimated that a ton each of cocaine and heroin passed through the ports of Mozambique every month on their way to the United States and Europe.[16]

Mozambique was once one of the most industrialized countries in Africa. Its factories produced clothing, textiles, furniture, processed cashews, and other commodities. Many farming families from Xai-Xai supplemented their sometimes precarious incomes by working in these industries. The Portuguese colonial government protected these businesses with import tariffs and subsidies, and other Portuguese territories provided a guaranteed market. But when the Portuguese entrepreneurs fled after independence in 1975, the inexperienced and poorly educated

Mozambicans who took their places could not maintain them. Local industries suffered even more after the onset of the bloody civil war in the 1980s.

The war, the lingering effects of the oil crisis of the late 1970s, a shaky global economy, and the development blunders of Mozambique's inexperienced new leaders all sank the country deeper into debt. Then, in the mid-1980s and again in the mid-1990s, the World Bank and the International Monetary Fund (IMF) informed the Mozambican government that they would continue to lend the country money only if it stopped protecting its struggling industries. The lenders, following the neoliberal development ideas of U.S. and western European leaders at the time, believed that developing countries would prosper if they reduced government spending and protectionist trading practices. Freer trade would, in theory, integrate these countries into the global economy so they would grow more quickly. This, in turn, would help ensure that countries like Mozambique would be in a better position to service their debts.

In theory, these policies made sense. In effect, they were so rashly implemented that they further impoverished large numbers of people.[17] By 2000, only about 600,000 of Mozambique's twenty million people had formal jobs. The rest worked mainly in the "informal sector," as subsistence farmers or petty traders. Meanwhile, throughout the 1990s, corrupt government cronies and shady businessmen "borrowed" from Mozambique's newly privatized banks hundreds of millions of dollars that might have been invested in the economy. This money was never repaid, and millions more were lost through accounting fraud.

Mozambique's banks also became notorious for illegal foreign-exchange deals, money laundering, and other criminal activities. Since 1997, two executives and one journalist investigating the banking system in Mozambique had been murdered, and several others shot at but not killed. While government officials were ultimately responsible for Mozambique's banking crisis, the World Bank and IMF may also bear some responsibility, because they put pressure on the government to privatize the banks quickly, before regulatory and accounting systems that might have reduced the risk of fraud could be put in place.[18]

Most Mozambicans now wore textiles from India and secondhand clothes imported from Western countries. The market was also flooded with manufactured goods imported, sometimes illegally, from neighboring countries, including South Africa. These imports often cost the same as, and sometimes even more than, the products Mozambicans used to make themselves.[19]

Mr. Uamusse and I drove past the ruins of buildings destroyed in the war and villages hidden among shady trees. Stout peasant women in kerchiefs and long skirts hammered the earth with their hoes, and goats trotted to and fro across the empty road. Mr. Uamusse wanted me to go back to America and find people to invest in southern Mozambique. "Now see here," he said, "we have been driving for nearly two hours, and we have not passed a single town. Why don't they put a town here?" I said I thought that was a good question. "Why don't they put up a factory in this area? We have mangoes, cashews, coconut. . . . We could make jam, we could make oils—oils for cooking, oils for beauty. . . . We could use the clay to make bricks."

THE FOLLOWING MORNING, Mr. Uamusse took me to a small clearing beside Xai-Xai's main road, where a table and chairs had been set up under a tree. About thirty people were waiting for us, mainly miners and former miners and the widows of miners. Mr. Uamusse made a speech in Portuguese, and then, with him as interpreter, I interviewed some of the women in the group, one by one. I wanted them to tell me how their community had been affected by HIV, what they thought they needed to confront the epidemic, and how they felt about condoms. But I soon realized these women did not want to discuss HIV at all. Although people in southern Mozambique were facing a terrible plague, what they wanted to talk about instead was money.

The women spoke softly, and when the wind blew through the trees you could hardly hear them. An old woman said her mine-worker husband had died in an ambush during the war in 1990. She believed that he had contributed to some sort of pension fund, and she had been trying to collect this pension for the past eleven years. Every few months she went to the local office in Xai-Xai that deals with mine workers' pensions to see if there was any money for her, but each time she was told that the money had not yet arrived. Sometimes she was told to go home and return with some document or other—perhaps a birth certificate, or a death record—but when she returned, the answer was always the same. "You come back later," they said.

The other women had similar tales. They all carried paper envelopes or plastic bags full of documents: birth certificates, death certificates, employment records, bankbooks, old bus tickets, receipts for things bought in South Africa—a stereo, a refrigerator, a mattress, some shoes. From what the women told me, it sounded as though some of their husbands might have died of AIDS—they had lost weight before they died, or had had tuberculosis that couldn't be cured. But the women all said they didn't know what their husbands had died of, and on the death certificates it was written that the cause of death was "undetermined." When I mentioned AIDS, the women said they had heard of it, but they knew nothing about it and looked away.

More people kept showing up while I was talking to the widows, and before long there were about fifty people in the clearing waiting to speak to me. I asked Mr. Uamusse whether any of them would be willing to discuss HIV, but when Mr. Uamusse addressed my question to the crowd in the clearing, everyone quietly left.

"Where are the AIDS widows and the sewing machines you told me about?" I asked Mr. Uamusse when we were alone again. The statistics from the Health Ministry and the women's own stories convinced me that AIDS was a serious problem in Xai-Xai, but the people who lived here clearly had other ideas about what their problems were. This is what they had come to tell me, but I did not understand them at first. Mr. Uamusse would say only this: "From our speeches, you will hear things that are true, and things that are not true. It is up to you to find out what is true."

While I pondered these mysterious words, a teenage boy approached us. He was wearing blue jeans, which gave him a more modern appearance than the other men, in their battered jackets and trousers. He told Mr. Uamusse he wanted us to meet his mother, and we followed him down a sandy lane to a small plot of land with a single concrete building on it, and a few shady papaya trees. Three little girls scampered in the yard and an old woman with bare feet as tough as tires dozed under a tree. A younger woman, who was the boy's mother, lay on a straw mat in the yard. Her name was Elisa, and she was very thin and coughed a lot and was clearly dying of what looked to me very much like AIDS. She said she had been sick for more than a year, but she found out only a month ago what the sickness was. "It is TB," she said. But if this was a case of simple TB, the hospital in Xai-Xai, which is equipped to deal with it, would not have waited a year to give her a diagnosis.[20] Her husband had worked in the South African mines for nearly twenty years until 1999, when he was sent home for "medical reasons."

Elisa sent one of her daughters to fetch something, and the girl emerged from the house a few minutes later with a snapshot of Elisa's husband. He was about fifty years old, smiling and handsome. He was leaning against a fence and looking right at the camera. He was supporting himself on a pair of crutches, and one of his legs was encased in a huge white cast. In the mines, he drove a "loco," a sturdy truck that runs along underground tracks hauling loads of rocks to the surface. He had been injured in an accident and sent home to Mozambique for several months to recover. Then he returned to South Africa, but within a week, he became very ill and collapsed at work. His friends found him and arranged for an ambulance to take him to the miners' hospital, but he was discharged almost immediately and sent home to Mozambique, where he died two weeks later, in July 2000.

When I asked Elisa what the doctors had told him about his illness, she said the doctors "did not discover the sickness. They only said he got it in South Africa." What did he look like before he died? "He got so thin," her son said. "Every day he seemed to get thinner and thinner." What do you think it was? "Maybe," he said, "it was the century sickness," which I would learn was a local euphemism for AIDS.

Like the other women, Elisa knew that her husband had put some money in a pension fund in South Africa. Shortly after he died, she went to the local mine workers' pension office to collect it but was told that if she wanted the money, she would have to go to South Africa to get a document from the mining company, stating that her husband had been employed there. So she applied for a South African visa and prepared to set off. But then she herself became ill and feared she might not survive the eight-hour bus ride. She returned to the pension office to ask whether she could send one of her children in her place, but she was told this would not be possible. And there the matter stood while she waited to recover. But she never did. In the meantime, the family was finding it increasingly difficult to make ends meet. One by one her children were being forced to drop out of school, but they could not find steady jobs, and those who remained in school could not afford books. Her mother-in-law, the old woman under the tree, earned some money for the family by laboring on a nearby farm, but she was paid less than a dollar for a ten-hour day. By now, more than a year had passed, and Elisa's only hope was that pension. "Many women around here are crying [because of poverty]," she said. Indeed, one of the other widows told me she was worried that if she didn't get her pension money, her daughters would fall into prostitution.

In 2000, the U.S. Agency for International Development funded an investigation into the AIDS crisis in southern Mozambique.[21] The researchers started in the usual way, by searching for groups with higher-risk behavior, meaning prostitutes and the people whom they serve, such as truck drivers and migrants. But they were able to identify relatively few real prostitutes in this region. They did discover, however, that many other women—farmers, market traders, housewives, and so on—form steady, sometimes clandestine relationships with relatively wealthy men in the hope that it will bring them some material benefit, the occasional chicken perhaps, school fees for the children, or favorable deals for a few cabbages.

These people are so poor, in other words, that sex has become part of their economy. In some cases, it's practically the only currency they have. A Mozambican doctor I met in Gaza explained it to me this way: "The railway line that goes through this town links Mozambique with South Africa and Zimbabwe. During the war in the 1980s, the trains were guarded by soldiers from those countries. There were shortages of food in those days and the relief supplies would come into Mozambique on those trains. Many of the women around here were starving, and they would sell their bodies just to eat. The problems started then."

AIDS has been described as a disease of poverty, but it might be more accurate to describe it as a disease of inequality, which settles along the ever-deepening chasm between rich and poor.[22] In southern Mozambique, returning miners with relatively high wages paid in the formal economy meet the staggering poverty of rural women struggling to make a living in the informal economy. The collision between these two worlds may disrupt the social ecology of those impoverished villages, creating favorable conditions for the spread of HIV, just as changes in weather patterns create new environmental niches for aggressive species that can destroy a forest or a lake. The poor themselves seem to know that money is at the root of their AIDS problem. Perhaps that is why, when I came to talk to them about HIV, they told me about money instead.

A few days before I met Elisa, I had visited the central office that deals with Mozambican mine workers' pensions in Maputo. The institution is called TEBA, which stands for "The Employment Bureau of Africa," and it was established in 1902 as the recruiting arm of the Chamber of Mines of South Africa. It is still associated with the chamber and is paid by the mining companies to recruit mine workers and disburse their salaries, pensions, and benefits. The director, an amiable white South African, explained the various pension and benefit funds that mine workers contribute to, and the many routes, through banks and ministries, that the money takes before it reaches his office, and then the beneficiaries.

On the way out, I passed through the section of the TEBA office where financial transactions take place. Some thirty women sat on benches in the waiting area, most of them in bright kerchiefs and long skirts like Elisa and the other farm women in Xai-Xai. A few clerks sat behind a transparent partition, surrounded by listing heaps of dusty paper. The clerks silently examined documents or filled out forms, and they moved so slowly, it seemed as though time in the TEBA office had nearly ground to a halt. The women in the waiting room were so quiet and still, and seemed so patient, it was almost as though they had been painted there. During the months after I left Mozambique, Mr. Uamusse and I contacted the TEBA office several times on Elisa's behalf, and also on behalf of another AIDS widow I met, and we were always reassured that the cases would be resolved very soon.

How many widows are in the same position as Elisa? In 2002, TEBA officials admitted that pensions and compensation money were owed to at least ten thousand Mozambican miners who lost their jobs during the past twenty years, or to their families, if the men had died. But, the officials claim, they have not been able to find the beneficiaries because of population movements caused by the war that had ended ten years earlier.[23] Why, in that case, was I able to meet at least fifty potential claimants during a single weekend? It is not known how much money is owed to the peasants of southern Africa by mining firms, insurance companies, government bureaucracies, pension funds, and other institutions, but it didn't take much effort for me to discover that about forty million dollars of unclaimed money has accumulated in the major pension fund to which most black, unskilled miners contribute, and that about two billion dollars is owed to hundreds of thousands of former mine workers who developed silicosis from dust exposure in the mines and are therefore eligible for compensation, but almost none of them had been paid either.[24]

The World Bank itself admits that the inefficiency of the basic institutions that should serve the poor, including banks, pension funds, insurance companies, courts, and real-estate transfer systems, are a major hindrance to economic development throughout the third world.[25] Making these institutions work requires government oversight, and so does rebuilding Africa's devastated economies. But donor policies emphasizing free trade and small government make regulation of such institutions more difficult.

Shortly after I returned from Mozambique, an article appeared in a medical journal by Peter Lamptey of Family Health International, an agency that implements AIDS programs for USAID. He wrote that HIV prevention programs must include awareness-raising to encourage people to use condoms and have fewer sexual partners, and improved treatment services for other sexually transmitted diseases that make HIV transmission more likely. He also conceded that the social conditions that make people vulnerable to HIV infection in the first place must be improved, including poverty, unemployment, and discrimination against women.[26] These recommendations had been in place for years, but even Dr. Lamptey admitted that they had not been as successful as he originally hoped they would be. The reasons why sexual behavior had been so slow to change in response to HIV in many developing countries were complex and mysterious. However, it is possible that by emphasizing HIV prevention among "groups with high-risk behavior," such as truckers, miners, and prostitutes, some development agencies recognized too late the risks faced by others. It is also possible that people in communities that have been broken by war, migration, and continuing economic hardship will be slow to take HIV awareness messages seriously. It is also possible that improving the social conditions that make the poor vulnerable to HIV is difficult when their fate is sometimes in the hands of remote economists, officials, and businessmen.

When I was in Mozambique, I couldn't escape the impression that there was something Victorian about the place—the women's long skirts, the hypocrisy about sexual matters, the absurd bureaucracy, the impoverished masses, and the misdirected charity that fails to help them. The Victorians also suffered from STDs, which they too blamed on prostitutes. The spread of STDs in Victorian times may have been similar to the spread of HIV in Mozambique today, in that it was driven partly by economic changes that created legions of impoverished women, and prevailing attitudes that made sex unspeakable, while tacitly pardoning men for adultery and punishing women for it.

CHAPTER SIX

A President, a Crisis, a Tragedy

ONE SUNDAY EVENING in early May 2000, shortly after I arrived in South Africa for the first time, I went for a walk in one of Johannesburg's wealthier suburbs. It seemed a world away from the dusty, jerry-built atmosphere of Uganda or Mozambique. The whitewashed stucco houses on well-tended lawns with hissing sprinklers and swimming pools, the twittering birds, the leaning jacaranda trees lined up on quiet streets—all reminded me of San Diego or Los Angeles, except for the barbed wire curled above the gates and the dogs that roared at me from behind each fence as I passed by. By the time I had walked half a block, it seemed as though all the dogs in Johannesburg were barking. I didn't go far. South Africa lives under a kind of self-imposed curfew. By sundown, the streets from the Cape to the Transvaal are eerily empty. Gates are bolted, alarms are set, and guards are on watch.

Everyone I met warned me to be careful. One acquaintance spent ten minutes listing all the people he knew who, in the past six years, had been shot, killed, or raped. One person had been hijacked in his car, robbed, thrown in the trunk, and then deposited, naked, by a roadside. Another South African told me that the bank in his middle-class neighborhood had been robbed five times in six months. A Johannesburg taxi driver said that, in his company alone, a driver is murdered every month. There are some fifty thousand reported rapes in South Africa each year, a number believed to represent a small fraction of those actually committed.[1]

Crime in South Africa affects everyone—black, white, Asian, rich, and poor. In 1999, someone walked off with an entire automatic teller machine that had been installed inside a police building in Johannesburg. In Cape Town, rapes and burglaries have been committed within the Parliament buildings themselves. Suspicion and paranoia seemed to me to pervade even the fancy shopping malls, tourist beaches, and expensive hotels. It even informs the country's policies, including its response to the greatest health threat in its history.

In 2000, the South African Ministry of Health estimated that roughly four million South Africans carried the HIV virus, and about seventeen hundred people were becoming newly infected every day. HIV had been present in the country for more than a decade but, as in much of the rest of Africa, the government and the general public had paid only desultory attention to the crisis. Prevention campaigns were episodic, newspapers and broadcasters largely ignored the subject, and even doctors in hospitals tended to attribute AIDS deaths to other causes, such as tuberculosis or meningitis.

Then, in 1999, President Thabo Mbeki began to solicit the opinions of a murky, informal network of scientists and activists known as "AIDS dissidents," including the University of California, Berkeley, molecular biologist Peter Duesberg and the former Georgia Tech biochemist David Rasnick. In their books and magazine articles, and on Internet Web sites such as virusmyth.com, the AIDS dissidents claimed that the disease is caused not by sexual behavior and HIV but by a vague collection of environmental and nutritional factors, including vitamin deficiencies, chemical pollution, and poverty.[2] They maintained that the tens of thousands of doctors and scientists who work on HIV and AIDS are, often unwittingly, part of a vast conspiracy to justify the market in anti-AIDS drugs, such as AZT and nevirapine, worth billions of dollars a year. During the 1980s, the views of some AIDS dissidents, including Duesberg, were briefly taken seriously by some AIDS researchers. Luc Montagnier, one of the discoverers of HIV, conceded that there was much about AIDS that was still unknown, including the mechanism by which the virus destroyed the immune system and the reasons some patients succumbed more rapidly to the disease than others. But as scientists learned more about the virus, and especially after powerful antiretroviral drug cocktails that both killed the virus and relieved AIDS symptoms were developed in 1996, the dissidents seemed to fade from the scene. Then, as the Internet took off in the late 1990s, their ideas began to circulate again in cyberspace. With a confused tangle of half-truths, inaccuracies, and outright falsehoods, the dissidents claimed that antiretroviral drugs were not only useless against AIDS, but also toxic—indeed, they claimed the drugs were a cause of, not a cure for, AIDS. The vast majority of AIDS scientists found their arguments highly unconvincing.[3]

Mbeki is the only head of state known to have taken the views of the AIDS dissidents seriously, and many doctors and AIDS activists in South Africa and in the West were beginning to wonder whether the president and his health minister had taken leave of their senses. By 1999, the evidence that HIV is the cause of AIDS was very strong indeed, and the implications for countries like South Africa were horrifying. Many people were surprised when President Mbeki invited a group of AIDS dissidents, including Professor Duesberg, to South Africa to present their views to a presidential panel on AIDS in Africa in May 2000. One scientist told me, "It's like the movie *Friday the 13th*. Just when you think you've finally killed the monster, it just keeps coming back to life." The interest Mbeki took in the AIDS dissidents was far more than an intellectual diversion. It was a public health disaster, because it distracted the Ministry of Health and other official institutions from addressing the epidemic and led to the unnecessary deaths of thousands of South African infants and AIDS patients.

Western pharmaceutical companies now sell a range of some twenty antiretrovirals that in combination can add many healthy years to the life of an HIV-positive person. But in 2000, the drugs were patented and expensive and the annual cost of treatment was more than ten thousand dollars per patient. However, researchers had found that a cheap, short course of some of these drugs, such as AZT or nevirapine, taken for a few weeks around the time of childbirth, could reduce by half the chances that an HIV-positive mother would transmit the virus to her baby. A small number of maternity clinics in developing countries had already launched programs to offer these drugs to HIV-positive pregnant women through the public health system, and in 1998 it looked as though South Africa would be doing so too. But suddenly, the then minister of health, Nkosazana Zuma, suspended public funds for these projects, because, she said, even these short courses of antiretrovirals were too costly.[4]

AIDS activists and doctors protested, claiming correctly that preventing HIV transmission in the womb was much cheaper than treating sick children with AIDS. But the Ministry of Health maintained its rigid policy. Then, in early 1999, the president stated in an address to Parliament that he had learned that antiretroviral drugs were not only expensive, they were also toxic, or so he had learned from speaking to the AIDS dissidents and reading their Web sites. These drugs would not, therefore, be administered to pregnant women attending public hospitals until they had been thoroughly investigated.[5]

The president and his circle were now on a crusade against antiretrovirals that grew more complicated and fanciful by the day. In 2000, Parks Mankahlana, Mbeki's spokesman—who died of AIDS shortly afterward—wrote in the newspaper *Business Day* that AIDS drugs were not only expensive and toxic, but part of a corporate conspiracy to exploit poor blacks:

> Like the marauders of the military industrial complex who propagated fear to increase their profits, the profit-takers who are benefiting from the scourge of HIV/AIDS will disappear to the affluent beaches of the world to enjoy wealth accumulated from a humankind ravaged by a dreaded disease. . . . Sure, the shareholders of GlaxoWellcome [the company that makes AZT] will rejoice to hear that the SA government has decided to supply AZT to pregnant women who are HIV-positive. The source of their joy will not be concern for those people's health, but about profits and shareholder value.[6]

At the time, about two hundred babies were being born in South Africa every day with HIV. Giving all of their mothers nevirapine or AZT around the time of delivery would spare as many as half of them.[7] In 1997, GlaxoWellcome had offered AZT at a discount to the South African Ministry of Health for use in public maternity wards, but the ministry turned the offer down.[8]

Have you ever seen a child dying of AIDS? When I worked at Mulago Hospital in Uganda, what always surprised me about the pediatric

AIDS wards was how quiet they were.* The thin, breathless children were too sick to cry. Before I left for South Africa, I had arranged to speak to some of South Africa's leading scientists and government officials about the government's anti-AIDS-drugs policy, which did not make sense to me. What I found when I got there was even more disturbing than what I had expected.

IN 2000, the only way a poor HIV-positive South African could obtain antiretroviral drugs was by participating in a clinical trial sponsored by one of the large Western pharmaceutical companies that make them. These companies test their drugs in Africa because there are so many HIV-positive people there who have never taken antiretroviral drugs before. Such patients are unlikely to have developed resistance to any of the individual drugs in the cocktails, and this gives the cocktails a better chance of success, which in turn allows the companies to obtain clearer results more quickly. In 2000, hundreds of such trials were under way across the country, and many HIV-positive South Africans were eager to sign up for them. "People are desperate," Florence Ngobeni of the Township AIDS Project in Soweto told me. "There is so much confusion and fear."

While I was in South Africa, a doctor named Costa Gazi, whom I was interviewing about the anti-AZT policy, told me about one clinical trial that seemed to have had disastrous results. I had read wire reports about the trial on the Internet in April.[9] Around five hundred HIV-positive people had been enrolled to compare two different cocktails of antiretroviral drugs at sixteen hospital clinics around South Africa. The reports claimed that since the trial began in September 1999, five participants had died, two of them from liver damage possibly caused by one of the drugs in the cocktails. According to subsequent news reports in the South African press, a sixth patient died in April.[10] Gazi told me that five of the six deaths on the trial had occurred at a single hospital in Pretoria, called Kalafong, out of only forty-two patients enrolled there. In addition, six other patients from the same hospital had experienced side effects so severe that some of them had had to be hospitalized.

*Because infants' immune systems are still developing, HIV produces symptoms in them more rapidly than it does in adults.

I wondered whether this could possibly be true. The reports that five out of five hundred patients died on the trial were disturbing, although perhaps the deaths could be explained by the occurrence of unexpected side effects or complications of AIDS. But if, in fact, eleven people out of only forty-two at one hospital had become very ill or died, something must have gone terribly wrong. For some time I tried to find out what happened to these people, but the truth seemed to be buried under endless evasions, innuendo, and rumors. However, the obstacles to finding out what happened were themselves revealing.

Shortly after I arrived in South Africa, the health minister, Manto Tshabalala-Msimang, gave a speech in which she said, "We place on record our determination [to fight the AIDS epidemic] with every means at our disposal." Certainly this was arguable. Not only were public hospitals not providing nevirapine to pregnant women; other evidence suggested that the government's response to AIDS was incoherent and disorganized. In fiscal year 1999–2000, the AIDS directorate in the Ministry of Health failed to spend 40 percent of its funds. In February, the government appointed a national AIDS council that included an athlete, a TV producer, numerous politicians, and two traditional healers, but did not include South Africa's most important scientists, doctors, activists, or representatives of nongovernmental AIDS organizations. At the time, fewer than 60 percent of South Africa's health facilities were able to carry out AIDS testing and counseling, and few community health-care clinics were equipped or staffed to manage AIDS patients. Some people with HIV reported being turned away, even for complaints not related to AIDS.[11] Ineffective and expensive campaigns to promote public awareness of AIDS had been mounted, including National Condom Week, during which free condoms that had unfortunately been stapled to cards were distributed.

I interviewed a doctor at a public hospital in the East Rand about what he had to offer people with AIDS. "We have no [antiretroviral] drugs here," he said. "Not even for needle-stick injuries." This shocked me. Doctors and nurses frequently stick themselves with bloody needles by accident, and in this way may expose themselves to HIV. If someone who is exposed to HIV through a needle stick takes a high dose of antiretroviral drugs immediately afterward, his chances of becoming infected are greatly reduced. These drugs, in kit form, are supposed to be available in all hospitals for health-care workers at risk of needle-stick injuries. But according to this doctor, they were not, at least "not since the president started talking to [the AIDS dissidents]." According to a Ministry of Health spokesperson, all hospitals were supposed to have antiretroviral kits for needle-stick injuries, but I still wondered why this large, well-known hospital failed to have them. Was the Ministry of Health too preoccupied with the president's inquisition into the causes of AIDS to ensure that routine hospital procedures were being followed?

Perhaps this distracted Ministry of Health had also failed to implement adequate ethical and safety guidelines for clinical trials. Patients taking any experimental medication need to be monitored to ensure that the drugs are not causing side effects. Perhaps those patients who, according to Gazi, became ill or died at Kalafong Hospital had been on a clinical trial that was poorly monitored. Maybe the patients got a bad batch of drugs from the pharmaceutical company or were particularly sensitive to them for some reason, and no one recognized it in time. Perhaps there were other explanations for what happened at Kalafong.

ABOUT SIX MILES west of Pretoria, the township of Atteridgeville blankets the tall grass and thorn bushes of the South African veldt. Like many of the townships on the outskirts of South Africa's cities, Atteridgeville was built to house Pretoria's black servants and factory workers. But as the grip of apartheid began to loosen, the population of Atteridgeville exploded, and the township spread over the brown hillsides. In 2000, the gap between rich and poor was greater in South Africa than in any other country except Brazil. As I turned into Atteridgeville from the main road from Pretoria, the inequalities of the new South Africa unfolded before me. On the hill stood rows of new houses, many of them built since the elections in 1994 for South Africa's emerging black elite, mainly lawyers, civil servants, and businessmen. The houses were two-story stucco structures, with tidy backyards and metal gates and signs indicating that the houses have alarm systems and that trespassers will be met with an armed response. At the foot of the hill lay the neat grid of streets and tiny brick houses built for the workers during the apartheid years, and just beyond this stretched the vast plain of Atteridgeville's squatter camp.

In the squatter camp, the listing shacks, made of sheet metal, wood, and heavy cardboard, were occupied by the overflow from the overcrowded township itself and by migrants from Zimbabwe, Mozambique, and other countries to the north. There were no municipal services. Garbage piled up by the roadside, and the squatters strung wires from power lines to steal electricity. Water was collected from communal taps, and sewage was ad hoc.

A tin shack I visited in the squatter camp was dark and cool and orderly. Its dirt floor was swept, and bright plastic jugs were lined up beside a small portable stove. The few pieces of furniture were draped with patterned cloth, and an ornamental mask hung on the wall. Andrew, the shack's resident, wore a sweater and button-down shirt, and looked very young, like a teenager about to have his yearbook photograph taken. He lost his job as a schoolteacher in Zimbabwe in the early 1990s, when the government imposed sharp cuts in the education budget to satisfy requirements for receiving a World Bank loan. After the change of government in South Africa, Andrew and his wife came here to look for jobs, but without a South African degree, he had little hope of finding work as a teacher. Instead, he picked up odd jobs as a plasterer or bricklayer on some of the new building sites on the hill.

In March of 1998, Andrew's wife gave birth to a daughter. The baby did not thrive. When she was about a year old, she became feverish and ill and her mother took her to Kalafong, the large, state-run hospital that serves the population of Atteridgeville. The child was tested for HIV and found to be positive. Then Andrew and his wife were tested as well. When they were both found to be positive, they were referred to Dr. Ingrid Steenkamp, who ran the HIV clinic at Kalafong. Dr. Steenkamp was also affiliated with the University of Pretoria, under whose auspices she conducted clinical research on AIDS patients.[12]

The University of Pretoria had recently been chosen by Triangle Pharmaceuticals, based in North Carolina, to be one of the sites for its clinical trial of an antiretroviral drug cocktail containing a new drug called emtricitibine. The university in turn had chosen Dr. Steenkamp to recruit HIV-positive people to participate in the trial. She would conduct blood tests to determine who was eligible to participate, give participants the trial drugs, counsel them about how to take them, and conduct follow-up examinations and lab tests to determine how well the drugs were working. She was supposed to report any side effects to Triangle and also to the Medicines Control Council, the South African equivalent of the Food and Drug Administration that oversees the safety of all pharmaceuticals in the country, including those undergoing clinical trials.

Because Dr. Steenkamp worked at Kalafong, she had access to a large and growing population of HIV-positive people, most of whom were very poor. She invited Andrew and his wife to sign up for the emtricitibine trial, to which they agreed, and gave each of them four bottles of pills that had to be taken at precise times.

To be eligible for the trial, the participants had to be HIV positive, but they also had to be healthy and not suffering from AIDS. Andrew had never been sick before, he told me, and it was only after his daughter's illness and death that he discovered he was HIV positive. However, almost as soon as he began taking the drugs, he felt very weak. He mentioned this to Dr. Steenkamp, but "she said it was not the tablets that made me sick, it was the HIV, and that I should keep taking the medicine." But Andrew's symptoms worsened. At the beginning of the trial he had been given a form with a telephone number to call in case of emergencies. The phone number was a fax number, of little use to someone feeling sick in the middle of an impoverished squatter camp. Within a month, Andrew had to be admitted to Kalafong Hospital with vomiting, rash, fever, and painful, bleeding sores that covered his entire body. Andrew stopped taking the trial drugs, and his wife, who did not experience any of these symptoms, also dropped out of the trial.

Molly also lived in Atteridgeville. She was about thirty years old and had been HIV positive since 1995. She was being treated for tuberculosis when, she says, Dr. Steenkamp enrolled her in a clinical trial at Kalafong. The TB treatment had been working, and Molly felt well enough to go to her job as a counselor at an HIV support center, and to care for her two children. However, soon after she started taking the drugs that Dr. Steenkamp had given her, her health deteriorated. She came down with pneumonia, severe constipation, and cramps, and her throat became very sore. Most frightening of all, her sight began to fade and she nearly went blind. "Dr. Steenkamp said, 'This is caused by the HIV, and you won't see for the rest of your life,'" Molly told me. But as soon as Molly stopped taking the drugs that Dr. Steenkamp had given her, her sight returned. When I met her, Molly was sitting on the edge of a bed in the TB hospital, before a plate of French fries and sausage that she seemed too weak to eat. She was extremely thin, found it difficult to talk, and would lean over at intervals and cough violently into a heap of tissue paper on the bed.

"They say it's TB," she said, "but I don't believe them. The treatment was working before. I don't know why it's not working now."

Confirming what Dr. Gazi had told me about what had happened at Kalafong proved extremely hard to do. He put me in touch with an opposition member of Parliament named Patricia de Lille, who was an outspoken critic of the ruling African National Congress's policies on AIDS—and other issues as well. De Lille told me what she had heard about the Kalafong trial, and she explained that she felt monitoring procedures on clinical trials were inadequate, and that the government was wasting time with the AIDS dissidents. De Lille then referred me to a lapsed Anglican priest in Johannesburg named Johan Viljoen.

That winter Viljoen had spent five months working at the Mohau Centre, an AIDS organization that ran support groups for HIV-positive people based at Kalafong Hospital. Around Christmas, a few months after he started working at Mohau, Viljoen began to hear disturbing reports from some of its clients who had been participating in the AIDS drug trial run by Dr. Steenkamp at Kalafong.

"Many of the people on the trial knew each other. I got involved when some of them started coming to me and telling me about this one that died, and then that one. People were really worried. There was this spate of four or five deaths right before Christmas." According to what the patients told Viljoen, four women who went on the trial in October were dead by Christmas, and a further five women and one man, including Andrew and Molly, became very ill after taking the pills they were given. Then, in April, another woman died.

Viljoen gave me copies of signed testimonies that he had collected from the six patients who said they had become ill on the trial, and from a man who said his mother had died. All these patients, including Andrew and Molly, testified that they were HIV positive; they all named Dr. Steenkamp, and all said that she had put them in a clinical trial. Only one of the testimonies specifically named the Triangle trial, however. The symptoms the patients described were very strange. "I developed severe headaches and fevers, I felt extreme stress, depression, and anger," testified one woman. Another woman said, "I began to experience muscle cramps, spasms, and fits. I also feel stress, to such an extent I feel I might get a stroke." Another wrote, "In February 2000, I began to have a serious rash, all over my body."[13]*

There was something about Viljoen's account that did not make sense. The patients' complaints seemed odd. Fits, mood swings, dizziness, muscle spasms, and stress were not known side effects of antiretroviral drugs—as far as I could find out. When I read the testimonies, I wondered whether the patients might have been suffering from hysteria. Most of the patients had only recently learned of their HIV status, and the diagnosis must have come as a terrible shock. Like their government leaders, who themselves were only now awakening to the disaster in their midst, they must have been casting around everywhere for answers, and the rumors issuing from the president's office that AIDS medicines were toxic can only have made things worse. They must have found it very hard to know where to turn and whom to trust.

But the more I learned about the Kalafong trial, the more South Africa's paranoid atmosphere began to get to me too. Were these patients really in a trial at all? I wondered. And if so, what sort of trial? And who was monitoring it to ensure it was safe? Was the government or any other institution doing anything to find out what had happened to these patients?

I HAD HEARD that a report on the Triangle trial had been drafted within the Ministry of Health, but that it had not been made public. I very much wanted to speak to someone who had read it. In addition, I wanted to discuss the other controversies surrounding AIDS and its treatment in

*Some of these testimonies were later retracted. In addition, three of the trial subjects became the plaintiffs in a defamation lawsuit against Patricia de Lille and her biographer who had revealed their names in a book. In April 2007, South Africa's Constitutional Court decided in the plaintiffs' favor. See "Privacy, Confidentiality and Stigma: The Case of NM, SM, and LH v. Patricia de Lille, Charlene Smith and New Africa Books Publishers"; details are on the Web site of the AIDS Law Project, www.alp.org.za.

South Africa, such as antiretrovirals for pregnant women and Mbeki's relationship with the AIDS dissidents. But one by one, most of my appointments were canceled.

One senior government scientist changed our appointment six times and then left on a trip to the United States. Many others never returned phone calls, e-mails, or faxes. Dr. Nono Simelela, the head of the AIDS directorate in the Ministry of Health, agreed to meet me in Pretoria on the Thursday after I arrived. When I turned up at her office, her assistant told me that Dr. Simelela had been called away suddenly, just fifteen minutes previously, to the director general's office. I was introduced instead to Cornelius Lebeloe, who is in charge of counseling, testing, and support of AIDS patients. He told me he was not allowed to talk about the AIDS dissidents, the government's position on antiretrovirals for pregnant women, or the trial at Kalafong. When Dr. Simelela appeared an hour later, she said she was too busy to talk to me.

"How about tomorrow?" I asked.

Dr. Simelela opened her diary.

"No."

"Saturday?"

"No."

"Sunday?"

"No."

"Monday?"

"No."

"Tuesday?"

"OK, call me at ten in the morning on Tuesday."

When I phoned Dr. Simelela the following Tuesday, I was told that she was out. Her assistant suggested I call again on Friday morning at nine. On Friday morning, Dr. Simelela was not in the office. I called several times the following week, but Dr. Simelela was either out of town, in a meeting, or otherwise unavailable. After I returned to New York I sent an e-mail requesting an interview by phone. She never replied.

I RESORTED to reading the president's speeches and the writings of his biographers. Mbeki had grown up in the anti-apartheid movement. His parents were prominent African National Congress members and movement organizers, for which his father spent years in jail. At Sussex University in the 1960s, Mbeki's politics were firmly on the left. He led anti-apartheid demonstrations, received military training in the Soviet Union, and was friends with Olof Palme, the future socialist prime minister of Sweden. But Mbeki's demeanor was conservative, even stiff. While his classmates smoked grass and wore miniskirts and jeans, Mbeki donned tweed caps and smoked a pipe, sporting what William Gumede, his biographer, calls "the Tory look." "He was very conscious that he was representing South Africa," a classmate explained to Gumede, "as if to say, look how good we are; look how civilized we are. How can people like us be discriminated against back home?"[14]

During the 1970s and '80s, Mbeki rose through the ranks of the then exiled African National Congress in Zambia, Botswana, and Swaziland. But as the apartheid regime began to crumble, this former revolutionary morphed into a global capitalist. He encouraged foreign investment, struggled to control government spending, and was very much at home debating international trade policy in Westminster, Washington, and Davos, where he was famously enamored of quoting Shakespeare and Yeats.

But underneath this cosmopolitan exterior, Mbeki remained deeply preoccupied with questions of African identity. During the 1990s, he helped establish the African Renaissance, an intellectual movement to bring cultural, spiritual, economic, and political renewal to the African continent in the wake of the Cold War and apartheid. In some respects, the African Renaissance was a revival of the idea of Negritude, the mid-twentieth-century philosophy associated with Leopold Senghor, Jean-Paul Sartre, and others that contrasted the organic strengths of African culture with the cold, analytical vulgarity of the West.

Observers often find the African Renaissance perplexing. How can anyone talk about an African Renaissance in the shadow of the Rwanda genocide and the wars that have broken out across nearly all of central Africa, from Sierra Leone to Angola, to the Democratic Republic of Congo, to Ethiopia—conflicts that seem to be pulling the rest of the continent down with them?

One of Mbeki's most famous speeches, given at the adoption of South Africa's new constitution in May 1996, movingly addressed this paradox:

> I am an African. I owe my being to the hills and the valleys, the mountains and the glades, the rivers, the deserts, the trees, the flowers, the seas and the ever-changing seasons that define the face of our native land. . . . I owe my being to the Khoi and the San whose desolate souls haunt the great expanses of the beautiful Cape—they who fell victim to the most merciless genocide our native land has ever seen. . . . I am formed of the migrants who left Europe to find a new home on our native land. Whatever their actions, they remain still part of me. . . . I am the grandchild of the warrior men and women that Hintsa and Sekhukhune led. . . . I have seen our country torn asunder as these, all of whom are my people, engaged one another in a titanic battle. . . . The pain of the violent conflict that the peoples of Liberia, Somalia, the Sudan, Burundi and Algeria experience is a pain I also bear. The dismal shame of poverty, suffering and human degradation of my continent is a blight that we share. . . . This thing that we have done today says that Africa reaffirms that she is continuing her rise from the ashes. Whatever the setbacks of the moment, nothing can stop us now! . . . However much we have been caught by the fashion of cynicism and loss of faith in the capacity of the people, let us say today: Nothing can stop us now!

Like the Negritude Poets looking toward independence, Mbeki hoped the end of the apartheid dark age would release a new spirit of confidence and creativity. Africa's legacy of suffering would generate the springs of this creativity and would also provide a great moral lesson for the world.

On a visit to Cape Town, I arranged to meet Dr. William Makgoba, then head of the South African Medical Research Council and editor of *African Renaissance*,[15] a volume of essays with a prologue by President Mbeki. Dr. Makgoba was an outspoken critic of Mbeki's policies on HIV and he considered the AIDS dissidents pseudoscientists. However, Makgoba was also personally acquainted with Mbeki; perhaps he would have some insight into the ideas and motivation of this complex man.

Makgoba also knew something about the scientific elements of the African Renaissance movement, which emphasizes the exploration of indigenous knowledge systems, such as traditional medicine. I wanted to ask him if he knew whether any South African scientists were looking for a cure for AIDS in the herbal pharmacopeia of Africa's indigenous medicine men and women. I was very eager to speak to Dr. Makgoba about this because, if such research was going on, it would not be the first time the government had become involved in unconventional AIDS research.

In 1996, the then health minister, Nkosazana Zuma, was approached by Olga Visser, a Pretoria-based medical technician who claimed to have discovered a treatment for AIDS. Visser said she had administered a substance known as dimethylformamide, or DMF, to a small number of South African AIDS patients, with, she claimed, great results. Minister Zuma quickly authorized further human trials of the treatment, which Visser called Virodene. When allegedly promising results were obtained from these further trials, Mbeki, then deputy president under Nelson Mandela, arranged for Visser and her colleagues to present their findings at a cabinet meeting, where the scientists reportedly received wild applause.[16]

The South African Medicines Control Council (MCC), which oversees clinical trials of all pharmaceuticals in the country, soon found out about Visser's trial and immediately put a stop to it, citing the lack of any evidence that DMF was anything other than a toxic chemical, useful for various industrial purposes including dry cleaning, but not as medicine. DMF was known to cause liver damage and skin rashes, and the trials were deemed unscientific and useless. The researchers went ahead anyway, apparently with Mbeki's blessing. When the MCC tried again to stop them in early 1998, its chairman and two other officials were sacked.[17]

Dubious AIDS cures abound, but few attract interest in such high places. Olga Visser continued to conduct trials of Virodene (now banned in South Africa) in Tanzania until 2001, when the government of Tanzania put a stop to them. In 2007, South African investigative journalist Fiona Forde reported that funding for the Tanzania Virodene trials passed though the President's office in Pretoria.[18] And Virodene wasn't the only AIDS cure the government was interested in. In 2003, South African government researchers were also discovered in Tanzania treating HIV-positive people with "oxihumate-K," another novel AIDS cure, derived from garden fertilizer.[19] Both the Virodene and oxihumate-K trials originated within the University of Pretoria, with which Kalafong Hospital was affiliated, and Dr. Steenkamp was involved in the oxihumate-K trial while she was also working on the Triangle trial.[20] There is no evidence that oxihumate-K is harmful, but questions inevitably arose in my mind, especially since no one was talking.

The African Renaissance was beginning to look more and more like the European one. The European Renaissance saw great advances in anatomy, physics, and navigation, but also the flourishing of astrology, alchemy, fortune-telling, and other forms of quackery. Just as in South Africa, much of this came at a time when a great plague was raising profound scientific and philosophical questions.

Dr. Makgoba arrived an hour late for our meeting and had to leave almost immediately to catch a plane. As I waited in his office, his secretary told me that she had reminded him of our meeting that very morning, and he had said he would be able to make it. But then he had gone to see his dietitian, and as far as she knew, he had been detained there. This seemed odd. Why suddenly consult a dietitian? And then be detained there? I began to feel as though I had landed in a fairy tale where everybody is evasive and ignores appointments.

When Dr. Makgoba finally appeared, he didn't want to talk about the president, the AIDS dissidents, the African Renaissance, the European Renaissance, or Virodene. He did tell me that research on traditional African medicine for AIDS was under way in South Africa, but when I asked for details, he said he didn't want to talk about that either. After fifteen minutes he asked me to leave.

BACK IN JOHANNESBURG, I finally found someone who would talk to me about the Kalafong trial. Professor Geoffrey Falkson was a retired oncologist who also ran the ethics committee at the University of Pretoria, which approved Dr. Steenkamp's application to conduct the clinical trial on behalf of the Triangle pharmaceutical company. As we sat in Falkson's small, sunny office in the academic hospital, he said, in answer to my questions, that five patients out of forty-two had died on the trial at Kalafong.

"Isn't that rather a lot?" I asked.

"They had full-blown AIDS!" he said.

"No, they didn't."

He took the protocol book off his shelf and turned to the page where the inclusion criteria for the trial were listed. Clearly, patients with advanced AIDS were not allowed on the trial.

Professor Falkson seemed confused about many of the details of the trial, and he didn't seem to appreciate the gravity of what he was telling me had happened: that five apparently healthy HIV-positive people suddenly died after receiving medications that were supposed to extend their lives. He talked about the difficulty of conducting trials in South Africa, the high ethical standards that prevail there, the selflessness of investigators like Dr. Steenkamp. He also wrote down a Web address for me, where, it turned out, some of his oil paintings could be viewed.

Finally I asked Dr. Falkson to tell me who was ultimately responsible for examining and caring for people like Andrew and Molly, who might have been harmed in a clinical trial, and for all the people who died.

"Clindepharm are the ones to talk to about that," he said. Clindepharm, a private company based in Pretoria, served as an intermediary between pharmaceutical companies wishing to conduct clinical trials using South African patients, and South African doctors and scientists wishing to carry out the work itself. Clindepharm packaged the drugs, distributed them to the doctors, and managed the data that came in from the laboratories and doctors' offices. The medical director of Clindepharm refused to speak to me, but he did tell me that all adverse events on clinical trials are reported immediately to the MCC, at which point they cease to be Clindepharm's responsibility.

During my last week in Johannesburg, I tried without success to reach Dr. Helen Rees, the new head of the MCC. By now, of course, I was not surprised when Dr. Rees did not return my calls. However, just as I was leaving South Africa, I spotted Dr. Rees in the departure lounge of the airport in Johannesburg.

"You have your facts wrong," she said, when I told her I had heard that five people died in the Kalafong trial.

"Well, how many people did die at Kalafong, then?" She did not remember. I asked Dr. Rees who was responsible for following up adverse events on clinical trials, and examining patients like Molly and Andrew who might have been harmed by experimental drugs.

"We refer the matter to the local ethics committee. We take these things very seriously," she said.

I said I thought that sounded strange, because Professor Falkson, the head of the ethics committee at the University of Pretoria, had told me that Clindepharm was responsible for following up adverse events; Clindepharm had, in turn, referred me to her, and now she was referring me back to Professor Falkson. The responsibility seemed to have gone full circle.

Dr. Rees told me that new legislation governing the ethics of clinical trials was now in draft form, and had been under negotiation for more than two years. It would be presented to Parliament soon, she said. I wondered whether the legislation had not come too late for the patients at Kalafong. Clearly it would be important to have such legislation in place before clinical trials of drugs that the government itself alleges can be toxic should be allowed to proceed. If Mbeki and his health minister were really so concerned about the toxicity of AIDS drugs, why wasn't the government doing more to regulate clinical trials of those drugs?

WHEN I RETURNED to New York, I called the Triangle pharmaceutical company and asked an executive there how many patients had died at the Kalafong site. I was surprised to learn that, contrary to Viljoen's account, only one patient in the trial had died at Kalafong. I called Dr. Steenkamp in South Africa, and she told me that none of the patients Viljoen claimed had died were, in fact, in the trial. She would say nothing about the patients who were sick but still alive because, she said, that would violate their privacy. When I told Dr. Steenkamp that all of these patients seemed to think they were in a trial, according to signed testimonies given to me by Viljoen, and all of them claimed to have come regularly to receive drugs from her, Dr. Steenkamp told me she had certainly been treating some of those patients, but she would not say whether they had been in a trial. What was going on?

Maybe it was hysteria. Maybe some of the patients were screened for the trial, but because they were already sick with AIDS, they were not eligible. Dr. Steenkamp may have given them some medication, but the patients may have misunderstood and thought they were actually in the trial. Perhaps these people became much sicker after their appointment with Dr. Steenkamp, simply because the disease was taking its course. When they died, their families blamed the doctor because they, like their president, could not accept the reality of AIDS, and they were looking for a culprit. Maybe whispers began circulating in the townships about a doctor at Kalafong. Maybe rumors were fueled by reports of the controversy in the president's office over whether AZT and other antiretroviral drugs were part of a Western plot to exploit and kill Africans. This would not have been an unreasonable fear. The apartheid government did support research into race-specific germ warfare agents right up until the early 1990s.[20] In the eyes of the surviving patients and the families of the dead, Dr. Steenkamp may have seemed like part of the broader conspiracy the president was warning everyone about.

But details of the story still perplexed me. Why would six patients and the families of five others think they were all in a clinical trial if they had not been? Why did Professor Falkson, who was admittedly weak on details, tell me that five patients had died in the Kalafong trial if in fact there was only one death there? Why did one of the patients who received drugs from Dr. Steenkamp write in her testimony, "[Steenkamp] told me not to talk to anybody else about [the trial] because it was our secret"?

Why did the patients who became ill report such strange symptoms? When Andrew described his symptoms to me, they sounded a lot like Stevens-Johnson syndrome, a potentially fatal, but rare, side effect of one of the antiretroviral drugs used in the Triangle trial. But a Triangle representative told me that no cases of Stevens-Johnson syndrome at the Kalafong site had been reported to him. If any cases had occurred there, he assured me, he would have known. So if Andrew's symptoms were not drug-associated Stevens-Johnson syndrome, what were they?

Molly testified that she was put in a "drug trial," but she had tuberculosis, which would have excluded her from the Triangle trial. Why, after Molly got sick, was she prevented from looking at her own medical file by the authorities at Kalafong? A friend of Viljoen's had sneaked into the hospital disguised as a nun and stolen the file, but when it was opened, Viljoen told me, the most recent three months of notes were missing. And why did Molly say she went temporarily blind? Temporary blindness is not a known side effect of any antiretroviral drug. Blindness does occur in AIDS patients, but it does not get better.

Clinical trials are often surrounded by secrecy. South African politics and evasion obscure matters even further. In early June, I was leafing through old copies of *The Lancet* and came across an editorial criticizing Mbeki's anti-AZT policy.[22] "Is there some other agenda," the author speculated, "such as the promotion of locally developed drugs?" Perhaps South Africa's paranoia was still getting to me, but I thought of Virodene, and of the persistent rumors that whites were still trying to kill blacks, now with AZT. I thought of the African Renaissance and the quest for African solutions to African problems. I also thought of Dr. Makgoba's reluctance to tell me about South African research into traditional African medicine for AIDS. I began to wonder whether some accident might not have occurred at Kalafong. This seemed unlikely, but what did happen remained mysterious.

PRESIDENT MBEKI arrived in the United States in late May, on the same day I did. During his visit, he was interviewed on *The NewsHour with Jim Lehrer*, and he was asked about his controversial AIDS policies. His replies were evasive. He claimed that he had never said that HIV was not the cause of AIDS, but he did not deny that he had questioned the link between the virus and the disease. When he was asked why he refused to make antiretrovirals available in public maternity wards, he answered that the state could not afford to make the drugs available for life to all HIV-positive people in South Africa. But he had not been asked why he didn't provide all HIV-positive South Africans with antiretroviral therapy for life. He had been asked why he didn't provide the drugs to HIV-positive women for a few weeks around the time of childbirth. That would cost about fifty million dollars a year, which the Ministry of Health could well afford.

The interviewer, seemingly beguiled by Mbeki's suave charm, did not try to pin him down, but as I watched him dodging every question, I felt that he wasn't being straight with his American audience, or with his own people. Here was a man who was allying himself with the AIDS dissidents and accusing the medical establishment of exploiting Africans in order to profit from the sale of toxic drugs, while he was himself aware of further trials of Virodene, a substance that really was toxic.[23]

In 2002, the South African government began to shift its AIDS policy. That year, the Cape Town–based Treatment Action Campaign successfully sued the government in South Africa's Constitutional Court over its refusal to offer antiretroviral drugs in public maternity clinics. Technocrats in the Ministry of Health soon developed plans to abide by the court order. By then, competition from generic-drug manufacturers in Asia and moral pressure from activists the world over had forced pharmaceutical companies to steeply lower antiretroviral drug prices. Offering these drugs to all AIDS patients through the public health system was now affordable and morally necessary, and shortly before the 2004 elections, the Ministry of Health launched a program to make antiretroviral drugs available to all South Africans with AIDS.

After the policy shift, Mbeki seldom spoke publicly about AIDS, but observers speculated that his personal views about the epidemic remained unchanged. Perhaps he had merely bowed to pressure from the activists and an astonished international community, including investors who may have wondered whether investing in such a country was prudent.[24] Even after antiretroviral drug programs were under way across the nation, the health minister, Dr. Manto Tshabalala-Msimang, continued to recommend unorthodox AIDS treatments, including olive oil, beets, and a vitamin mixture marketed by a California AIDS dissident named Matthias Rath.[25]

Mbeki's silence, his minister's confusing recommendations, and the mounting death toll from AIDS would fuel a vicious cycle of fear, rumor, and denial in the country for years to come. Why had this otherwise sensible president, who had done so much to fight for the dignity and rights of his people, been so wrong on AIDS? Who was this African chauvinist in tweeds, this dreamy intellectual with the steely, globalist economic outlook and the strange ideas about medicine? I knew I would never figure it out, but at the turn of the century, he seemed to embody all the tortured pride and shame of his conflicted continent.

CHAPTER SEVEN

AIDS, Inc.

IN RESPONSE to government prevarication over HIV treatment, a vigorous AIDS activist movement emerged in South Africa and a fierce public relations battle ensued. The Treatment Action Campaign, or TAC, along with other activist groups, accused the South African health minister, Manto Tshabalala-Msimang, of "murder" for denying millions of South Africans access to medicine for AIDS. A spokesman from the ANC Youth League then called the activists "paid marketing agents for toxic AIDS drugs from America."[1] An official in the Department of Housing accused journalists who defended the AIDS activists of fanaticism, and quoted Lenin on how the "press in bourgeois society . . . deceive[s], corrupt[s] and fool[s] the exploited and oppressed mass of the people, the poor."

Meanwhile, across the nation thousands of people were becoming infected daily, from the rural homesteads of the former Bantustans to the peri-urban townships and squatter camps to the formerly all-white suburbs, now home to a growing black middle class. By 2005, the death rate for young adults had tripled.[2] Surveys showed that nearly everyone in South Africa knew that HIV was sexually transmitted and that it could be prevented with condoms, abstinence, and faithfulness to an uninfected partner. Children were receiving AIDS education in school and condoms were widely available, but these programs made little difference. In the din of the battle between the activists and the government, the deeper message, that HIV was everyone's problem, was lost.

In 1999, a group of public health experts sponsored by the U.S.-based Kaiser Family Foundation stepped into this fray. They were concerned about the worsening AIDS crisis in South Africa and wanted to launch a bold new HIV prevention program for young people. They also knew they had to take account of the South African government's attitudes toward AIDS and AIDS activists. Their program, called loveLife, would soon become South Africa's largest and most ambitious HIV prevention campaign. It aimed both to overcome the limitations of similar campaigns that had failed in the past and, at the same time, to avoid dealing with the issues of AIDS treatment and care that had become so controversial.

Could this work? I wondered. Was it possible to reduce the spread of HIV without involving HIV-positive people and the activists and community groups that supported them? LoveLife had been endorsed at one time or another by the archbishop of Cape Town; Nelson Mandela; the king of the Zulu tribe; Jacob Zuma, South Africa's former deputy president; and even Zanele Mbeki, the wife of the president. In 2003, loveLife's annual $20 million budget was paid for by the South African government, the Kaiser Family Foundation, UNICEF, the Bill and Melinda Gates Foundation, and the Global Fund to Fight AIDS, Tuberculosis and Malaria. At least South Africa's leaders were beginning to take AIDS seriously, I thought, but what kind of program was this?

WHAT WE WANT to do is create a substantive, normative shift in the way young people behave," explained loveLife's director, David Harrison, a white South African doctor, when I met him in his Johannesburg office. The average age at which young South Africans lose their virginity—around seventeen—is not much different from the age at which teenagers in other countries do. What's different, Harrison said, was that many of the young South Africans who were sexually active were very sexually active. They were more likely to start having sex at very young ages, even below the age of fourteen—well below the national average. Those vulnerable young people were more likely to have more than one sexual partner, and they were less likely to use condoms. South African girls were more likely to face sexual coercion or rape, or to exchange sex for money or gifts, all of which placed them at greater risk of HIV infection. For Harrison, the trick was to "get inside the head-space of these young people . . . we have to understand what is driving them into sex—they know what HIV is, but they don't internalize it," he said.

LoveLife's aim was to get young people talking, to each other and to their parents, so they would really understand and act on what they knew. But to reach out to them, you had to use a special language that young people could relate to. According to Harrison, traditional HIV prevention campaigns were too depressing: they tried to scare people into changing their behavior, and this turned kids off. LoveLife's media campaign, on the other hand, was positive and cheerful, and resembled the bright, persuasive modern ad campaigns that many South African kids were very much attracted to.

In the past couple of years, nearly a thousand loveLife billboards had sprouted all along the nation's main roads. They were striking. For example, on one of them, the hands of four women of different races caressed the sculpted back and buttocks of a young black man as though they were appraising an antique newel post. The caption read, "Everyone he's slept with, is sleeping with you." On another, a gorgeous mixed-race couple—the boy looked like Brad Pitt, the girl like an Indian film star—lay in bed, under the caption "No Pressure." Some people told me they found these ads oversexualized and disturbing, but it is hard to see why. On the same roads, there are torsos advertising sexy underwear and half-naked actresses advertising romantic movies. Sex is a potent theme in marketing all sorts of products; loveLife, according to its creators, tries to turn that message around to get young people thinking and talking about sex in more responsible ways and convince them of the virtues of abstinence, fidelity, and the use of condoms.

Harrison calls loveLife "a brand of positive lifestyle." The sexy billboards and similar ads on TV and radio, as well as newspaper inserts that resemble teen gossip magazines, with articles and advice columns about clothes, relationships, and sexual health, were designed, Harrison says, to persuade young people to avoid sex in the same way a sneaker ad tries to seduce them into buying new sneakers, because the players in the ads look so cool. The idea is "to create a brand so strong that young people who want to be hip and cool and the rest of it want to associate with it," Harrison told an interviewer in 2001.[3]

The concept of a "lifestyle brand" originated with the rise of brand advertising in the 1960s, when ads for such products as Pepsi-Cola and Harley-Davidson began to promote not only soft drinks and motorcycles, but also a certain style or aesthetic. People were urged to "join the Pepsi generation" or ride a Harley-Davidson not just to get around, but to embrace a certain attitude. A Harley wasn't just a bike; it was a macho rebellion, an escape from the workaday world to the open road. In the 1970s, family-planning programs also tried to promote contraceptives in developing countries by tapping into poor people's aspirations for a glamorous Western lifestyle. Campaigns depicted small, well-dressed families surrounded by sleek new commodities, including televisions and cars. Harrison predicted that young South Africans would readily respond to this approach too.

"Kids have changed," Harrison explained. Today's young South Africans weren't like the activists who risked their lives in the anti-apartheid demonstrations at Sharpeville and Soweto. "Seventy-five percent of South African teenagers watch TV every day," Harrison informed me. "Their favorite program is *The Bold and the Beautiful*"—an American soap opera in which glamorous characters struggle with personal crises while wearing and driving some very expensive gear. "They are exposed to the global youth culture of music, fashion, pop icons, and commercial brands. They talk about brands among themselves, even if they can't afford everything they see."

The Kaiser Foundation's Michael Sinclair told me that loveLife drew much of its inspiration from the marketing campaign for the soft drink Sprite.[4] In the mid-1990s, sales of Sprite were flagging until the company began an aggressive campaign to embed Sprite in youth culture by sponsoring hip-hop concerts and planting attractive, popular kids in Internet chat rooms or college dormitories and paying them to praise or distribute Sprite in an unobtrusive way. Sprite is now one of the most profitable drinks in the world because it managed to exploit what marketing experts call "the cool effect"—meaning the influence that a small number of opinion leaders can have on the norms and behavior of large numbers of their peers. So far, corporate marketers had made the greatest use of the cool effect, but there was speculation that small numbers of trendsetters could change more complex behavior than shopping, such as criminality, suicide, and sexual behavior.[5]

For this reason, loveLife had established a small network of recreation centers for young people, known as Y-Centers, throughout the country. At Y-Centers, young people could learn to play basketball, volleyball, and other sports, as well as learn break-dancing, radio broadcasting, and word processing. All Y-Center activities were led by "loveLife Ground-Breakers"—older youths, usually in their early twenties, who, like the kids who made Sprite cool, were stylish and cheerful and enthusiastic about their product, in this case, loveLife and its program to encourage safer sexual behavior. If abstinence, monogamy, and condoms all happened to fail, each Y-Center was affiliated with a family-planning clinic that offered contraceptives and treatment for sexually transmitted diseases such as syphilis and gonorrhea. The centers offered no treatment for AIDS symptoms, however, and when I visited, none of them offered HIV testing either.

Any young person could become a Y-Center member, but in order to fully participate in its activities, he or she had to complete a program of seminars about HIV, family planning, and other subjects related to sexuality and growing up. The seminars emphasized the biological aspects of HIV and its prevention, but not the experience of the disease and its effects on people's lives. Members also received training to raise their self-esteem, because, as Harrison told an interviewer in 2001,

> there is a direct correlation between young people's sexual behavior and their sense of confidence in the future. Those young people who feel motivated, who feel that they have something to look forward to—they are the ones who protect themselves, who ensure that they do not get HIV/AIDS. . . . It's all about the social discount rates that young people apply to future benefits.[6]

Dr. Harrison arranged for me to visit a loveLife Y-Center in the archipelago of townships in the flat scrubland south of Johannesburg known as the Vaal Triangle. Millions of people live in these townships, many of them recent migrants from rural South Africa or from neighboring countries. The Vaal, once a patchwork of white-owned farms, is now a residential area for poor blacks. At first, only a few families moved here, because the apartheid government used the notorious pass laws to restrict the tide of impoverished blacks seeking a better life in Johannesburg. But when the apartheid laws were scrapped, people poured in. Today, the roads and other services in the area are insufficient for its huge and growing population, and many people have no electricity and lack easy access to clean water and sanitation. Unemployment exceeds 70 percent and the crime rate is one of the highest in South Africa.[7]

The loveLife Y-Center was a compound of two small lavender buildings surrounded by an iron fence and curling razor wire. Inside the compound, a group of young men in shorts and T-shirts were doing warm-up exercises on the outdoor basketball court, while girls and barefoot children looked on. Inside the main building, another group of boys in fashionably droopy jeans and dreadlocks practiced a hip-hop routine, and two girls in the computer room experimented with Microsoft Word.

Valentine's Day was coming up, and the Y-Center had organized a group discussion for some of its members. About thirty teenagers, most of them in school uniforms, sat around on the floor of a large seminar room and argued about who should pay for what on a Valentine's Day date. A GroundBreaker in a loveLife T-shirt and with a loveLife kerchief tied pirate-style on her head officiated. "I go with my chick and I spend money on her and always we have sex," said a husky boy in a gray school uniform. "And I want to know, what's the difference between my chick and a prostitute?" As we have seen, long-term transactional relationships—in which money or gifts are frequently exchanged—may not be the same as prostitution, but they nevertheless put many township youths at risk of HIV.[8]

"Boys, they are expecting too much from us. They say we are parasites if we don't sleep with them," said a plump girl in the uniform of a local Catholic school.

"The girls, they ask for a lot of things," another boy chimed in.

"Me, I think it is wrong. If most of the boys think Valentine's Day is about buying sex, the boys must stop," a girl said. "We girls must hold our ground."

These young people were certainly talking openly about sexual relationships all right, just as Harrison prescribed. Nevertheless, I felt something was missing. "Do you ever talk about AIDS in those discussion groups?" I asked the GroundBreaker afterward. "We do it indirectly," she replied. "We know that if we just came out and started lecturing them about AIDS, they wouldn't listen. They would just turn off. So we talk about positive things, like making informed choices, sharing responsibility, and positive sexuality."

Was this true? Do young people in South Africa, like their politicians, really want to avoid the subject of AIDS? I wanted to meet young people outside the Y-Center and ask them what they thought about that. A few hundred yards away from the Y-Center stood the headquarters of St. Charles Lwanga, a Catholic organization that carries out a number of activities in the township. Their AIDS program, called Inkanyezi, meaning "star" in Zulu, provides counseling to young people about AIDS and also brings food and other necessities to some four hundred orphans and people living with AIDS in the Vaal.

St. Charles Lwanga was independent of loveLife, and its budget was modest, less than a tenth of what loveLife spent on its billboards alone. The Inkanyezi program was staffed almost entirely by volunteers, whose only compensation was that they were allowed to eat some of the food—usually rice and vegetables—that they prepared for the patients. Lack of funding greatly limited the help that Inkanyezi was able to provide. Although Inkanyezi nurses were able to dispense tuberculosis medicine, antiretroviral drugs were as yet unavailable. Indeed, many of the patients they visited lacked some of the most basic necessities for life and human dignity. Sometimes destitute patients had their water and electricity cut off. But the worst thing was that many of the patients were socially isolated and lived alone in flimsy shacks. The doors were easily broken down and at night neighborhood thugs sometimes came in and stole what little they had. Sometimes the patients were raped.

Justice Showalala, who ran Inkanyezi, organized a meeting for me with a group of about twenty-five young people from Orange Farm. The HIV rate in the area was not known, but several people explained to me how their lives had been changed by the virus. They said they had witnessed extreme prejudice and discrimination against people with AIDS, and they did not know where to turn when they learned that a relative or friend was HIV positive. "People say you shouldn't touch someone with HIV," said one girl. "I have a friend at school who disclosed she has HIV, and the others won't even walk with her." Justice explained how he had offered to introduce some teachers from a local school to some of his HIV-positive clients. "They said, 'If you want me to meet people with AIDS, you better give me a rubber suit.'"

The loveLife Y-Center did little to help young people deal with such confusion, stigma, and shame. "I learned basketball at the Y-Center," one girl told me, "and at meetings we talked about resisting peer pressure, [like when] your friends advise you to break your virginity, to prove you are girl enough. But I was afraid the people there would find out my sister had HIV. We talked about it as though it was someone else's problem."

In general, although sex was openly discussed at the Y-Center, the experience of AIDS was not. The Y-Center offered individual counseling for a small number of young people with HIV, but those who were hungry, homeless, or destitute, or were suffering from the symptoms of AIDS, were told to consult other organizations, including Inkanyezi.

It turns out that talking about the pain, both physical and emotional, that the disease creates is far more difficult than getting over the embarrassment of talking about sex. "I had heard about HIV before," said an Inkanyezi girl, wearing a bright blue T-shirt and matching headband. "But then I found out my mother was HIV positive. I was so shocked, so shocked. I even talked to my teacher about it. She said it can happen to anyone; it must have been from mistakes my mother made, and that I shouldn't make those mistakes in my own life."

"Sometimes, women have no choice," said the older woman sitting next to the girl in blue. She was thin, with intense dark eyes and a deep, wry smile. She was dressed entirely in black, except for a baseball cap with a red ribbon on it—the universal symbol of solidarity with HIV-positive people. "They get infected because of their husbands, and there's nothing they can do.

"It happened like this," the older woman went on. "It was back when we were living in Soweto, before we moved here. One day my daughter and I were washing clothes together," she said, nodding at the girl in blue. "She said she'd had a dream that I was so sick, that I had cancer and I was going to die. I waited until we were done with the washing, and then I told her that I was HIV positive. She said, 'I knew it, you were always sick and always going to support groups.' She was so down, she just cried all day and all night after that. I told her, 'Only God knows why people have this disease. Don't worry, I won't die right away.'

"Once I visited the loveLife Y-Center," the woman continued, "but I just saw children playing. I sat and talked with them, and they were shocked when I said I was HIV positive. I told them about what it was like, and one of them said she would ask the managers whether I could come and talk to a bigger group. But that was about six months ago and they haven't called me. I haven't moved and my number hasn't changed. I don't know why they haven't called."

"I think there should be more counseling and support groups for people who find out their parents are HIV positive," the girl in blue said. "It puts you down, it really gets to you, it haunts you. When you are standing in class and you have to recite a poem or something, I find I can't get anything out of my mouth. I can't concentrate. [The problem] here is ignorance. I didn't care about HIV until I found out about my mother. Then I started to care about these people. I wish many people in our country would also think like that."

IN 2003, the only African country that had seen a nationwide decline in HIV prevalence was Uganda. Since 1992 the HIV rate had fallen by some two-thirds, a success that saved perhaps a million lives. The programs and policies that led to this success will be discussed in later chapters, but the epidemiologists Rand Stoneburner and Daniel Low-Beer have argued that a powerful role was played by the ordinary, but frank, conversations people had with family, friends, and neighbors—not about sex, but about the frightening, calamitous effects of AIDS itself.[9] Stoneburner and Low-Beer maintain that these painful personal conversations did more than anything else to persuade Ugandans to come to terms with the reality of AIDS, care for the afflicted, and change their behavior. This in turn led to declines in HIV transmission. The researchers found that people in other sub-Saharan African countries were far less likely to have such discussions.

In South Africa, people told Stoneburner and Low-Beer that they had heard about the epidemic from posters, radio, newspapers, and clinics, as well as from occasional mass rallies, schools, and village meetings; but they seldom spoke about it with the people they knew. They were also far less likely to admit knowing someone with AIDS or to be willing to care for an AIDS patient. It may be no coincidence that the HIV rate in South Africa rose higher than it ever did in Uganda, and has taken far longer to fall.

When I was in Uganda during the early 1990s, the HIV rate was already falling, and I vividly recall how the reality of AIDS was alive in people's minds. Kampala taxi drivers talked as passionately about AIDS as taxi drivers elsewhere discuss politics or football. And they talked about it in a way that would seem foreign to many in South Africa because it was so personal: "my sister," "my father," "my neighbor," "my friend."[10]

Ugandans are not unusually compassionate people, and discrimination against people with AIDS persists in some families and institutions. But Ugandans do seem more willing to openly address painful issues in their lives. This courage owes much to the AIDS information campaigns launched by the government of Uganda early on in the epidemic. But it may have other sources as well. Maybe the difference between the ways South Africa and Uganda have dealt with AIDS has historical roots. Both South Africa and Uganda have bitter histories of conflict. But while Uganda was terrorized for decades by a series of brutal leaders, they could not destroy the traditional rhythms of rural family life. Uganda is one of the most fertile countries in Africa; there is enough land for everyone, and most people live as their ancestors did, as peasant farmers and herders. No large settler population displaced huge numbers of people or set up a system to exploit and humiliate them, as happened in South Africa and in many other African countries. This means Ugandans are more likely to know their neighbors and to live near members of their extended families. This in turn may have contributed to what sociologists call "social cohesion"—the tendency of people to talk openly with one another and form trusted relationships. Perhaps this may have facilitated more realistic and open discussion of AIDS, more compassionate attitudes toward infected people, and pragmatic behavior change.

Perhaps many attempts to prevent the spread of HIV fail because those in charge of them don't recognize that the decisions people make about sex are usually a matter of feeling, not calculation. In other words, sexual behavior is determined less by what Dr. Harrison called "discount rates" that young people "apply to future benefits" than by emotional attachments. I thought of the South African girls who said they had lost a sister or a friend to AIDS. If one of them was faced with a persistent, wealthy seducer, what would be more likely to persuade her to decline? The memory of a loveLife billboard, with its flashy, beautiful models? Or the memory of a person she had known who had died?

ON THE MORNING before I left South Africa, I attended a loveLife motivational seminar at a school not far from Orange Farm. "These seminars help young people see the future, identify choices, and identify the values that underpin those choices," Harrison had told me. "We help them ask themselves, 'What can you do to chart life's journey and control it as much as possible?'" The seminars were based on Success by Choice, a series devised by Marlon Smith, a California-based African-American motivational speaker. How was Mr. Smith's message of personal empowerment translated to South Africa, I wondered, where children have to contend with poverty, the risk of being robbed or raped, and a grim future of likely unemployment?

About twenty-five children aged ten to fourteen were in the class, and the GroundBreaker asked them to hold their hands out in front of them, pretend they were looking in a mirror, and repeat the following words:

"You are intelligent!"

"You are gifted!"

"There is no one in the world like you!"

"I love you!"

The children spoke quietly at first, then louder, as though they were being hypnotized. The GroundBreaker urged them to talk more openly with their parents, to keep themselves clean, and to make positive choices in their lives, especially when it came to sexuality. There was little mention of helping other people, nor was there much advice about how to avoid being raped or harassed by other students as well as teachers, relatives, or strangers, or how to plan a future in a country where unemployment for township blacks was so high.

Then something really odd occurred. One of the GroundBreakers asked the children to stand up because it was time for an "Icebreaker." "This is a little song-and-dance thing we do, to give the children a chance to stretch. It improves their concentration," another GroundBreaker told me. The words of the song were as follows:

Pizza Hut
Pizza Hut
Kentucky Fried Chicken and a Pizza Hut
McDonald's
McDonald's
Kentucky Fried Chicken and a Pizza Hut.

In the dance, the children spread their arms out as though they were rolling out a pizza, or flapped their elbows like chickens.

What kinds of choices was Dr. Harrison really referring to? I wondered. The techniques of marketing attempt to impose scientific principles on human choices. But it seemed a mad experiment to see whether teenagers living through very difficult times could be persuaded to choose a new sexual lifestyle as they might choose a new brand of shampoo, or whether children could be trained to associate safe sex with pizza and self-esteem.

Afterward, I spoke to some of the children who had participated in the seminar. They all knew how to protect themselves from HIV, and they were eager to show off their knowledge about condoms, abstinence, and fidelity within relationships. But they all said they didn't personally know anyone with AIDS; nor did they know of any children who had lost parents to AIDS. They did mention Nkosi Johnson, the brave HIV-positive twelve-year-old boy who became world-famous in 2000 when he stood up at an International Conference on AIDS and challenged the

South African president, Thabo Mbeki, to do more for people living with the virus.

In fact, their principal would tell me later, more than twenty children at the school were AIDS orphans, and many more had been forced to drop out because there was no one to pay their expenses after their parents died. The children I spoke to seemed not to know why some of their classmates wore ragged uniforms or had no shoes or stopped showing up at all.

The week before, I had met some teenage girls in Soweto and I had asked them the same question. They answered in the same way: the only person they knew with AIDS was Nkosi Johnson, the famous boy at the AIDS conference. Just as Harrison had warned me, these girls said they were tired of hearing about AIDS. The girls were orphans, although they said their parents had not died of AIDS. I later discovered that, in another part of that same orphanage, there was a nursery where thirty babies and small children, all of them HIV positive, all abandoned by their parents, lay on cots or sat quietly on the floor, struggling for life. No wonder those girls were tired of hearing about HIV. It was right in their midst, within earshot, but the world around them was telling them to look the other way.

A COUPLE of years later, I would meet a group of primary-school students in Kigali, Rwanda. By then, the HIV infection rate in Rwanda had fallen steeply, just as it had in Uganda years earlier. The school was a typical single-story line of classrooms in one of the poorest sections of Kigali. I spoke to the principal first, and he showed me the government-issued manual used for teaching about AIDS, which contained the usual information about abstinence and condoms. The school day had just ended, and he went outside and asked a few students to stay behind and chat with me.[11]

The Rwandan students had no idea in advance what I wanted to talk to them about. But when I asked them the same question I had asked the South African children, "Do you know anyone with AIDS?" their answers floored me. Every one of them had a story about someone they knew who was HIV positive or suffering from AIDS. "I knew a man who had bad lips [sores] and tears all over his skin," said a fourteen-year-old boy. "People stigmatized him and he died because no one was caring for him." Another boy described a woman who was "so thin, she almost died." But then her relatives took her to the hospital, where she was given AIDS treatment. "She got better because people cared for her," he said.

When I asked the Rwandan children whether they had any questions for me, all they wanted to know was what they could do to help people with AIDS. The responses of the South African children were strikingly different. When I asked them if they had questions for me, they quickly changed the subject from AIDS and asked me what America was like and whether I knew any of the pop stars they admired on TV.

The persistent denial of AIDS in South Africa was deeply disturbing. People liked the colorful, frank advertising and the basketball games sponsored by loveLife. But its programs seemed to me to reinforce the denial that posed so many obstacles to preventing HIV in the first place. In 2005, the Global Fund to Fight AIDS, Tuberculosis and Malaria would come to similar conclusions and terminate its multimillion-dollar grant to loveLife.[12]

Epidemiologists are equivocal about whether loveLife had any effect on HIV transmission in South Africa, but during the program's first seven years, HIV infection rates continued to rise steadily.[13]

A more realistic HIV prevention program would have paid less attention to aspirations and dreams unattainable for so many young people, and greater attention to the real circumstances in people's lives that make it hard for them to avoid infection. It would also have been more frank about the real human consequences of the disease. But that would have meant dealing with some very painful matters that South Africa's policymakers seemed determined to evade.

It was heartening that Western donors were now spending so much money on AIDS programs in Africa. But the problem with some large foreign-aid programs was that distributing the funds often involved negotiating with governments with a poor record of dealing with AIDS. In addition, the huge sums of money involved were often very difficult to manage, so that small community-based groups that need thousands of dollars, rather than millions—like Inkanyezi in Orange Farm—were often overlooked in favor of overly ambitious megaprojects, whose effectiveness had not been demonstrated and whose premises were open to question. It seemed clear to me that more could be learned from Inkanyezi's attempt to help people deal with the reality of AIDS than from loveLife's attempt to create a new consumerist man and woman for South Africa.

CHAPTER EIGHT

Why Don't They Listen?

EVERYWHERE I WENT in southern Africa, AIDS-related shame and denial seemed to hang over the region like a spell. Many AIDS patients suffered and died in their houses, cared for with compassion but in silence, their condition shrouded in euphemisms. Occasionally, those known to be HIV positive would be thrown out of their houses, scorned by their relatives, or quietly fired from their jobs when their status became known or even suspected. On World AIDS Day in 1998, Gugu Dlamini, a South African AIDS counselor, announced to her community that she was HIV positive. A few days later, a group of teenage boys spotted her in a neighbor's yard and stoned her to death. In court, they said they had done it to punish her for bringing "shame on the community."

In KwaZulu-Natal, the province with South Africa's highest HIV infection rate, the hush surrounding the epidemic was so spooky that it surprised even me. KwaZulu-Natal is the homeland of South Africa's Zulu people, a fiercely independent tribe whose ancestors were famous for their skills at warfare and their defiant battles against white settlement in the nineteenth century. Today, most Zulus live in desolate rural homelands or impoverished urban townships. Staggering levels of unemployment and poverty have further hardened these tough people. In village bars, drunk and rowdy men listen to booming rap music, fight about women, and sometimes kill each other. Even small children greet each other with gangster hand signals. A study conducted in the area found that among adults in their twenties, around a third of all men and half of all women were HIV positive.[1] By the time I arrived, in December 2004, virtually everyone must have seen a case of AIDS. But no one talked about it.

An antiretroviral drug program, run by the Catholic church with funds from the U.S. PEPFAR (President's Emergency Plan for HIV/AIDS Relief) program, had been under way for more than a year at a local hospital. "Home-based care" teams set out each day to bring porridge, soap, and other necessities to the sick and try to encourage people to be tested for HIV and, if necessary, join the treatment program. I spent a week following these volunteers on their rounds, and as we went from one homestead to another and sat with dying patients and their families, no one, not once, said the word "AIDS." Patients told us they were suffering from "ulcers" or "tuberculosis" or "pneumonia."[2] Orphans said their parents had "gone away" or had been "bewitched" by a jealous neighbor.

One day, I was taken to the house of an old woman whose two daughters had recently died, almost certainly of AIDS. She was looking after eight orphaned grandchildren, aged eighteen months to eleven years. I asked her why there were so many orphans in the area. "Because," she said, "when a girl meets a boy, the boy doesn't have enough love."

"That's very sad," I said, "but why does that create orphans?"

"I cannot explain," she replied.

"They all know it's AIDS, but they won't say it," said Thulani Zuma, one of the home-care volunteers. "And their families won't say it either. It's very hard to deal with a problem you can't even name."

Some people chose to die rather than admit they had the disease. The Africa Centre for Health and Population Studies, a research institute in the region, had for years offered free antiretrovirals to all employees who needed them, but four workers had recently died because they refused to come forward for testing and treatment. The Africa Centre also launched a door-to-door HIV testing program in which nurses visited every household in the area and asked whoever was at home to undergo a quick, simple HIV test. The nurses described to me how people would flee when they saw the Africa Centre vehicle drive up. Only 7 percent of the population wished to know their results.[3]

Denial seemed to be the unofficial policy of the nation, even much of the continent. During the late 1990s, as Western governments faced mounting popular pressure at home to do something about the AIDS crisis in developing countries, they ran into a curious roadblock. Many African leaders simply did not seem interested in fighting the epidemic. They seldom, if ever, mentioned it in speeches and they left AIDS policy-making largely to foreign consultants. In 1999, when African leaders were invited to a UN-sponsored AIDS meeting in Zambia at which it was hoped they would make common cause against the epidemic, none of the leaders showed up, even for the opening and closing ceremonies. Instead, lesser bureaucrats delivered stultifying speeches in "abstract planning language, with promises to organize, decentralize, and base the work within the community," reported the Australian demographer John Caldwell in the journal *Population and Development Review*. But unlike government responses to other public health crises, "there was no desire among government representatives to discuss precisely what would work in the local setting and why. This was jarringly different from the down-to-earth language and examples offered at family-planning conferences and immunization workshops."[4]

That same year, the South African activist group Treatment Action Campaign launched a courageous movement to demand government action on AIDS. But their protests were mainly held in large cities, outside the offices of South African government officials and pharmaceutical-company executives. In townships and rural areas throughout the country, ordinary South Africans approved of the activists, but relatively few of the five million HIV-positive people, or their millions of relatives, saw it as a cause of their own.[5]

When antiretroviral drug programs were launched in southern Africa in 2004, some people theorized that the programs would naturally eliminate stigma and denial by making an AIDS diagnosis seem less frightening.[6] By reducing AIDS symptoms—the sores, rashes, and coughing—antiretroviral drugs do help reduce the fear of touching an HIV-positive person. But AIDS-related stigma also arises from the association of the disease with what is locally considered "immoral behavior," and antiretrovirals offer no protection against this.[7]

"They think that if you have AIDS, you must be some kind of prostitute and have sex recklessly," Thulani, the home-care worker, told me. "That's why they deny it."

Deborah Posel, a sociologist at the University of the Witwatersrand in Johannesburg, discovered this too when, in 2002, she set out to study attitudes to AIDS in South Africa's Limpopo province, not far from KwaZulu-Natal:[8]

"AIDS is a disease of shame," said one respondent in a focus group.

"AIDS is disgusting," said another.

"It means you were practicing prostitution, which means you have been sleeping around with many men," said a third.

"People are afraid that if they reveal that someone died of AIDS, it will be a shame on the whole community that she was a prostitute or he was fooling around with girls. It is not just sex. It is something that is morally unacceptable to the people."

Some of the people in Posel's focus groups—including those who held the deepest prejudices against people with AIDS—were almost certainly HIV positive themselves: AIDS is common in Africa not because African people have so many sexual partners, but because they are more likely than people in other world regions to have a small number of concurrent long-term partners. This places them, along with their partner or partners, within a vast network of ongoing sexual relationships that is highly conducive to the spread of HIV. Some of the people Posel interviewed would have been men supporting a wife and one or two mistresses; some would have been young women with only one boyfriend or husband who had another girlfriend as well. Perhaps a small number of these women had more than one boyfriend. Many people would have been in monogamous partnerships, but one member may have had an unfaithful partner in the past. Most likely, none of the women in this rural area were prostitutes and very few of the men would ever have had sex with a prostitute. Few of these people would have had more than five or ten sexual partners in a lifetime, hardly outrageous behavior in this day and age. But because they were linked up in a network of concurrent partnerships, they would all have been at high risk.

One source of confusion may have been the region's AIDS campaigns.[9] Until 2006, no public health campaign in southern Africa had informed people of the dangers of long-term concurrency and how this sexual system puts all sexually active people at risk, even though most people have few sexual partners. The topic of concurrency was absent from school-based AIDS education curricula, media and billboard AIDS campaigns, national government AIDS strategic plans, and the policy documents of virtually every single international public health organization working on the epidemic in the region.

Instead, for years the main sources of AIDS information in southern Africa were the flashy but vague loveLife campaign and condom promotion programs carried out by a small number of nonprofit organizations based in Washington, D.C., London, and other European capitals, including Population Services International (PSI), and Marie Stopes International. These organizations had been established during the heyday of the population control movement in the 1970s, when experts warned that the "population explosion" threatened economic growth, the environment, and global security much as AIDS does now.[10] With funding from USAID and other bilateral aid agencies, these organizations developed an approach called "social marketing" to encourage the use of a variety of contraceptives—all initially unpopular—in developing countries, by using private-sector advertising and marketing techniques. They had found that when condoms and other contraceptives were distributed free of charge in bland medical packaging, people found them unappealing. But when packaged in bright, colorful sleeves and advertised on billboards and radio spots as sexy and fun, they were much more popular. Selling condoms in shops, even at very low prices, rather than distributing them for free also added to their cachet.[11]

In towns and cities throughout southern Africa, cheap condoms were made available in clinics, shops, and bars, and they were advertised on billboards and the radio. Condom social marketers also sponsored impromptu musical and comedy performances, fashion shows, soccer matches, golf tournaments, and other events.[12] These campaigns often had a ribald tone. In Mozambique, billboards displayed a cartoon of "condom-man" slurping and winking at passersby. Radio ads broadcast at midday, when families were sitting down to lunch, advised, "When you have sex next time with your lover, do not forget to use JeitO condoms!"[13] In South Africa, a loveLife billboard displayed a naked girl with her arms draped over a boy's bare shoulders with a condom in her hands. The phrase "roll-on" in the caption—"The one roll-on every girl wants"—is township slang for "secret lover." Some campaigns bordered on the misogynistic. In Botswana, roadside billboards posted next to a cheerful beer ad depicted a red boxing glove, a condom, and the slogan "It can take the fiercest punches!" Another depicted a basketball, a condom, and the slogan "Even the best ballers take a safe dunk with it!" In Angola, condom packs carried a logo in the shape of a machine gun.

The condom campaigns were intended to encourage frank discussion about sex among normally reticent African populations and reach out to high-risk populations with the message that casual sex was nothing to worry about as long as condoms were used.[14] But it is possible to imagine how they might have had the opposite effect.[15] By associating AIDS with beer drinking, premarital sex, prostitution, and—in the case of the boxing glove and basketball ads—womanizing and rape, the lusty condom ads might well have clashed disastrously with local sensibilities concerning decency and self-respect and further inflamed the prejudice, denial, and rumormongering that have featured so strongly in the AIDS epidemic, and in virtually all epidemics since biblical times.

"The campaigns were totally wrong," said Nkosazana Ngcobo, who works with a South African organization that helps orphans. "The message was you had to be a prostitute or a truck driver to get AIDS."

"We knew AIDS was there," Lindiwe Dlamini, an HIV prevention worker from Swaziland, explained when I asked her why her country's HIV prevention programs had failed so dismally in the 1990s. "We all knew about it, but it was 'on the other side,' somewhere 'over there,'" she said, gesturing with her hands to a faraway place. "I thought I was in a secure relationship, that since my partner and I were faithful, we were OK."

A detailed study of newly infected male factory workers in Zimbabwe found that the vast majority contracted the virus not from prostitutes or onetime flings with people met in bars, but rather from steady partners whom they assumed to be "nice" or "clean" or "not the type to be infected."[16]

In African AIDS-related shame and denial are partly a defensive reaction to centuries of racist stereotypes about African sexuality. The condom campaigns were a reminder that these stereotypes persist.

"To some extent, AIDS stigma was brought to Africa from the West," Maxine Ankrah told me. "There was this assumption that AIDS was due to 'bad behavior' and you avoided it with condoms. But that meant condom-users or people with AIDS were automatically considered prostitutes."

The condom campaigns are gradually being replaced with "ABC" messages, including loveLife's PRD—Protect (with condoms), Reduce (your partners), Delay (your sexual debut)—but these messages still fail to explain to people why they themselves are at risk, and need to do A, B, or C, even if they have few partners and their partners have few partners. Thus the stigma and denial persist and remain the greatest obstacles to AIDS prevention in this region.

What the people who designed Africa's early condom social-marketing programs may not have understood is that Africa is not the Sodom and Gomorrah depicted by nineteenth-century missionaries. Just as everywhere else, sexual behavior on the continent is governed by strict moral rules. They may not be the same as Western rules—polygamy and other forms of long-term concurrency are considered acceptable to many people—but they are rules all the same.[17]

Young people across Africa still undergo highly secret coming-of-age rituals, where they learn the specific sexual practices of their tribe. Much of Africa's sculpture and dancing is a symbolic exploration of the powers of sexuality, which is seen to forge a supernatural connection between the realm of the ancestors and the future of the clan. Even traditional African "praise songs"—ritual poems concerning spiritual matters, of which one missionary said "no decent person could even speak"—testify to the rule-bound nature of African discourses about sex. In *The African Genius*,[18] his fascinating introduction to African culture, Basil Davidson describes the praise song of a Zulu girl, which begins: "He mounted me on the mons veneris because he knows me very well." Davidson recognized that the song signified not a free-spirited, "anything goes" attitude to sex, but rather the girl's promise to the community that she would go so far and no further. In Zulu culture, it was appropriate for young unmarried people to fool around, but penetrative sex was forbidden. So when the girl says, "He knows me very well," she means "He knows the rules."

In Uganda, I once spent an afternoon reading through some of the thirty thousand letters that young people send annually to Straight Talk, a media organization that answers young people's questions about love, sex, relationships, and AIDS. It was striking how many of the letters were concerned with matters of proper behavior. "Straight Talk has improved my social character and my behavior in the community," wrote one teenage boy. "Being smart"—meaning "well-dressed"—"is always a problem," wrote a girl. "Because of your smartness you become attractive to everyone, so it's better to put on a T-shirt, wash it, iron it, and make sure it isn't transparent." When a Straight Talk radio quiz asked young listeners to send in answers to the question "What is 'good sex'?" many parents feared that it would invite a torrent of lewd responses, but this did not happen. "'Good sex' is sex after talking about it," ventured one respondent. "'Good sex' is sex you wait for," wrote another. "'Good sex' is sex within marriage."

IN HER 1987 book *Illness as Metaphor*,[19] Susan Sontag described how, when people don't understand the causes of a disease—why some people get it and others don't—they tend to imbue these afflictions with moral or metaphysical significance. As HIV spread rapidly throughout the 1990s and early 2000s and people began to see others dying all around them, they couldn't believe the cause was AIDS, because the sick were not prostitutes or philanderers. How could people they respected and cared for have such a "sinful" disease? So they denied the disease's existence, attributed it to dark forces beyond their control, or searched the cosmos for answers.

All over Africa, bizarre rumors about AIDS swirl through townships and rural areas: AIDS is caused by witchcraft, a CIA-backed germ-warfare campaign against blacks, or some poison in the food.[20] "It seems this thing is like magic," an old man told Deborah Posel. "Nothing can stop it."

Many people attribute the epidemic to condoms themselves. "With JeitO"—the local condom brand—"we are teaching people to live a bad life," a Mozambican pastor told the Case Western Reserve University anthropologist James Pfeiffer in 2004. When Pfeiffer asked young people in Mozambique where AIDS came from, several respondents repeated a rumor, widespread in southern Africa, that is symbolically consistent with the view that condoms "cause" AIDS. "AIDS came from JeitO," explained one young man. "If one hangs a JeitO condom up to dry in the sunlight for a day, one can eventually see the HIV virus squirming inside."[21]

AIDS prevention workers despair when they hear such rumors.[22] After all, if you believe AIDS is caused by the CIA or witches, why would you use a condom or abstain? But perhaps it's not their beliefs but our messages that are wrong. Witchcraft beliefs are not rigid and unchanging; they derive from thought patterns whose purpose is to interpret events that don't make sense.

Perhaps the South African who was most confused about AIDS was the current president, Thabo Mbeki. He publicly questioned the relationship between HIV and AIDS, claiming the disease was not caused by a virus, but by a mysterious syndrome resulting from poverty and malnutrition; it was more common in Africa because African people had been physically weakened by centuries of humiliation and oppression. It was no wonder they were more susceptible to tuberculosis, wasting, and other symptoms that looked like AIDS. To Mbeki, HIV tests were meaningless and AIDS drugs were toxic poison, foisted on Africa by a venal pharmaceutical industry bent on exploiting the poor. Well-meaning AIDS doctors were themselves in denial about the horrors of the legacy of colonial oppression.

Mbeki's views about AIDS confounded even the most sympathetic observers of his presidency. They were variously attributed to insanity, to an inability to confront his own sexual behavior, to a secret desire to forestall AIDS treatment programs until local researchers could come up with an "African solution" to the crisis, and to economic calculation: after all, AIDS was concentrated among the poor, who were a drain on the economy.[23]

But it is also possible that Mbeki was struggling with some of the very epidemiological issues discussed above. In 2000, he convened a panel of AIDS experts, including distinguished scientists and doctors from South Africa, the United States, and Europe, and asked them to engage in a debate with a group of AIDS dissidents who maintained that HIV was not the cause of the disease. The meeting was held in a Pretoria hotel; consensus was never reached and a final report was never issued. But in 2003, a ninety-three-page essay titled "Castro Hlongwane, Caravans, Cats, Geese, Foot & Mouth and Statistics: HIV/AIDS and the Struggle for the Humanisation of the African" appeared on the Internet.[24] The anonymous author of this angry, rambling document is assumed to be Mbeki himself, although this has not been proven. Amidst the rage, bombast, and wild digressions lies a simple question that the international scientific community had thus far failed to answer. "Why does the same Virus behave differently in the US and Western Europe from the way it behaves in Southern Africa!" he writes. The author refuses to believe what he has been told about high-risk behavior and high-risk groups. According to this theory, Africa had "the highest incidence of HIV infection and AIDS deaths, caused by sexual immorality among our people. . . . As Africans, we are prone to rape and abuse of women and . . . we uphold a value system that belongs to the world of wild animals. . . ."

In other words, if AIDS was a disease of "promiscuity," as Western experts with their condom campaigns and "high risk" group models were claiming, and a third of South Africans carried the virus, then that third were "promiscuous." The implications of this line of reasoning must have struck this African chauvinist right in the heart.

Europeans had always justified their presence in Africa with the claim that Africans could not govern themselves because they occupied a lower rung on the evolutionary ladder and were more subject to elementary animal drives. Dispelling the racial contempt that shaped such ideas has been a vital mission for generations of intellectuals of African descent, from Léopold Senghor to James Baldwin, and so it is for Mbeki. Essentially, what he's saying is that if you believe that HIV is the sole cause of AIDS, you must also believe the entire infrastructure of racist myth and ideologies that have held Africa back for centuries. "The HIV/AIDS thesis . . . ," he writes, "is . . . informed by deeply entrenched and centuries-old white racist beliefs and concepts about Africans and black people," and makes "a powerful contribution to the further entrenchment and popularisation of racism." In a speech given at the University of Fort Hare in 2001, Mbeki railed against those who were "convinced that we are but natural born promiscuous carriers of germs, unique in the world. They proclaim that our continent is doomed to an inevitable mortal end because of our unconquerable devotion to the sin of lust."[25]

Albie Sachs, a former African National Congress freedom fighter who now sits on South Africa's Constitutional Court, has described how political and social life in South Africa is shaped by something that cannot be measured or captured in research studies, but which is nevertheless forever bubbling to the surface. It is the experience of being told that "you are savage, barbaric and that your culture is nothing. It is the experience of having been compelled physically to live on the outskirts of the city and the margins of the country and having been poor, without the vote, having your language disregarded and having government take all decisions for you and subjecting you to countless humiliations."[26]

Mbeki's response to AIDS suggests that you can change all the laws, design a new flag, and install black leaders, but the shame, doubt, and self-hatred that racism evokes will linger for generations.

For whom was "Castro Hlongwane" written? The author seems to have given up on trying to convince the medical establishment of his views. Instead, he may have been reaching out to his own South African constituents. As Deborah Posel discovered in Limpopo, it had not escaped notice that AIDS cases began increasing in South Africa in the early 1990s, just as the apartheid regime was crumbling and black politicians, including Mbeki, were promising that with the yoke of colonialism finally thrown off, they could now deliver a better life for everyone.

Nor had it escaped notice that many of these promises had been broken. For many of South Africa's poor, life was harder now, not easier. Although the national GDP had grown, the new wealth was highly concentrated in a small number of hands, and unemployment and inequality had soared. The nation's vast underclass had entered a period of crisis similar to that which occurred in 1970s America, in the aftermath of the civil rights movement. In his 1987 book *The Truly Disadvantaged: The Inner City, the Underclass and Public Policy*,[27] the Harvard sociologist William Julius Wilson described how, as the black middle class embraced its hard-won freedoms and moved out of the ghetto, poor, unskilled blacks became consolidated in redlined slums. Without the social and economic anchor of a middle class, they descended into a mire of drugs, crime, and family breakdown.

Something similar was now under way in townships and rural areas throughout South Africa. As middle-class blacks decamped to formerly all-white suburbs, the people left behind became even more marginalized than they were before. The humiliations of poverty and exclusion and residual feelings of resentment against whites gave rise to a frightening subculture of street gangs, prostitutes, and thugs who fought, stole, abused women, and treated elders with contempt.[28] When AIDS emerged, many people came to associate it with the unruly, "disrespectful" behavior of these newly "liberated" young people. They blamed not the legacy of racism and the vicissitudes of globalization, but "freedom."

As an older man in one of Deborah Posel's focus groups explained, "1994"—the year the African National Congress came to power—"brought out the worst in this country."

"People think they have freedom, whereas the freedom they have is leading them to death," said another.

"Thabo Mbeki gave them"—meaning women—"too much freedom to sell sex and this kills them," said another.

"Now children are chasing money. A young girl can have more than two boyfriends just because they will give her money. Before 1994, this was not happening," said another.

"People are misusing these rights," said a younger man.

"Rights have made life difficult because we no longer respect each other," said another.

It's as if these people had come to see AIDS sufferers as living symbols of all that had gone wrong in their country during the preceding decade. The epidemic was leading them to question their government, their future, and themselves. They were even repeating the most pernicious apartheid-era narratives about African sexual behavior and disparaging the very rights they and their leaders had fought and died for. This was something that their president, Thabo Mbeki, who had devoted his life to upholding the dignity and promise of African people, must have found very hard to bear.

The author of "Castro Hlongwane" may have misled people about the causes of AIDS, but so did the condom campaigns and the high-risk-group model. But that wasn't the point. The question South Africans really wanted answered was not about epidemiology. It was the question black intellectuals have been asking since the dawn of colonial times. Not "What is AIDS?" or even "Why is this disease more common in Africa than in the West?" but "Who are we?"

WHAT HAPPENED IN UGANDA AND WASHINGTON AND GENEVA

CHAPTER NINE

The Invisible Cure

THE FIRST THING that struck me when I arrived in Bukoba—a dusty Tanzanian town of some sixty thousand people on the shores of Lake Victoria—was how devout everyone seemed. The steeples of the churches of seven different denominations poke above the town's dense tree line, and the pageantry of the Sunday-morning congregants—the men in dark suits, the women in magnificent Easter hats, and the streams of children in ties and jackets and lacy dresses—resembles a royal procession. People name their children Moses, Deus, and Augustine. Prayers are recited before work, meals, bedtime, and trips out of town, and the most ordinary conversations are sprinkled with blessings. I was not surprised when a group of boys at the local high school told me they aspired to be pastors or bishops.

But if you hang around Bukoba for a while, you learn that those future bishops have been known to purchase condoms from the kiosks in town, and the born-again Christian hotelier rents rooms to couples by the hour. Bukoba is the capital of Kagera Region, a lush green strip that lies in the rugged hills of the Rift Valley, between the western shore of Lake Victoria and the borders of Rwanda and Uganda. During the 1970s, the global AIDS pandemic was probably first ignited here, in Kagera Region. Researchers theorize that HIV evolved somewhere in West Africa sometime in the early twentieth century and then spread slowly across central Africa for decades, unnoticed by any public health authority. Then, in the late 1970s, the first explosive epidemic occurred in Kagera and quickly spread to Rwanda, Burundi, and southern Uganda.

From there, the virus made its way east to the rest of Tanzania, to Kenya, south to Zambia, Malawi, and Zimbabwe, and then to the rest of the continent.

The explosion of HIV in Kagera was probably no accident. The women of this region have a long history of prostitution, dating back to colonial times, and they still have a bawdy reputation in East Africa today. Kagera is unusually fertile, and during colonial times it became a center for the cultivation of cotton and coffee, which were much in demand by world markets in the early twentieth century. The cash-crop boom made some families rich, but it also had a downside, especially for women. According to the customs of the Haya—the main tribe in Kagera—women performed most of the agricultural labor, but received none of the profits and, unlike women in neighboring tribes, were not allowed to inherit land from their fathers; their in-laws sometimes took everything, including their children, when their husbands died.

As colonial trade increased, women became virtual slaves of their husbands. A colonial official in the 1930s wrote that Haya men "regarded a wife as an agricultural machine, and a domestic drudge. Having worked all day while her husband engages in the more dignified pastime of drinking and gossiping, the woman returns home to cook the evening meal. But the lord and master is still thirsty at a neighbor's house, and she herself is not allowed to eat until he returns much later." Wife beating was common, as was abandonment, often on the charge that a wife was too "lazy."[1]

Prostitution in the growing railway towns of colonial East Africa provided Haya women with a route to freedom in this male-dominated world. In Nairobi and Kampala, Haya prostitutes were free agents. There were no pimps, and the colonial police looked the other way most of the time.[2] After a few years a woman might earn enough to return home and purchase land of her own. Back in Kagera, returned prostitutes formed an elite group. They wore fashionable clothes, kept their money in bank accounts, and had their own gramophones and sewing machines. Some drove motorbikes, a luxury in this region even today. In the 1950s, when the colonial authorities tried to forbid a group of Haya prostitutes to travel to Nairobi, the women chartered a plane. Today, the stone houses the prostitutes built are among the largest in Bukoba.

But by 1920, these prostitutes had brought a terrifying epidemic of syphilis back to Kagera, and during the first half of the twentieth century, sexually transmitted diseases became so widespread that the Haya began to describe themselves as "a dying people."

Then, in the 1950s, syphilis rates began to decline. Penicillin was being introduced into African hospitals, but the historian Birgitta Larsson has argued that people's behavior was also changing. Beginning in the 1940s, a powerful religious revival had attracted thousands of East Africans back to the Protestant church. Larsson and others have described how the revival radically changed gender relations in Kagera and brought about a new sense of equality between men and women. This revival was led in part by a generation of newly empowered returned prostitutes, who used their personal wealth to start small businesses and welfare organizations. They helped other poor women escape abusive marriages and paid tuition for legions of children. Some former prostitutes even became church elders. For the first time, women, normally silent in the presence of men, were standing up in church and addressing large congregations. They urged men to stop philandering and beating their wives and squandering all their money on beer. For a while, some men appear to have taken this advice: "Where the Revival has been, the men begin, happily and voluntarily, to assist in the daily work," wrote the Swedish missionary Barbro Johansson in 1949. "They are eager to go together with their wives to gatherings and tea-parties; they want to know their views and they ask for their participation in deliberations, testimonies and prayer fellowship. They set their 'slaves' free!"[3]

Larsson acknowledges that it is hard to know what was going on in people's homes, behind this "pious façade," but syphilis rates did fall, as did reports of divorce and abandonment. Then, a generation later, disaster struck. In the 1970s, the price of coffee, the main cash crop produced by the Haya people, was at an all-time low, and then came the banana weevils, termite-like insects that temporarily wiped out most of the banana trees and with them, people's main source of food. Meanwhile, rising world oil prices, declining sources of credit, and Tanzania's socialist economic policies combined to make Tanzania one of the poorest countries on earth. All trade was state controlled and all goods were sold through government shops. People waited in line all day to buy things;

toothpaste was a luxury, even for the middle class. Corruption flourished, and a clandestine black-market trading center near the Ugandan border attracted large numbers of smugglers and prostitutes from both countries. Then, in 1978, Idi Amin, claiming that part of Kagera rightfully belonged to Uganda, sent bombing raids over the border in an attempt to take over the region.

To defend Kagera against Amin, the Tanzanian government raised a large volunteer army, which massed in Bukoba. Before long, the soldiers, smugglers, and prostitutes began returning from the military posts and trading centers at the border not only with syphilis, gonorrhea, and other STDs, but with strange symptoms that no one had ever seen before. The new disease soon spread rapidly through the region's complex networks of sexual partnerships—concurrent and otherwise—and by 1987, nearly a quarter of all adults in Bukoba were HIV positive. Across the border, in the southern towns of Uganda—Masaka, Rakai, Kampala—the HIV infection rate was almost as high.

Then something remarkable occurred. Sometime during the late 1980s the HIV infection rate in this entire region began to fall. By 1996, Bukoba's HIV rate had fallen by half and by 2003 it was down 80 percent from its peak fifteen years earlier. Declines of similar magnitude occurred in southern Uganda at around the same time. Millions of lives were saved as a result.[4]

The declines in the HIV infection rates in Uganda and Kagera were first announced at scientific meetings in 1995 and 1996.[5] I was not in Africa at the time, but when I read about the findings in newspapers and conference reports, I assumed, as did many others, that the decline was due to the natural course of the epidemic. The most susceptible people—the prostitutes and the promiscuous men—succumbed to the disease first. As they became sick and died, HIV prevalence naturally fell. As people witnessed their suffering, they took heed and changed their sexual behavior, and this ensured that the HIV rate remained low.

But as the HIV rate continued to soar nearly everywhere else in the eastern and southern arc of the African continent, some public health experts began to wonder. In 1992, epidemiologists reported that 20 percent of pregnant women in Francistown, a city in the southern African nation of Botswana, were HIV positive—a rate similar to that in Kagera and southern Uganda at the time. While the HIV rate in southern Uganda fell by half during the 1990s, the HIV rate in Francistown nearly doubled. In Zambia, Zimbabwe, and Malawi, the HIV rate remained high throughout the 1990s, even though the epidemic struck these countries around the same time as it did Uganda and Kagera.[6]

As the 1990s drew to a close, journalists began returning from Africa with photographs and stories of dying women and children that stirred the conscience of the world. The African AIDS crisis, virtually ignored for years outside the health field, finally began to attract the attention of world leaders. In 2001, the UN General Assembly convened a special session on AIDS in New York, at which thousands of government and civil-society leaders and AIDS experts from around the world came together to identify what they believed it would take to fight the epidemic. Soon, prime ministers and presidents, tycoon philanthropists, star Christian evangelists, famous singers and actresses, and other celebrities were joining forces with public health experts who had been working on AIDS for years. Billions of dollars were raised to fight the pandemic, mostly for AIDS treatment, but everyone knew that stopping the virus's spread was at least as important.

A few months after the UN meeting, a group of AIDS experts writing in the British medical journal *The Lancet* put a price tag on the General Assembly's prescriptions. They calculated that millions of HIV infections could be prevented with a "package" of public health interventions including condom promotion programs; mass media campaigns on radio, TV, and billboards; AIDS education programs for schools, factories, and other businesses; HIV testing services; and STD treatment services. Many of these programs were already under way in some countries, but to make them available throughout the developing world by 2010 would cost some twenty-seven billion dollars. This did not include the cost of medical treatment for AIDS patients, which amounted to many billions more.[7]

Meanwhile, behind the scenes, other AIDS researchers were scrambling to find out what had happened in Uganda and Kagera a decade earlier to bring the infection rate down. Few international public health officials had been working in the region when the decline occurred, and little had been written about it. Nevertheless, it was clear that both places lacked many of the elements of the twenty-seven-billion-dollar "package" prescribed in *The Lancet*. At the time the HIV infection rate began falling, few people used condoms, HIV testing services were not widely available, and there was only one clinic in Uganda that specialized in the treatment of STDs.[8] Mass-media campaigns, limited by the fact that Amin and Obote's cadres had stolen most of the TVs and billboards, consisted mainly of rudimentary hand-painted signs and radio announcements.

During the early 2000s, many AIDS experts traveled to Uganda to try to find out why the HIV rate there had fallen. Billions of dollars in funding for global AIDS programs were at stake, and the question soon became mired in controversy. Most public health officials attributed it to government commitment and condom programs. Evangelical Christians attributed it to abstinence programs in schools and churches, World Health Organization officials attributed it to new bureaucratic structures designed by WHO consultants, and so on.[9]

While all of these factors certainly mattered, they didn't seem to fully explain the decline, and eventually I would draw my own conclusions. It seemed to me that what mattered most was something for which public health experts had no name or program. It was something like "collective efficacy"—the ability of people to join together and help one another. Felton Earls, the sociologist who coined the term, was trying to explain varying crime rates in American cities, but the phenomenon is present everywhere there is a spirit of collective action and mutual aid, a spirit that is impossible to measure or quantify, but that is rooted in a sense of compassion and common humanity.[11]

During the 1980s and early 1990s, while people in most African countries were ignoring the AIDS crisis, hundreds of tiny community-based AIDS groups sprang up throughout Uganda and Kagera to comfort the sick, care for orphans, warn people about the dangers of casual sex, and address the particular vulnerability of women and girls to infection. Yoweri Museveni's government developed its own vigorous prevention campaigns and the World Health Organization provided funding, but much also came from the pockets of the poor themselves. Their compassion and hard work brought the disease into the open, got people talking about the epidemic, reduced AIDS-related stigma and denial, and led to a profound shift in sexual norms. This process was very African, but it was similar in many respects to the compassionate, vocal, and angry response to AIDS among gay men in Western countries during the 1980s, when HIV incidence in this group also fell steeply.[12]

Why did this social movement emerge in Uganda and Kagera, but not elsewhere in Africa until much later? It is hard to know for certain, but it may have had something to do with the fact that the people in this region understood earlier than others that in this part of Africa, AIDS was not just a disease of prostitutes, truck drivers and other stigmatized high-risk groups. The word "concurrency" would have been unknown to those who joined this social movement, but even so, government campaigns made one thing clear: everyone was at risk. This in turn may have created a sense of collective urgency that roused people into action.

The Ugandan response to AIDS was vastly different from that taken in southern Africa. However, as we shall see, people in southern Africa have the capacity to respond to AIDS just as Ugandans did, and governments and foreign-aid programs can support them. But as we shall also see, they can sometimes undermine them.

In 1984, a Ugandan government official from the southern district of Rakai informed the Ministry of Health in Entebbe that young adults in the area were dying of a mysterious new disease that the locals called "Slim." He noted that the symptoms resembled those of AIDS, the disease that was killing homosexuals in the West.[13] When a group of Makerere University professors arrived to investigate the situation in Rakai, they were accosted by people in the streets, desperate to know what was causing Slim. Some people, noticing that polygamous families were especially susceptible, wondered whether jealous co-wives were not casting spells on each other. Others noticed that many of the victims were smugglers who worked at the illegal border marketplaces, and some people wondered whether a Tanzanian who had been cheated in a business deal had cast a spell on anyone who came into contact with the money he had lost. The houses of the afflicted stood abandoned, and banknotes fluttered in the road; no one in this impoverished place dared to pick them up.

But many Ugandans already suspected the truth. By 1983, doctors at Mulago Hospital were already tentatively diagnosing patients with the disease.[14] "We suspected the disease came from sex even before the missionaries and doctors came to tell us," a farmer in Kagera who had been a young woman at the time told me years later. "When we saw a husband and wife getting the disease together, we wondered why. Was it from eating the same food? Then why weren't all their children getting sick too? We knew it was a disease of young people. We learned about syphilis from our grandmothers. They told us there was a disease that could kill the eggs in your stomach, so you shouldn't go around with different men."

Uganda's civil war continued and the government fell twice in the following year. Then, in January 1986, Yoweri Museveni's National Resistance Army took power. Museveni quickly recognized the gravity of the AIDS crisis. Many of his own soldiers had succumbed to the disease, and he saw the threat to the future of the country he had just taken over. At the time, there were few Western health experts in the country, but Museveni assembled a team of Ugandan health experts who launched a vigorous AIDS education campaign of their own. Warnings about AIDS were broadcast on the radio each day at lunchtime, accompanied by the beating of a drum in the traditional rhythm of warning. "When I was young, I'd lie awake all night if I heard a drum beating that way," a middle-aged Ugandan told me. "It meant a thief or a murderer was on the loose."

The slogans "Love Carefully" and "Zero Grazing"—meaning, in the words of the head of Uganda's AIDS Control Program, "avoid indiscriminate and free-ranging sexual relations"[15]—were posted on public buildings, broadcast on radio, and bellowed in speeches by government officials. Teams of AIDS educators trained by the Ministry of Health fanned out across the country and held all-day meetings with women's groups, village elders, teachers, and church congregations.[16] Religious leaders scoured the Bible and the Koran for quotations about adultery. Newspapers, theaters, singing groups, and ordinary people spread the same message.[17]

Condoms were hotly debated in newspaper letters to the editor, church gatherings, and everyday conversation. Some said they promoted sin; others said sinful or not, condoms were necessary.[18] Before long, a nationwide conversation about formerly taboo sex-related topics was under way. In 1993, *The New Vision*, Uganda's government-owned newspaper, began distributing a newsletter called *Straight Talk*, which provided frank, non-squeamish information about sexual feelings, puberty, AIDS and other STDs, contraception, sexual abuse, drugs and alcohol, and many other topics that had never been aired publicly before.

In 2004, the UN launched a campaign to raise awareness about the links between women's rights violations and the spread of HIV, but Ugandan women had recognized these links two decades earlier.[19]*

Uganda's women's rights movement is one of the oldest in Africa, and it flourished in the politically liberal atmosphere allowed by the government in the late 1980s. For decades, the movement had been suppressed by the paranoid dictatorships of Idi Amin and Milton Obote, but in 1985 a small number of Ugandan women attended the UN Conference on Women in Nairobi, Kenya, and returned with new energy and ideas. When the young coup leader Yoweri Museveni came to power in 1986, he promoted community organizing and self-help, which encouraged the women even more. Before long, at rallies throughout the country, women were being urged to keep their daughters in school, start small businesses, and challenge discrimination. As a result, a number of laws regarding rape, divorce, and women's property rights that previously favored men, were changed.[20]

HIV was always on the agenda. "There was not a single workshop or meeting where the subject of AIDS did not come up," says Mazine Ankrah, who helped establish Action for Women in Development, Uganda's largest women's rights organization at the time. "We told women, if your husband is unfaithful and is going to kill you with AIDS, you divorce him." There was even a Ugandan Association of Co-wives and Concubines that policed the behavior of polygamous men, encouraging them to avoid the casual affairs that could endanger all their wives and future children. Meanwhile, the eloquent sadness of women throughout the country who nursed the sick and helped neighbors cope was a further harsh reproach to promiscuous men. So was their gossip, a highly effective method of spreading any public health message.

During the late 1980s and early 1990s, the fraction of Ugandan men with multiple partners sharply decreased, and as a result—as will be described in more detail in the next chapter—the HIV infection rate fell by

*Jonathan Mann, head of the World Health Organization's Global Program on AIDS between 1986 and 1992, also understood these links, but when he left WHO, the women's rights agenda in the organization left with him and would not return for another decade.

roughly 60 percent. In bars and discos once mobbed with men and single women, men now sat drinking among themselves and went home early. Some bars closed down completely. Attendance at sexually transmitted disease clinics also fell sharply.

Gender-related attitudes also shifted. The enrollment of girls in school increased sharply, as did the participation of women in the economy. In the early 1980s rape was generally considered an excusable crime in Uganda, and some Kampala lawyers and officials even joked about it.[21] But then women's rights activists began speaking out about the double horror of rape and AIDS. They organized marches against rape in the city streets and warned women across the country to band together and confront abusive men. In the early 1990s, Miria Matembe, a member of the Ugandan parliament, declared that "rapists, defilers and all those who in one way or another commit sexual offenses are in possession of potentially dangerous instruments which must be taken away from them if they can't use them properly." Her remarks rocked the nation, even though this was not a statement of a policy. But you don't hear many jokes about rape in Uganda anymore.[22]

Most ordinary Ugandans, accustomed to helping each other through war and other hardships, responded to AIDS with compassion. Throughout the country, neighbors and extended families pooled their meager resources to comfort the sick, help families cope, and ensure that orphans had someone to care for them. "We started with one child," Wilberforce Owori, the founder of one such organization, explained to me in 2006. "My wife and I were in a meeting at our church, and we were challenged to care for orphans. We found out we didn't have the money, so we joined with three others and started a bank account, and each of us made a monthly contribution to pay the child's school fees. Then other people joined us. We'd just collect any amount of money, three hundred shillings [about twenty U.S. cents], whatever. The first year, we took care of one child, the next year, eight children, then eighteen, then thirty."

By 1991, there were hundreds of community- and church-based AIDS care and support groups in Uganda and more than a dozen in Kagera, a much smaller region. Medically, there wasn't much that could be done for people with AIDS, since Uganda's health-care system had been all but destroyed during the war, and drugs to effectively treat the disease had yet to be developed in any case. But Ugandans pioneered the concept of home-based care, which is now a central activity of AIDS organizations throughout Africa.

"You just go out and get water, go and sweep someone's house, plant pineapples for the patients, take care of the children. It doesn't take much money," Owori told me. "There were many people with that desire to give care. I didn't want to miss the chance to do something. You couldn't just do nothing. Just to be there and converse with the person. Anyone can do that."

The AIDS Support Organization, or TASO, which is now one of the largest indigenous AIDS organizations in Africa, was started in much the same way as Owori's group, when AIDS patients and their relatives began holding meetings at Mulago to support each other and share information. They soon realized that many supplies and medications could be more easily delivered to people's homes than to the overcrowded, dilapidated hospital. By the late 1980s, TASO, along with a number of mainly Catholic hospitals throughout the country, was providing home-based care services to thousands of AIDS patients and their relatives throughout Uganda.

In *We Miss You All*,[23] her memoir about the founding of TASO, Noerine Kaleeba, a former physiotherapist at Mulago who was widowed by AIDS in 1986, recalls her first encounter with an AIDS patient in 1983:

> I had gone to one of the medical wards at Mulago to locate a paraplegic patient for a practical demonstration for physiotherapy students on the techniques of transferring a paraplegic from a bed to a wheelchair. I located a young man who couldn't have been more than 30 years old. I introduced myself and explained what I required of him. He was very receptive and gave permission for my students to learn from him for that afternoon. His medical notes indicated that he had paraplegia due to Immunosuppression Syndrome, but I did not know what that was. I went to the ward sister to get permission to teach the students on her ward that afternoon. She came closer to me and said,

"I wouldn't touch him if I were you. He has AIDS. We don't touch him, we only show his mother what to do."

I did not use him for the demonstration. Neither did I go back to him and explain that I would not be coming. I canceled the class and arranged for another patient from the orthopedic ward.

I did not think about him again, until the diagnosis of AIDS came through my front door. Today there isn't a day that passes that I don't wonder what happened to him. With whom did he carry the burden? With whom did his mother carry the cross? What friends did she have to share her emotions? How much did he know about AIDS? What support did he have: God, children, loved ones? I suppose I will never know.

When her own husband died of AIDS three years later, Kaleeba saw for herself what it was like to be on the receiving end of AIDS-related discrimination. She was shunned by her own friends. "They would stop conversation as soon as I made an appearance. . . . They would hold their hands behind their backs while greeting me. . . . The toilet key [at work] would go missing as soon as I needed to use it."

"There was a lot of stigma at first," said Sister Ursula Sharp, the Catholic nun who founded Kitovu Mobile, a home-based care program in Masaka district, in 1987. "It was hard to get nurses to work with me. There was fear of contamination and also fear of witchcraft. Some of our volunteers' huts were burned down because there was a rumor that we were poisoning people in the community. But we kept going back and going back and going back," she said. "We were there every time. We'd never miss an appointment with a patient. They knew we'd be there if we promised to come, rain or shine."

Throughout the region, home-based care counselors taught millions of people that it was safe to touch and care for AIDS patients, and that the affliction was neither a curse from God nor a punishment for sin, but a terrible disease than no one deserved.[24]

Before long, a new generation of Ugandan AIDS activists emerged, most of them women, most of them openly HIV positive, including Beatrice Were, the founder of the National Community of Women Living with HIV/AIDS, and Milly Katana, cofounder of the National Guidance and Empowerment Network of People Living with HIV/AIDS. They would combine the best elements of the two campaigns of the 1980s: the fight for women's rights and the fight for better care and treatment of people living with AIDS. "As a woman living with HIV," says Were, "I am often asked whether there will ever be a cure for HIV/AIDS, and my answer is that there is already a cure. It lies in the strength of women, families and communities who support and empower each other to break the silence around AIDS and take control of their sexual lives."[25]

Through the 1980s and 1990s, officials from the World Health Organization, USAID, and other development agencies largely dismissed Uganda's AIDS programs. "It seemed like chaos," Gary Slutkin, a WHO official who worked in Uganda in the late 1980s, told me much later. "For many of my colleagues, the problem was there was no 'theory' behind Uganda's approach."[26] Public health programs were supposed to be "rational," "budgeted," and targeted at those groups thought to be most at risk. They were not supposed to be a free-for-all. But what WHO officials did not understand at the time was that there was a theory. It just wasn't their theory. The intimate, personalized nature of Uganda's early AIDS campaigns—the open discussions led by government field workers and in small groups of women and churchgoers, the compassionate work of the home-based care volunteers, the courage and strength of the women's-rights activists—helped people see AIDS not as a disease spread by disreputable high-risk groups or "others" but as a shared calamity affecting everyone. This made discussion of sexual behavior possible without seeming preachy or prurient. Behavior change then became a matter of common sense. Maybe foreign public health officials missed this at the time because such "social mobilization" is actually quite hard to program. It is a spirit that flourishes when people come together to face a common threat. It is not something that can be packaged and paid for and then shipped around the world.

In 2003 I visited Botswana. This vast, underpopulated country in southern Africa, with its bleached salt-pan deserts, natural mineral wealth, and peaceful democratic government, is an African paradise. Shortly after independence from Britain in 1966, large diamond reserves were discovered within its borders, and the country's economy would soon grow faster, for longer, than almost any other in the world. Its benevolent government invested heavily in free, universal health-care services and education. Corruption is rare, the crime rate is low, and the nation has never been at war. The Batswana, as the people of Botswana are called, are exceedingly loyal to their country. I quickly learned that even mild criticism of anything related to Botswana is considered impolite. But why, then, did Botswana, given all its advantages, have the highest HIV infection rate in the world at the time?

It was not that the nation's highly efficient government had failed to respond to the epidemic. I was amazed at how well organized Botswana's AIDS programs were. Botswana was the first to introduce free antiretroviral drug treatment for all citizens with AIDS in 2002, and it had had a vigorous program to promote condoms since 1992. The main university even had "condom police" at one time, who ensured students were carrying them. There were programs to encourage HIV testing and treatment for STDs, there were AIDS billboards on every major road, and every schoolchild received education about the disease. There was a National AIDS Council, a National AIDS Coordinating Agency, a National Strategic Framework for AIDS, and "multisectoral partnerships" with bilateral and multilateral donors, the UN, and international nongovernmental organizations. When I was in the country, I attended a condom rally in a dust-blown marketplace, where some two hundred people had gathered to watch a dance troupe perform a hip-hop routine to promote safe sex. I visited a spotless HIV testing kiosk and a clinic where dozens of AIDS patients were waiting for their medicine. I saw the lab block at the main hospital in Gaborone, where all the blood samples from the entire country were sorted and screened, and I had to admit it seemed cleaner and better run than many of the British and American labs I had worked in during my scientist days.

But no one talked about AIDS. Until the end of the 1990s, Botswana's politicians made virtually no reference to the epidemic in their speeches; newspapers were largely silent on the issue; few community-based AIDS organizations even existed, and those that did received very little support from donors, churches, or the government. When patients went to hospitals to die, health workers informed them that they were suffering from tuberculosis or pneumonia and never gave them, or their families, the true diagnosis.[27]

By the time Festus Mogae, Botswana's newly elected president, declared AIDS a national emergency in 1999, nearly a third of all adults were HIV positive, the highest HIV rate in the world at the time. In one city, the figure had reached 70 percent.

In an article in the *Financial Times* of London, Daniel Low-Beer, of the Global Fund to Fight AIDS, Tuberculosis and Malaria, described how stunned he was by the silence surrounding the disease when he toured Botswana's AIDS programs in 2003. "Do you talk to a patient who comes in with AIDS about AIDS, do you confront it?" he asked a health worker. "'No,' a six-week counseling course had told him not to. . . . I asked about the village chief—he does not feel qualified to talk about AIDS. I asked about the church, no one mentions it at funerals."[28]

Perhaps this explains why the infection rate in Botswana in 2003 was nearly six times higher than it was in Uganda, a much poorer country—even though Botswana seemed to have all the elements of the "package" recommended by public health experts. Perhaps Uganda's early AIDS campaigns, though technically simple, possessed a quality that Botswana's lacked. Uganda's campaigns built upon the personalized, informal, intimate, contingent, reciprocal nature of African society, while Botswana relied mainly on mass-media campaigns, the distribution of condoms and other commodities, and hospital-based services. These services undoubtedly benefited many individuals, but they failed to stir the nation's conscience.

When I was in Botswana, I met a social scientist who had worked on AIDS for years. I asked her why she thought the HIV rate in Botswana was still so high and had not fallen as Uganda's had. There were many reasons, she said. For one thing, in Botswana AIDS has always been seen as a disease of the poor, marginalized, and immoral. The nation's many admirable programs never conveyed the crucial message that here HIV was everyone's problem. In Uganda, many middle-class families were affected by AIDS early on, and they bravely spoke out and gave a human face to the disease. Few prominent Batswana were willing to do that.

Then she said something that surprised me. "You know, in Uganda, they had home-based care. Here, if you are sick, you go to a hospital with clean sheets and three square meals a day. In my mother's time, people were born at home and died there. Now to do that is a sign of poverty. Development is good, but we have to ensure we don't lose the ability to care for one another." The government was now supporting programs to counsel and care for AIDS patients, she said, but they had been slow to get off the ground. "Now they are sending out ladies in white dresses to teach us the things we used to know." What the social scientist was trying to tell me was that sexual behavior change may require more than a mere cognitive understanding of risk. It may require an emotional jolt, and home-based care programs can spark it by bringing people closer to the reality of AIDS.

In 2005, Busisiwe Ncama, a researcher in the School of Nursing at the University of KwaZulu-Natal in South Africa, measured the effects of a home-based care program on sexual behavior. She found that where the services were offered, people spoke more openly about the disease and patients disclosed their HIV status to more people. Strikingly, the social contacts of the patients—their friends, relatives, and coworkers—were more likely to say they had changed their sexual behavior and were now being faithful, compared to the social contacts of patients on a waiting list for the services. They were not more likely to say they used condoms, but since condom use in South Africa is often a marker for high-risk behavior, this could be a good sign. "It's a beautiful model," Ncama told me. "We wanted to show that home-based care benefited the whole community, not just the people receiving the services."[29]

On the way back to the United States, I stopped in South Africa, where the HIV rate was almost as high as it was in Botswana at the time. There I met Nkululeko Nxesi, then head of the Johannesburg-based National Association of People Living With HIV/AIDS, and I asked him the same question I had asked the Batswana social scientist. Why was the HIV rate so high, and why wasn't behavior changing, as it had in Uganda?

The problem was history, Nxesi explained. The upheavals of apartheid and the migrant labor system had destabilized the southern African family, and this made the epidemic much harder to fight. Uganda was different, he said. Whites never settled there in large numbers, never threw large numbers of poor blacks off their land, never subjected people to the degrading conditions of migrant labor or the racist contempt that stifled discussions of sexuality.

Uganda's climate is rainy and the soil fertile, and although this is changing, many Ugandans still make their living on the same small farms where their ancestors lived. As a result, Ugandans are more likely to live near their families and know their neighbors, and this probably enabled greater communication and a more compassionate, open response to AIDS. In southern Africa, drought and competition from commercial farms have pushed most Africans off the land and into anomic cities, and this had the opposite effect. It weakened people's sense of trust and undermined their relationships, their sense of community and their faith in themselves.

"I met a Ugandan AIDS worker a few years ago," Nxesi said, "and he told me, 'In Uganda we may not have highways and tall buildings, but we take care of our people.'" Nxesi had been thinking about that lately. "Down the line," he said, "we will realize that development is not only about how good your infrastructure is; it's also about the heart."

CHAPTER TEN

Forensic Science

IT WASN'T EASY to find Maxine Ankrah. Ankrah, an African-American woman of about seventy, lives in Mukono, a small town about thirty miles outside of Kampala. Her compound stands atop a steep hill covered in dry grass and tangled forest that some of the locals believe to be inhabited by ghosts. It took my taxi driver some time to find the place. When we stopped to ask directions, some people told us the house was in one direction, while others sent us the other way. We traversed Mukono's ramshackle main avenue several times and made a few hopeful detours up dirt tracks that dead-ended in the bush.

Eventually we arrived at the Ankrah Foundation, a vast conference center and hotel that sprawls across several steep terraces overlooking Mukono, Lake Victoria, and the smoky blue hills of Kampala in the distance. Ankrah's large one-story house stands on a ridge above the conference center. With its gravel driveway and well-groomed lawn it would not be out of place in a suburb in the United States. But the view that afternoon—the sun flashing off the lake, the clouds like giant blossoms, the first lights of the city shining through the haze of wood smoke and diesel fumes—could only be African.

I had come here to settle a score. For years, I had been trying to figure out how people's behavior had changed to bring down the HIV infection rate in Uganda. According to the public health literature I had read, this was supposed to be an agonizing process.[1] Deciding whether or not to use a condom or to have sex at all was said to be based on an individual risk-benefit calculation—with lust and social pressure in one column, and fear in the other.[2] This is what the textbooks said, but it didn't sound to me like what happened in Uganda. When millions of people changed their sexual behavior in the late 1980s and early 1990s, the process was sudden and highly coordinated, more like a phase transition in nature—when water turns to ice, for example, or when clouds condense and produce rain.

Ankrah had studied this mysterious process in great detail. In the late 1980s, the World Health Organization's Global Program on AIDS set out to study sexual behavior in different populations around the world. This giant "Kinsey-like" project was intended to determine the types of behavior that fuel the spread of HIV and predict the future course of the epidemic. Ankrah, then head of the department of social work and social administration at Makerere University, was chosen to conduct the survey in Uganda.

It was 1989, and Uganda had the highest HIV infection rate in the world at the time. Ankrah's research assistants fanned out into villages throughout the country and interviewed thousands of people about their sexual behavior: they asked them how many partners they had, whether they used condoms, and what they were doing to protect themselves from HIV.

Ankrah did not know it, but her timing was perfect. In 1989, the incidence of new HIV infections in Uganda had probably reached its peak and was just about to start falling. Her study was like a snapshot taken right at the start of Uganda's miraculous "phase transition" in behavior.

Ankrah wrote a report on her findings and presented it to WHO in 1993. I first heard about it some ten years later, but when I tried to find it, its whereabouts seemed shrouded in mystery. The results had never been published, and the report was not referred to in the scientific literature on AIDS in Uganda.[3] A small number of other researchers had copies of Ankrah's report, but they had been strangely reluctant to share it with me. Ankrah herself had retired from Makerere more than a decade previously, and had published little since then. I had almost given up hope of finding it before I finally managed to obtain a copy from a specialist research library in Canada.

When I read it, I felt as though a small stick of dynamite had gone off in my head. For years, a storm had been brewing about the Uganda AIDS "miracle." In 1995, epidemiologists at the Ugandan Health Ministry reported that the HIV rate in Uganda had been falling steadily for several years.[4] That same year, WHO commissioned a second "Kinsey-survey" of sexual behavior in Uganda. This survey was very similar to Ankrah's, but it provided a snapshot of Ugandan sexual behavior after the HIV decline had been under way for some time. By comparing the two surveys, it was now possible to figure out what behaviors had changed. Were people using more condoms? Were they abstaining from sex? Or what?

The answer could not have been more important. In 1995, there was no treatment for AIDS. Preventing the spread of the virus was the only hope for millions of poor people in Africa. Uganda was the only African country where the infection rate had declined, and the results of these two behavior surveys would potentially show how this had happened. This in turn could inform the design of prevention programs for other countries and determine the fate of hundreds of millions of dollars in donor funds for global AIDS programs.

The task of analyzing the two surveys fell to Michel Carael, a suave Belgian medical anthropologist who had worked for WHO's AIDS program for many years. In 1996, WHO closed down its AIDS program, and many former staff moved to the newly created Joint UN Program on AIDS (UNAIDS). In 1997, Carael, now head of UNAIDS's evaluation-and-monitoring unit, published an article in the prestigious medical journal *AIDS* describing the results of the Ugandan "Kinsey" surveys. He concluded that there had been steep rises in condom use and in the age of sexual debut, but almost no change in the proportion of people with multiple sexual partners.[5]

This article made few waves. After all, it seemed to confirm what many AIDS experts suspected at the time: condoms were the key to HIV prevention in Africa, and HIV infection rates would soon fall in other countries as condoms became increasingly available. International donor agencies, including USAID, were already pouring millions of dollars into condom programs in Africa, and UNAIDS and the World Bank had devoted considerable resources of their own to encouraging African governments to expand these programs, especially for so-called high-risk groups. Carael's article on the Uganda "Kinsey" surveys only seemed to provide further support for this policy.[6]

But by the end of the 1990s, some AIDS experts were beginning to worry. Condom sales in Africa were indeed soaring, but the HIV infection rate was soaring too.[7] Admittedly, HIV prevention programs in Africa were patchy, but even where condoms were heavily advertised and freely available, the HIV rate rose steeply, year after year.[8] Everywhere, that is, except Uganda. What had happened in Uganda? And why hadn't it happened anywhere else? A storm was brewing, and Maxine Ankrah's 1989 "Kinsey" survey was right in the eye of it.

Rand Stoneburner, an independent consultant who had worked as an epidemiologist with the World Health Organization in the early 1990s, became interested in the Uganda surveys at around the same time as UNAIDS did. He obtained a copy of Ankrah's report, along with the original data from the 1995 survey. But when he compared the results, he found something different from what Carael was finding. According to his calculations, partner reduction, not condoms or abstinence, was the most pronounced change in sexual behavior in Uganda during the 1990s.[9] Clearly, someone had made a mistake, either Ankrah or Carael. To get to the bottom of this, Stoneburner tried to obtain Ankrah's original data so he could do the analysis again. Ankrah had turned it over to UNAIDS officials, and Stoneburner claims he could not obtain it from them.

In 2001, anthropologist Daniel Halperin, joined USAID's Global Health Program as a senior HIV-prevention advisor. He immediately began scrambling to pull together every bit of data he could find on sexual behavior and HIV in Uganda. He hired consultants and organized seminars and flew out to Africa and interviewed health officials, researchers, and ordinary Ugandans. He read through academic journals and dug up old reports and surveys, including the original data from the Uganda "Kinsey" studies. Perhaps because he worked for the US government, he had little trouble obtaining them from UNAIDS. He immediately gave them to Stoneburner and to another statistician, and they both soon discovered that the mistake had been Carael's. The Uganda HIV decline had coincided not with a uniquely marked increase in condom use, but rather with a plunge in the proportion of people with casual sexual partners—meaning girlfriends, boyfriends to one-night stands, and visits to sex workers.[10]

Although condom use had risen in Uganda during the early 1990s, few people used them consistently, and in 1995 the fraction of people using them at all was similar to that in other countries such as Zambia and Zimbabwe, where the HIV infection rate had not fallen.

Halperin wasn't entirely surprised by these findings. Condoms weren't even widely available in much of Uganda until the mid-1990s, and the Ugandan government banned condom advertising until 1994. Uganda's AIDS campaigns emphasized Zero Grazing and avoiding "indiscriminate sexual relations," so it would be reasonable that many people would heed this advice.[11] Other surveys conducted in Uganda at the time had found that most people said they didn't trust condoms—they were afraid they would come off or break and might even become lodged inside a woman and kill her.[12] Instead, most respondents said they were protecting themselves from HIV by reducing their partners or "sticking to one."[13]

When I first heard about Halperin's research, I thought of Martina Morris's concurrency hypothesis and realized why condom promotion had had so little impact on the epidemic in East and Southern Africa. It's not that condoms don't work—they do—but that they are seldom used in long-term relationships. But in this part of Africa, that is where most transmissions occurs.

While condoms probably played some role in reducing HIV transmission in Uganda, it stood to reason that partner reduction would have had a more powerful effect. If the network of concurrent relationships serves as a superhighway for HIV, partner reduction would be like a sledgehammer, breaking up the highway into smaller networks, and destroying the "on-ramps"—the casual relationships that let HIV onto the superhighway in the first place. In theory, condoms could have created "roadblocks" on the superhighway, if only people used them consistently. But most condom use in Africa is inconsistent, especially in the longer-term relationships in which so much HIV transmission takes place.[14]

It turns out that partner reduction has played a key role wherever HIV rates have fallen—from the market towns of East Africa to the red-light districts of Asia to the gay enclaves of the United States.[15] In Thailand, HIV infection rates declined steeply during the 1990s. While condom use increased significantly, visits by men to sex workers also fell by 60 percent. Among gay men in the United States, HIV incidence fell by 75 percent during the 1980s. Part of this decline was attributable to the increased use of condoms, but partner reduction was even more important. In San Francisco, the proportion of gay men with multiple anal-sex partners fell by 60 percent between 1984 and 1988, and similar changes were recorded in New York, Chicago, and other cities.[16] In Zimbabwe and Kenya, the HIV rate began to decline in the late 1990s. Rates of condom use had been increasing throughout the decade, but it was not until rates of multiple partnerships began to decline that the HIV rate in these countries also fell. Meanwhile, in such countries as Botswana, South Africa, and Lesotho, where no partner reduction occurred in the 1990s and where condoms were emphasized as the main method of prevention, HIV rates rose. In all three countries, condoms were used more frequently than in Uganda when the HIV rate was falling.[17]

THROUGHOUT the 1990s and well into the 2000s, programs to encourage partner reduction were all but nonexistent in Africa—Uganda's Zero Grazing campaign and Kagera's more informal community-based counseling programs being among the few exceptions. Elsewhere, government planning documents, United Nations agency reports, AIDS awareness campaigns, and AIDS education curricula were strangely silent on the subject.[18] Even the Bush administration's "ABC," or "Abstain, Be Faithful, or Use Condoms," policy was weak on partner reduction. Although the fifteen-billion-dollar President's Emergency Plan for AIDS Relief earmarked $1 billion for abstinence-and-faithfulness programs, PEPFAR-funded programs on the ground in Africa overwhelmingly emphasized abstinence for unmarried youths; very few addressed adults or multiple partnerships directly. In 2004, Halperin and his colleagues put it this way in the *British Medical Journal*: "Partner reduction has been the neglected middle child of the ABC approach."[19]

In 2004, I sent the UNAIDS executive director, Peter Piot, an e-mail message in which I asked, among other things, why the agency had not done more to promote partner reduction, given the strong evidence for its effect on the epidemic in Uganda and elsewhere. He answered my other questions, but he didn't answer that one. When I asked Michel Carael about the silence on this topic, he denied that the agency played down fidelity in favor of condoms, but when I read through every UNAIDS document I could find that had been produced in the decade since the agency was established in 1996, I found almost no mention of partner reduction and none whatsoever of Zero Grazing. When independent consultants, some of them hired by UNAIDS itself, reported to the agency that partner reduction, not condoms, was largely responsible for Uganda's HIV decline, their reports were ignored or never made public.[20] The agency's "Best Practice" collection of briefing documents contains issues on condom programs, voluntary testing and counseling, STD treatment services, and many other things, but as of this writing, there was no Best Practice document about encouraging partner reduction or fidelity. It was only in 2006 that UNAIDS officials began to stress that the reduction of multiple sexual partnerships should be a key goal for AIDS prevention programs in southern Africa.[21]

BECAUSE OFFICIALS at UNAIDS refused to talk to me about it, I can only imagine why the agency overlooked the importance of partner reduction for so long. Admittedly, the subject of fidelity would not have been an easy one for Western advisors like Piot to broach. Perhaps the UN and USAID officials who helped design AIDS programs for African countries feared the topic implied racial stereotyping and moral judgment; perhaps they also felt it would be futile to try to change deeply rooted patterns of behavior. Playing down the role of infidelity—particularly on the part of men—in the spread of HIV may also have been politically expedient. For years, most African governments did little to address the AIDS crisis in their countries. Outside experts struggled to get African leaders to care about it at all. Perhaps recommending an AIDS policy that implied criticism of adult sexual behavior—behavior the elite policymakers might well have engaged in themselves—would have pushed these African bureaucrats further into denial.

The din of the culture wars in America was undoubtedly also a factor. The main proponents of faithfulness programs were conservative lobby groups such as Focus on the Family or Americans for a Sound AIDS Policy that were dogmatically opposed to contraception, comprehensive sex education, and abortion rights. As the political influence of these groups increased, along with the most conservative elements of the Republican party, the entire field of reproductive health became polarized between those calling for a return to "family values" and those, including most public health experts, who supported the right of every individual to determine his or her own sexual behavior. As the pitch of these disputes rose, sober scientific debate was often drowned out. At the fifteenth International AIDS Conference, in Bangkok, researchers presenting evidence about the importance of fidelity for HIV prevention were accused of "moralizing" and practically booed off the stage. Meanwhile, other participants engaged in a rowdy celebration of sexuality, safe and otherwise. In the corridors, actors in giant condom costumes twirled through the crowds and a trained elephant passed out free condoms with its trunk. Off-site, a topless go-go bar for the "HIV positive and proud to be sexy" had to close when another elephant trampled a conference-goer to death.

Shortly after the Bangkok AIDS conference, I spoke by phone to Malcolm Potts, former CEO of Family Health International, a U.S. government contractor that had been running condom campaigns in Africa for decades. He admitted that part of his own resistance to the idea of partner reduction or fidelity programs had been ideological.

"AIDS produces so much emotion," he said. "It's hard to look at the evidence. We've never really been on an even keel with respect to strategy. There was a sense that promoting fidelity must be totally wrong if it was a message favored by the Christian Right. We've made an emotion-based set of decisions," he lamented, "and people have suffered terribly because of that. And they will go on suffering. Everything we learn about the epidemic goes in slowly and is resisted on the way. I don't believe in God, but it is as though this virus was created by the devil himself."

Some experts maintain that encouraging partner reduction in Africa is pointless because most women are faithful anyway, and their fear of abusive partners prevents them from confronting men about their behavior.[22] While this is true for many women, some do have multiple partners, and partner-reduction messages are, in any case, an appropriate message for men. Obviously, if your one partner is HIV positive, you are in trouble unless you use condoms consistently. But when even a relatively small fraction of people reduce their partners, it can slow the virus down considerably. Only very high rates of consistent condom use would have a similar effect.

Encouraging partner reduction may even improve gender relations, since so much domestic violence involves accusations of infidelity. In Uganda and Kagera, men treated women differently in the wake of the Zero Grazing campaign. Reports of desertions and divorces declined, and one study suggested that domestic battery there, though frequent, was half as common as it was in Johannesburg, where no such behavior change had occurred.[23] Something similar took place during the 1980s in the gay communities of the United States; as rates of casual sex declined, gay men came to relate to one another differently, placing far more emphasis on friendship and commitment in sexual relationships than before.

WHEN I FIRST READ Daniel Halperin's report on the Uganda "Kinsey" surveys, conspiracy theories churned through my head. Here were two groups of scientists—Carael's group, based at the UN, and Halperin's, based within the U.S. government. Both groups had the same data, but had come to radically different conclusions. It was 2003, and the administration of George W. Bush was preparing to launch PEPFAR, a fifteen-billion-dollar program that would reserve one billion dollars for "abstinence and faithfulness" programs, to be carried out in part by the very evangelical Christian groups that had supported Bush's campaign. Were Halperin and USAID part of a government plot to cook up scientific evidence to support this policy? Or was Halperin correct, and it was Carael who had made the mistake?

In an effort to get to the bottom of this, I obtained the Uganda "Kinsey" surveys and asked Anne Case, a respected Princeton University economist, to analyze them again. She easily reproduced the finding of steep declines in casual partnerships, but could not reproduce Carael's results.[24]

When I finally obtained a copy of Maxine Ankrah's report on her 1989 "Kinsey" survey of Uganda, there was only one figure I wanted to check. The discrepancy between Carael's results and those of other groups could be traced to his calculation of the proportion of people with casual partners in 1989. Carael's figure was much lower than those of the other groups, and this made the drop between 1989 and 1995 seem much smaller than it was. Sure enough, Ankrah's figure was high—similar to Daniel Halperin's, Anne Case's, and Rand Stoneburner's—and it differed markedly from Carael's. The right answer had been in UNAIDS's hands all along. When I asked Michel Carael in an e-mail why his calculation differed so markedly from those of four other researchers working with the very same data, his reply suggested that he was as perplexed as I was.[25]

In his 2003 book *Rethinking AIDS Prevention*,[26] the anthropologist Edward C. Green attributes the neglect of partner-reduction campaigns like Zero Grazing to the bureaucratic inertia of the mainly European and American health experts who advise governments about how to draw up policies to fight AIDS. Many of today's vast international health bureaucracies were established in the 1970s, when rich governments, fearing a population explosion in developing countries, poured money into programs to market and distribute contraceptives in those countries. When AIDS began to spread, this approach was rapidly deployed. Public health officials quickly identified a package of programs and commodities that their organizations could deliver and foreign donors could pay for, including condoms, HIV testing kits, and STD services.[27]

When UNAIDS was established in 1996, the fledgling organization's most pressing concern was fundraising. But since the breakup of the Soviet Union, funding for all UN agencies had fallen sharply, as industrialized nations strove to secure bilateral alliances with developing countries, bypassing the UN altogether in many cases. The UN needed to convince donors that its own programs were necessary to fight the AIDS crisis, and it is possible that the implications of the findings from Uganda—that Africans had fought this epidemic on their own with frankness and common sense, compassion for the afflicted, and a shift in norms and attitudes surrounding sexual behavior and the rights of women—were the last thing UN bureaucrats would have wanted to hear. It would mean that fighting AIDS would require an approach with which they were quite unfamiliar, and for which their existing expertise might not be paramount.

The mid-1990s were a tumultuous time for the field of reproductive health. Since the 1950s, most work in this area had focused narrowly on population control and the promotion of contraceptives in developing countries, but during the 1980s, a global movement emerged that linked family planning to women's rights, including the right of women everywhere to determine their sexual and reproductive lives and to protect their sexual health. Many of the people who supported this movement were also working on the control of sexually transmitted diseases and AIDS. In September 1994, thousands of delegates came together at the UN population conference in Cairo, to call for more funding for family planning and other women's health programs, including AIDS programs. It was a hopeful time. Most funding for reproductive health programs traditionally came from the US government, and President Bill Clinton pledged to increase it.

Then in November 1994, just two months after the Cairo population conference, the Democrats lost control of Congress to a cadre of highly conservative Republicans whose very first act was to slash USAID's family planning budget by thirty-five percent. They then proceeded to launch a crusade to curtail abortion rights, install abstinence-only programs in schools, and otherwise promote what they considered "family values" but what many others considered an attack on women's rights. Until recently, few people outside of the reproductive health field realized how threatening the rise of the Christian right in Washington was to the future of the reproductive health and rights movement. But UNAIDS officials must certainly have been aware of this, because many of them had moved into the AIDS field from family planning. The new political tone in Washington threatened both their funding and the programs they believed in. It is possible that these officials, desperate for evidence to support programs involving contraceptives, including condoms, saw something in the Uganda data that simply was not there.

If so, they made a grave error, but as we will see in the next chapter, they were right to be worried. In 2003, the Bush administration began investing millions of dollars in evangelical Christian groups that disparage condoms and promote abstinence-until-marriage programs in Africa, even though research has consistently shown that these programs have no effect on the spread of sexually transmitted diseases. Meanwhile, African people were having to figure out how to prevent HIV for themselves.

Over dinner at Ankrah's house in Mukono, she told me about her life. She grew up in North Carolina at a time when black elites were at the center of the liberal Christian intellectual movement that would soon produce such civil rights leaders as Rosa Parks, Martin Luther King, Jr., and Ralph Abernathy. But Ankrah was looking to Africa. As a teenager in the 1940s, she had read *Cry the Beloved Country*, Alan Paton's stirring novel about a Zulu pastor in South Africa, and she set her sights on becoming a missionary. She eventually met and married a fellow theology student from Ghana. He took a job working with refugees for the World Council of Churches, and the couple, along with their two children, eventually settled in Uganda in 1974. Idi Amin was in power, and it was not uncommon to find bodies lying in the road, or to hear that friends had disappeared. The family would start worrying if everyone wasn't home by five. But they stayed on through that dark period, and Maxine eventually became head of the social work and social administration department at Makerere University. A remarkably popular professor, she trained thousands of Uganda's managers, NGO officials, and researchers. She also established Makerere's first women's studies department and helped lead Uganda's flourishing women's rights movement during the 1980s.

I asked Ankrah whether she had ever read Carael's 1997 article about the Uganda "Kinsey" surveys. She told me she had looked at it once or twice. But when she saw that her own report was not mentioned in it, even in the footnotes, she just put it aside. "It was as though I had been written out of history," she said. "It was the worst thing that ever happened to me in my professional career."

"Did you ever look at the results in Carael's paper and compare them to your own?"

"You know," she said, "I guess it's just my personality, but when bad things happen to me, I just put it out of my mind. I don't think I've even thought about that paper but once or twice in the past eight years."

I explained to her that three different statisticians, working independently, had been unable to reproduce Carael's results, and that the source of the problem could be found in his analysis of her own data from the 1989 "Kinsey" survey.

Ankrah was genuinely surprised. "I have no evidence that this was anything other than an honest mistake," I said, "but it's possible that the reason the WHO and UNAIDS never released your report or made any reference to it was that they did not like your results."

Ankrah shook her head. "You know, for a long time, I wondered whether there was something wrong with that study. But I was so careful. Some researchers just sit in their offices and shuffle papers, but I went out into the field to check on things myself all the time."

It was dark now, and the lights of the city in the distance seemed to merge with the stars like a shower of sparks. "If those people really were protecting their preconceived notions, they will have a lot to answer for," she said.

As evidence for the importance of partner reduction in the control of HIV has accumulated from studies all over the world, some public health officials have endeavored to shroud the history of the Uganda HIV decline in a fog of uncertainty. In 2005, the UNAIDS director, Peter Piot, told a reporter from the PBS *NOW* program that we may never know what happened to bring the HIV rate down in Uganda.[28] Even after USAID released its report on Uganda in 2003, UNAIDS documents continued to maintain that the main reason for the HIV decline in Uganda was condom use, not partner reduction. To make this argument, agency officials cited a study of sexual behavior conducted between 1994 and 2003, years after the decline in HIV incidence actually began.[29]

Some academics have even questioned whether any decline in infection rates actually occurred in Uganda.[30] Others claimed that the Ugandan surveys of sexual behavior—including Ankrah's—were flawed and impossible to interpret.[31] Still others suggested the decline may have had nothing to do with conscious changes in behavior at all. They speculated that the HIV decline was an inevitable consequence of the deaths of AIDS patients, or the end of Uganda's civil war in the mid-1980s, which brought greater social stability to the country.[32] But the fighting in southern Uganda ended in 1979, years before the AIDS epidemic exploded there during the early and mid-1980s. Although fighting continued farther north, the AIDS-affected districts in the south were relatively peaceful throughout that time. In any case, the relationship between war and the spread of HIV is far from simple. It is likely that war, rather than exacerbating the spread of HIV, can break up the sexual networks that sustain the spread of the virus. HIV infection rates tend to be higher in peaceful, prosperous countries such as Botswana and South Africa, and lower in such war-torn countries as the Congo and Somalia. The HIV rate soared in Mozambique when the civil war ended there in 1992, and the HIV rate fell in the Democratic Republic of Congo during the civil war between 1997 and 2003.[33] It does seem unlikely that the end of the war in Uganda would have been a more important factor in Uganda's HIV decline than the activism and compassion of the Ugandan people themselves, and the wisdom of their government, their doctors, and academics like Ankrah.

The view that the HIV decline in Uganda defied comprehension, and the dismissal of the work so many people in Uganda did to bring it about, was striking. Adriana Petryna, an anthropologist at the University of Pennsylvania, used the phrase "socially constructed nature of the unknown" to describe the response of Ukrainian government officials to the Chernobyl disaster—first suppressing statistics about the number of casualties, and then, after 1989, when the casualties could be blamed on the now defunct Soviet Union, inflating them into the millions.[34] Petryna's insights into the ways in which health statistics are sometimes fudged for political reasons is relevant to the AIDS crisis as well. "A catastrophe whose scale was unimaginable, difficult to map, and 'saturating' became manageable" through a particular dynamic of "non-knowledge," which enabled specialized authorities to deploy whatever programs they wished and obscure the mistakes they made.*

*In June 2007, the UNAIDS Program, which for years maintained that condom use, not partner reduction was the main reason for Uganda's HIV decline, posted a response to this book on its website, which stated:

"When solid evidence is presented, it informs publications released by UNAIDS. For example, Uganda's success in partner reduction was highlighted in the June 2004 technical report which has been on the UNAIDS website for three years."

But evidence for Uganda's success in partner reduction had been in UNAIDS hands since 1995. Why did the agency wait until 2004 to put this evidence on its website?

CHAPTER ELEVEN

God and the Fight Against AIDS

IN 2003, President George W. Bush asked Congress for fifteen billion dollars to fight AIDS in developing countries. The United States had long been criticized for not doing enough to fight the epidemic, and when the bill passed, many Americans, moved by images in the press of dying women and children, praised the administration.[1] But some were not sure. Much of the money was to go to church-affiliated charities or faith-based organizations, including some evangelical Christian groups that had very little experience with AIDS.

Traditional Catholic and Protestant churches had been running exemplary AIDS programs in Africa since the 1980s, but few evangelical Christian groups did so until much later. Indeed, as the deadly virus spread around the world, many evangelical Christians were silent or worse. Jerry Falwell called AIDS "God's judgment on promiscuity," and former senator Jesse Helms, a longtime congressional ally of the evangelicals, told *The New York Times* in 1995 that AIDS funding should be reduced because homosexuals contract the disease through their "deliberate, disgusting, revolting conduct." When lawmakers moved to amend the Americans with Disabilities Act to protect people with HIV from discrimination, some evangelical Christians lobbied against them. In a 2001 poll, only 7 percent of American evangelicals said they would contribute to a Christian organization that helped AIDS orphans.[2]

Shortly after the 2000 election, evangelical Christians began to change their tune. "We cannot turn away," Helms wrote of the global AIDS crisis that had by then killed twenty million people over two decades. "It is true," wrote Ken Isaacs of Samaritan's Purse, an evangelical charity run by Billy Graham's son Franklin, "that when we choose to act outside of God's mandate for sexual purity, we should be prepared to deal with the consequences. . . . However," he went on, "God calls Christians to tell others of the redeeming love of Christ and the eternal life they can have through him." Moreover, with so many people on the verge of death, "AIDS has created an evangelism opportunity for the body of Christ unlike any in history."[3]

It is worth noting that during the 2000 campaign, Bush, a born-again Christian, received considerable financial and popular support from evangelical Christian groups, including a number of those that would soon be receiving money from the President's Emergency Plan for HIV/AIDS Relief. Thus it may be no coincidence that some of the same people who once treated the issue of AIDS with indifference and scorn suddenly seemed so concerned about it. Do evangelical Christian groups have a role to play in fighting the AIDS epidemic? Maybe they do, but during the PEPFAR years, they were engaged in an unseemly battle with secular AIDS organizations over U.S. government contracts that threatened to derail what little progress had been made in combating the epidemic.

MOST OF THE $15 billion in the AIDS plan was to be spent on medical treatment for people with AIDS, but $1 billion was earmarked for HIV prevention programs that encouraged sexual abstinence. Many of the programs that received funding under the earmark were modeled on U.S. programs that strictly promote "abstinence-only until marriage." Since 1996, the U.S. government had spent hundreds of millions of dollars on such programs in American schools. These programs teach children that heterosexual intercourse within marriage is the only safe and acceptable form of sexual behavior. Teachers are barred from mentioning condoms and birth control—except their failure rates.

To date, every abstinence-only program that has ever been evaluated has failed to reduce rates of teen pregnancy or sexually transmitted diseases, and many experts feared that abstinence-only programs funded by the $1 billion earmark would have similarly dismal results in Africa.[4] Human Rights Watch maintained that such programs were not only ineffective, they also violated the right of young people to information about sexuality, condoms, and other methods of contraception that could save their lives.[5]

In justifying the $1 billion earmarked for abstinence programs, the U.S. administration cited Uganda's successful HIV prevention campaigns of the 1980s and early 1990s. When researchers at USAID began asking why HIV infection rates had fallen so rapidly in Uganda and not elsewhere in Africa, they concluded that these other countries had relied too heavily on condom promotion, while Uganda had a range of programs that encouraged abstinence, partner reduction, and faithfulness as well as condoms—a strategy that Bush administration officials named "ABC"—for Abstain, Be Faithful, or Use Condoms.[6]

During the congressional debates over the president's fifteen-billion-dollar AIDS bill, the virtues of ABC were hotly debated and, unfortunately, distorted. Right-wing Republicans argued in favor of earmarking funds for abstinence programs, while Democrats tried to defend funding for existing condom programs.

In the midst of the congressional debates, Uganda's first lady, Janet Museveni, flew to Washington and presented a formal letter to Republican lawmakers stating that abstinence was key to Uganda's success.[7] Her involvement helped secure the $1 billion abstinence-and-faithfulness earmark that appears in the final bill.

The Republicans justified the earmark by citing the work of a then little-known public health consultant named Edward C. Green, who, along with a small number of other experts, had been arguing for years that abstinence, faithfulness, and reductions in casual sex had been more important than condoms in Uganda.[8] The public health community largely ignored them, but now Green was a voice in the wilderness no longer. He had the ear of powerful evangelical Christians, who in turn had the ear of key congressmen and Bush advisors. Republican congressmen such as Joseph Pitts of Pennsylvania and Henry Hyde of Illinois claimed that Green's research supported abstinence-only-until-marriage programs, but it didn't. Green's claim that the battle against HIV in Africa could not be won with condoms alone was almost certainly correct. The role of abstinance, however, was not supported by the evidence.

While faithfulness and partner reduction were crucial to Uganda's success, abstinence probably had little to do with it. Between 1988 and 2001, as the national HIV rate fell by some 70 percent, the average age at which young Ugandan women started sexual activity rose by less than a year.[9] During the early 1990s, when the HIV decline was most rapid, Uganda's teenage-pregnancy rate, which even today is among the highest in the world, did not change at all. If abstinence among teenage girls had increased significantly, it would be expected that the teenage pregnancy rate would have fallen.[10] When I asked epidemiologists about this, they explained that abstinence among unmarried teenage girls did increase significantly in the early 1990s, yet marriage rates for that group also increased at the same time. Thus the proportion of all teenage girls who were sexually active changed little, but more girls were in committed relationships. This could explain why fewer of them became HIV positive even though roughly the same number became pregnant. Thus the HIV decline in this group resulted not from abstinence, but from increased faithfulness on the part of their male partners.

Some researchers theorize that early sexual debut is dangerous for girls because the immature genital tract is particularly vulnerable to infection,[11] but the evidence for this is unclear. In Western countries, girls who lose their virginity at young ages are more prone to STDs, but in Uganda, the age of sexual debut seems to have little effect on a young woman's risk of HIV. One study found that young women who abstain from sex until age twenty have the same risk of HIV at age twenty-four as young women who first had sex in their teens.[12] Young girls are probably placed at risk less by their fragile genitals than by who they are. In America, girls who have sex at young ages are often troubled runaways or victims of abuse. In Uganda, early sexual debut is more normative and is not necessarily a marker for promiscuous or "deviant" behavior.

WHILE AMERICA'S congressmen were ironing out the details of the new AIDS bill, Uganda's leaders were gearing up to launch a moral purity campaign of their own.

In 2004, First Lady Janet Museveni sponsored a march for virginity through the streets of Kampala, and the king of the Baganda, Uganda's largest tribe, pledged that all female virgins would receive a free washing machine on their wedding day. Not to be outdone, leaders of the Karimojong tribe called for a ban on miniskirts, even though Karimojong people traditionally wear no clothes at all. In a 2001 speech, President Yoweri Museveni claimed that abstinence until marriage was a traditional African value. Before colonial times, if an unmarried girl became pregnant, "the punishment then for the boy and girl was death," he told an audience of AIDS researchers. "The girl would be tied in dry banana leaves, set on fire, and rolled down a cliff, and the boy speared." These traditions broke down when the Europeans took over and society became permissive, he said. This is when syphilis, gonorrhea, and eventually HIV began to spread.[13]

Tyrannical African leaders—from Kenya's Daniel arap Moi to Malawi's Hastings Banda to Zimbabwe's Robert Mugabe—have long blamed Western decadence for Africa's problems. Even Idi Amin took time out from murdering cabinet ministers and religious leaders to crack down on miniskirts and makeup and lecture the nation about morality.[14] Therefore, it was worrying that Museveni, whose undemocratic tendencies have been noted, was drawing increasing attention to the personal morality of others.[15]

The renewed emphasis on abstinence was puzzling for other reasons. While virginity until marriage may have been valued in the old days, faithfulness in marriage never was. Uganda's traditional chiefs and kings had hundreds and sometimes thousands of wives and concubines; polygamy, of both a formal and informal nature, remains extremely common in Uganda; and the sexual affairs of President Museveni himself are a frequent subject of gossip, as are those of other government officials, including the men and women who set the nation's AIDS policy. Among members of Parliament, sexual harassment by male colleagues is a fact of life for many female MPs,[16] and prostitution, though officially illegal, flourishes in Kampala's good hotels, including those owned by close associates of the president and his wife. Traditional herbal "sexual activators" are sold openly on the street, along with pornographic magazines featuring serialized novellas such as *The Randy Professor* and *Angela the Sugar Mummy*.[17] Sexual matters such as breast implants and premature ejaculation are fervently discussed in mainstream newspapers and on the radio. According to police reports, among the most frequent culprits in cases of defilement—or sex with a minor—are Christian pastors, along with teachers and policemen. In 2004, a local nongovernmental organization urged pastors to use condoms because they were endangering their congregations.

The preaching about abstinence in Uganda thus seemed at odds with the culture. But Africa's masks and secrets are often impenetrable to outsiders. Was this a charade to impress the right-wing bureaucrats in the office of the U.S. global AIDS coordinator who would oversee the spending of the $1 billion earmarked for abstinence programs?

I ARRIVED IN Uganda in September 2004 with this question in mind. As I usually do, I stayed at Makerere University in Kampala. It was the beginning of the school year and students were arriving from all over the country. The freshmen dressed in the formal way of 1940s American college men and women, in long skirts or slacks and buttoned-up white shirts with collars. Each year, upperclassmen at Lumumba Hall, a men's dormitory, welcome the freshmen by displaying their dorm mascot on the grass in front of the building. The mascot is a life-sized sculpture of a man, made from scrap metal, with a large drainpipe for a phallus. In order to educate their peers about HIV, the students dress the phallus in a new condom every day, and a box of fresh condoms—free for the taking—is placed at its feet. "He symbolizes the culture of our hall of residence," one of the students explained to me. "He has girlfriends, but he always uses a condom." One afternoon shortly after I arrived, a pastor from a nearby church marched up to the statue, removed its condom, set a match to the box of free condoms, and then prayed over the fire: "I burn these condoms in the name of Jesus!" he boomed, and then promised each student a free Bible.

Uganda is in the throes of a born-again Christian revival. With the arrival of the first missionaries in the nineteenth century, most Ugandans became either Catholic or Protestant, but during the past ten years, thousands—perhaps millions—of them have been swept out of their dusty, austere churches into bright new amphitheaters that even on weekdays are filled with music and prayer and swaying worshipers speaking in tongues. Born-again Christianity is catching on throughout sub-Saharan

Africa, from the slums of South Africa to the windswept plains of Masailand, but Uganda's Christian traditions, and its position bordering heavily Muslim Sudan, Kenya, and Tanzania, have made it a magnet for American evangelical missionaries, who have poured huge sums into the country during the past ten years.

In the major towns, "crusades"—massive religious gatherings—are held nearly every week, often attended by thousands of people. At one of these events, I watched a pastor in a silk suit and patent-leather shoes warn an enormous crowd against the sins of fornication, homosexuality, pornography, and "nude dancing"—the striptease shows that had recently become popular in the capital. He healed people's livers, backaches, and broken legs, passed around gigantic collection baskets, and jitterbugged vigorously to Christian rock hymns, accompanied by a chorus of Ugandan youths. Around one-third of the Ugandan population has been "born again" in the past decade, and new churches were springing up in warehouses, shacks, school auditoriums, and village clearings. At traffic circles in the center of Kampala, men in black suits waving Bibles preached through glimmering exhaust fumes to stalled commuters. Two of Uganda's four TV stations beamed in religious programs from around the world, twenty-four hours a day, and quotations from scripture were becoming part of everyday speech.

SHORTLY AFTER I arrived in Uganda, I paid a visit to Martin Ssempa, the pastor who burned the condoms at Makerere. He is an authority on abstinence education in Africa and has given presentations at USAID and led the prayer at Mrs. Museveni's March of Virgins. Ssempa ran a church and sponsored a Billy Graham–style sex-and-alcohol-free abstinence rally every Saturday night on Makerere's campus. In his sermons, he condemned homosexuality, pornography, condoms, certain kinds of rock music, and women's rights activists, who, he said, promoted lesbianism, abortion, and the worship of female goddesses.[18] He told me that Satan worshipers held meetings under Lake Victoria, where they were promised riches in exchange for human blood, which they collected by staging car accidents and kidnappings. In his headquarters, just down the hill from Makerere, there was a special room for exorcisms.

Ssempa was stocky and bald, with a broad, avuncular smile. He wore colorful Hawaiian-style shirts and wire glasses. Although born in Uganda, he had spent years in the United States and his Ugandan accent had a warm American twang. We talked about Satan, homosexuals, pornography, and other sins, and he asked me whether I had any idea where he could obtain a million dollars to buy land for his church. Our meeting was interrupted by numerous phone calls. As I listened and took notes, he shouted in English and Luganda. There had been some sort of crisis. Population Services International, the U.S.-based contractor that had been running condom campaigns in Uganda and other African countries for years, had recently received U.S. government funding to carry out an abstinence program. PSI had used the money to produce a new comic book in which the main characters, a teenage boy and girl, flirt with each other, make out on a couch at her parents' house, and then decide to abstain from sex. In one of the frames, they walk by a condom billboard on the street.

"Look at this!" Ssempa yelled, pointing at the drawing of the condom billboard. "It's horrible. You can't promote condoms and abstinence at the same time!" It would only confuse young people, he said, and send the message that it was really OK to be promiscuous.

"They won't get away with it. I have spoken to the first lady's office," he told me. "We need to ensure that George W. Bush's money gets into the right hands, those who are doing abstinence-*only*, as determined by the legislation."

In the fall of 2004, Ssempa and his congregation prayed together for a Bush victory in the U.S. presidential election. I was reminded of the African bureaucrats who played the United States and the Soviet Union off against each other during the Cold War. This time, it was a battle over moral rather than political ideology but, just as in the Cold War, a rich country was using foreign aid to fight its battles in developing countries. Now that there was finally a huge amount of money for AIDS programs in Africa, a scramble for it appeared to be under way in Uganda, and faith-based groups like Ssempa's were going to considerable lengths to get rid of the organizations that had been receiving U.S. government contracts for years, especially organizations like PSI that promoted condoms.

This was worrying because condoms did help to control Uganda's epidemic. HIV infection rates fell most rapidly during the early 1990s, mainly because people had fewer casual sexual partners. However, since 1995, the proportion of men with multiple partners had increased, but condom use increased at the same time, and this must be why the HIV infection rate remained low.[19]

But condom programs in Uganda were now threatened. Under pressure from both the Ugandan and U.S. governments, billboards advertising condoms, for years a common sight throughout the country, were taken down in December 2004. Radio ads with such slogans as "Life-Guard condoms! Ribbed for extra pleasure!" were to be replaced with messages from the cardinal of Uganda and the Anglican archbishop about the importance of abstinence and faithfulness within marriage. In October 2004, Engabu, a highly popular Ugandan condom brand, was pulled from the shelves when a faulty consignment was discovered. The government then insisted that all condoms entering the country be subjected to additional quality-control tests. However, Uganda did not have the equipment to carry out such tests, and this resulted in a shortage of condoms throughout the country.[20] Then, in 2005, PSI's U.S. government contract was not renewed.

Meanwhile, American evangelical Christian magazines such as *Citizen*, published by Focus on the Family, a Washington, D.C., organization that lobbies against gay rights and abortion, and *World*, edited by Marvin Olasky, a Bush advisor, claimed that USAID was pouring money into condom programs in Uganda and ignoring abstinence and monogamy, which, according to the articles, are the only interventions that really work.[21]

CONDOMS HAVE a controversial history in Uganda, and official attitudes toward them have tended to shift with the ebb and flow of U.S. government funds. During the 1980s and early 1990s, condoms were not widely available in Uganda, and many people did not believe they really worked. Religious leaders denounced them as immoral and "un-African." The Zero Grazing campaign launched by the Ugandan Ministry of Health in 1986 did not promote condoms.[22]

Then, in the early 1990s, health experts at USAID, the World Bank, and other international agencies, skeptical that the Zero Grazing campaign would work, set out to make condoms more appealing, not only to ordinary Ugandan citizens, but also to policymakers and religious leaders. The agencies began funding condom social-marketing programs, and at the same time they increased funding for the Ministry of Health, the Uganda AIDS Commission, and various church-affiliated organizations run by some of the leaders who most vocally denounced condoms. This new funding had the effect of toning down public criticism of condoms. Meanwhile, the Zero Grazing campaign was gradually phased out.

By the late 1990s, international contractors that specialize in social marketing, such as PSI, the publishers of the comic book that Ssempa complained about, were selling hundreds of millions of condoms each year in Africa. Organizations like PSI don't profit directly from the condoms they sell, but they do obtain lucrative government contracts to carry out social-marketing programs. Uganda's social-marketing campaigns were especially dynamic, and, as the Makerere student informed me, condoms had become part of Ugandan culture.

Then, shortly after Mrs. Museveni returned from Washington in 2003, where she had helped Republicans lobby for the $1 billion appropriated for abstinence programs, Ugandan officials resumed denouncing condoms after a ten-year hiatus. In a speech at an international meeting of AIDS experts in 2004, President Museveni said AIDS was "a moral problem" caused by "undisciplined sex," and that condoms should be reserved for prostitutes. Mrs. Museveni even accused those who promote condoms of racism. "They think Africans cannot control their sexual drives," she said in a speech in 2004. "We will prove them wrong!" She warned young people that organizations that promote condoms are only after their money. On a similar note, the information minister, James Butoro, also a born-again Christian, accused condom social-marketing organizations of "profiteering."

Mrs. Museveni's Uganda Youth Forum (UYF) began receiving U.S. funding to promote abstinence-only in 2004.[23]

WHEN I WAS IN UGANDA, a large number of new faith-based abstinence organizations like Ssempa's Campus Alliance to Wipe Out AIDS (CAWA) and Mrs. Museveni's UYF were springing up around the country, including the Glory of Virginity Movement (GLOVIMA), the Family Life Network (FLN), and American groups such as True Love Waits. Like Ssempa, officials of these organizations were hoping to receive U.S. funding from the $1 billion abstinence-and-fidelity earmark. U.S. law forbids organizations receiving federal funds from evangelizing, but every abstinence event I attended involved much praying and discussion of Jesus. As Human Rights Watch pointed out, it was sometimes hard to tell what the aim of these organizations actually was—preventing AIDS or saving souls.[24]

While I was in Uganda, I met Emily Chambers, the attractive twenty-six-year-old woman in charge of AIDS programs in East Africa for Samaritan's Purse, the charity run by Franklin Graham that had just received a multimillion-dollar U.S. government contract to carry out HIV prevention programs. Among other things, the organization planned to train African Christian pastors to promote abstinence.

I knew that Samaritan's Purse was in favor of abstinence-only education, but inevitably some of the pastors they planned to train would be approached by people wanting to know more about condoms. I asked Ms. Chambers whether Samaritan's Purse would recommend that pastors refer such people to other organizations. "We don't know about that yet," she said. But when I asked her about the role of faith in abstinence programs, her eyes opened wide. "It's *huge*," she exclaimed. "Abstinence is near impossible without the helping hand of the Lord."

Later, I met a group of girls who were members of GLOVIMA, a Ugandan abstinence club run by an evangelical church. When I asked them how they intended to ensure that their future husbands would be faithful to them, only one hand went up. A little girl in a tartan dress stood up very straight and said, "I will pray for him."

I WAS SORRY that no American or Ugandan was trying to revive the Zero Grazing campaign, because that program probably contributed more to the decline in Uganda's HIV rate than either abstinence or condoms. The Zero Grazing message recognized the vital importance of partner reduction but also the difficulty of promoting lifelong monogamy in a culture in which polygamy and informal long-term concurrent relationships were common. Ugandan health officials knew that it would have been unrealistic to insist that all men abandon their extra wives and mistresses, many of whom depended on the men for the opportunity to work on the land and for money and consumer goods for themselves and their children. Zero Grazing was a compromise, and its real message was this: "Try to stick to one partner, but if you have to keep your long-term mistresses, concubines, and extra wives, at least avoid short-term casual encounters with bar girls and prostitutes. Also, you mustn't casually seduce and exploit young women, who may be susceptible to your charms and wealth."

Even religious leaders embraced the Zero Grazing slogan. In the 1980s, a Catholic church van was seen around the capital with "Zero Grazing in the Diocese of Kampala" emblazoned on the side. Unlike the Catholics, the evangelicals would make no such concessions to the culture.

In 2004, I asked David Apuuli, the affable head of the Uganda AIDS Commission, why the government did not revive the Zero Grazing campaign, which seemed to have been so effective. He giggled, poked me with his elbow, and winked theatrically. "You know what that was all about, don't you?" What Dr. Apuuli meant, but did not say, was this: "What kind of an idiot are you? What do you think the Christians are going to say if we start talking about Zero Grazing? Zero Grazing recognized that polygamy, both formal and informal, was normative and legitimate. That would not fly in the current political and religious climate. Mrs. Museveni would have a fit, and the Bush administration, which pours billions of dollars a year into Uganda, would be very dismayed if the country they hold up as a triumph of abstinence education started promoting Zero Grazing."

THERE MAY BE other reasons why Zero Grazing had not been revived. For one thing, there was no multimillion-dollar bureaucracy to support it. For condoms, there were the large contractors like PSI, with headquarters in Washington and thousands of employees all over the world. Abstinence-only education was supported by a similarly well-endowed network of faith-based and abstinence-only education organizations, mainly in the United States. Zero Grazing was devised by Ugandans in the 1980s, when they were facing a terrible problem and had to deal with it largely on their own. Now that AIDS is a multibillion-dollar enterprise, donors with vast budgets and highly articulate consultants offer health departments in impoverished developing countries a set menu of HIV prevention programs, which consists of either abstinence education or condom social marketing or HIV testing and other services. Beleaguered health officials have no time, money, or will to devise programs that might better suit their cultures.

Another reason why abstinence programs are favored over Zero Grazing may have to do with the sexual hypocrisy common to all known societies. The revival of interest in virginity in Africa is not always driven by American money. In southern Africa, many communities have revived the custom of virginity testing, which has become so popular that it is sometimes carried out en masse, at football stadiums. Meanwhile, Swaziland's King Mswati III decreed in 2001 that all young, unmarried Swazi women should abstain from sex for five years and wear special tassels in their hair, as a signal to men to leave them alone. Fines were imposed on subjects who broke the rule.

Like other abstinence programs, Swaziland's was not a success. In 2004, three years after the decree, over 25 percent of all Swazi adults were HIV positive—the highest HIV infection rate in the world at the time. Shortly after these grim statistics were released, the government abandoned the virginity program, and young women were advised by the Ministry of Health to throw away their tassels.

One reason the program might have failed was that while the king frowns on premarital sex, he tolerates polygamy, which is far more dangerous. The king himself had thirteen wives at the time, and chose a new bride each August at the annual Reed Dance Festival, where thousands of topless girls in traditional grass skirts dance and sing his praises. In 2003, when the king chose a seventeen-year-old, he fined himself one cow, in line with his own ban on sex with underage girls.[25]

The South African anthropologist Suzanne Leclerc-Madlala attributes the revival of interest in virginity to an increasing sense among elders, especially men, that they are losing control of young people and women. All around they see worsening economic and social conditions and the horror of AIDS, and because they are only human, they blame this state of affairs on the loosening morals of increasingly educated, urbanized women and young people, rather than examining how their own behavior also contributed to these problems.[26]

AFTER PASTOR SSEMPA showed me the controversial PSI comic book, he unfurled a poster produced by the same group, depicting a young African woman singing in a choir. She was wearing a cassock and there were other young people singing in the background. The caption read, "Lucy is a beautiful girl. She's a good daughter and the best friend. She always makes her family proud. And she has HIV. Anyone can catch HIV, everybody can prevent it."

"I hate this poster," Ssempa sneered. "It says, 'If you want to make your parents proud, go out and get HIV.' Proud indeed! I'd like to meet that girl's parents."

The poster was part of PSI's Trusted Partner campaign. Studies had shown that one of the reasons people don't use condoms is that they trust their sexual partners and don't believe that they might be HIV positive. The poster was intended to remind people that everyone is at risk, even choir girls with loving parents, but it also sent a powerful message about the cruelty of AIDS-related stigma. This is what Ssempa objected to.

"AIDS is a disease of promiscuity," Ssempa said sternly. "Sure, there are minor exceptions. Some faithful women are infected by their husbands, but at the root of it, you always find the same thing: promiscuity! This thing of fighting stigma is a foreign concept," he went on. "It was brought to us by the UN for World AIDS Day. It has no relevance here."

"The evangelicals have that stigma," a Ugandan woman living with HIV told me later. "According to the way they preach, you feel they are cursing us sometimes. As if we got it because we wanted it."

When I spoke to Emily Chambers, the HIV/AIDS coordinator for Samaritan's Purse, I asked her how her organization reconciles the need to fight stigma with the tendency of pastors like Ssempa to associate AIDS with what they consider "sin." She explained that the philosophy of Samaritan's Purse was "forgiveness" and recounted Jesus' defense of the adulterous woman, "Let him who is without sin cast the first stone." But she admitted it was difficult. "We don't expect that"—meaning stigmatizing remarks—"won't happen."

How the Christian message about AIDS had changed, I thought. When I was in Kagera, where the HIV infection rate had fallen steeply during the early 1990s, I asked Sister Debora Brycke, the Lutheran missionary who founded Huyawa, the region's oldest and largest AIDS organization, what pastors had said about the epidemic then. "There were some sermons in the church," she explained, "but mostly we just did it with small groups, people waiting for a bus or in a market. Even in a bar—it is safe, if it is not too late. We told people that parents were dying and children were being left alone and behavior change was the only way out. The secret of teaching is that you can't scream at people," she said. "You have to use a special approach. I call it love. If people really feel you care for them, you can be quite open."

AFTER TWO WEEKS spent visiting pastors, watching the televangelist Joyce Meyer's sermons in my hotel room, and shopping at stores with names like Trust in God Hardware, I felt I needed a change of scene. One of the women's dorms on Makerere campus had a reputation. "Go there some Saturday night," said a professor I knew. "That's when the men in their big cars come and pick up the girls and take them out. Sometimes you just see men sitting in front of the entrance, waiting. They call it 'benching.'" The dorm in question wasn't far from where I was staying, so one Saturday night a friend and I walked over. As we approached, we saw some people sitting along the edge of the parking lot, facing the entrance of the building. At first we thought they were "benchers," but about half of them were women, their eyes glistening with tears. They were watching a Christian movie about a girl who has just told her boyfriend she is suffering from cancer. We watched as they prayed together, and then we spotted a couple walking away from the dorm. As we drew closer to find out what was going on, my friend realized they were discussing the Gospel according to John.

Afterward, we wandered over to Pastor Ssempa's abstinence rally at the Makerere campus swimming pool. There must have been three thousand people there and we couldn't get past the huge overflow crowd on the street outside. The show consisted of skits, comedy routines, testimonies from former sinners, prayers, and thundering Christian rock music sung in local languages by Ugandan stars. The entire audience swayed together, dancing and singing and waving at the night sky. The music was so powerful, the ground itself seemed to tremble.

As the music became increasingly ecstatic, a few members of the audience began to twitch and shake in a peculiar way. Then a woman some distance away from us began to writhe quite violently and, in a fit that might be described as orgasmic, she suddenly flew backward into the crowd and had to be pulled up by her friends.

"She was battling the spirits," one of the students explained to us.

Afterward, as I was walking back to my hotel alone, the rumble of the music still in my ears, I departed from the crowds of students and followed a dark road lit only by the moon and the occasional approach of slow-moving, yellow-eyed cars. Many of the sidewalks on campus are broken, and here and there the smashed concrete opens into dark, stinking sewage channels below, as if they had been torn open by some spasm of the earth. Flocks of bats hung from the jungly black branches of bottlebrush and eucalyptus trees, and giant scavenger birds loomed on the crests of the trees, their long, stiff beaks chattering like tom-toms. Disco music surged from numerous nearby bars, and images of nude dancers and homosexuals and pornographers and beer-addled prostitutes merged with the memory of the hysterical woman at the rally.

Sexuality truly does belong to the world of magic and unreason. It is impossible to plan and control it totally. We were made that way. If sex were an entirely rational process, the species would probably have died out long ago.[27] But the delirious, illogical nature of sex makes setting a realistic HIV prevention policy very difficult. Cheerful, sexy condom ads that fail to address the real dangers of AIDS may promote a fatal carelessness; but an exclusive emphasis on abstinence until marriage may well lead to an even more dangerous hysterical recidivism. The genius of the Zero Grazing campaign was that it recognized both the universal power of sexuality and the specific sexual culture of this part of Africa, and it gave people advice they could realistically follow.[28]

CHAPTER TWELVE

When Foreign Aid Is an ATM

On a visit to Uganda in February 2006, I stopped by the Kampala offices of the Global Fund to Fight AIDS, Tuberculosis and Malaria. The Geneva-based multibillion-dollar health agency had been launched with great fanfare in 2002, shortly after the first UN General Assembly Special Session on AIDS. It was hailed as a transparent, efficient aid mechanism that would deliver the elements of the AIDS prevention and treatment package prescribed at that meeting, including HIV testing services, condoms, and AIDS treatment with antiretroviral drugs. Donor governments, including the United States and the United Kingdom, as well as private philanthropists such as Bill Gates, had so far given roughly five billion dollars to the Global Fund to support some exemplary programs around the world. The funding was to be controlled by local actors, including officials from government and nongovernmental organizations, and would thus avoid both the inevitable politicization of bilateral programs like USAID and the occasionally shoelace-tripping bureaucracy of the UN agencies.

The Global Fund had thus far disbursed $54 million to Uganda, but in August 2005, the auditing firm PricewaterhouseCoopers concluded that the whereabouts of much of this money was unknown. No one knew exactly how much was missing, but grapevine estimates ranged into the tens of millions of dollars. According to the report and to local newspaper accounts, some ended up in the private bank accounts of government officials. Some was spent on bogus trips abroad to meetings and "workshops." Some was spent on campaign junkets by ministers seeking reelection. Some may have been spent on campaigns for the lifting of presidential term limits so that Uganda's President Yoweri Museveni could run in the country's upcoming elections. Some was simply disbursed to government cronies, "to spend as the need arose."[1]

Shortly after the Pricewaterhouse report was issued, the Global Fund temporarily suspended all disbursements to Uganda. Ugandan authorities responded promptly by sacking the entire project management unit, the local body overseeing the grant, including the receptionists and cleaning ladies. A new team was hired and a commission of inquiry was set up to find out how much money was stolen, who stole it, and what they did with it.

When I visited the local Global Fund offices in Kampala, four armed guards stood at the entrance, and the new receptionists were reading Bibles. It was heartening to see how seriously the Ugandans were taking the matter, but none of this could erase the fact that an enormous act of international goodwill that might not come again had been squandered. The shenanigans had fatal consequences. Programs to deliver treatment for the three diseases were behind schedule. One Ugandan complained on an Internet blog that his child almost died of malaria because all the health workers at the local clinic were at a "workshop" in the capital or out of the country. In Kampala, I heard the officials involved in the scandal referred to as "night dancers," evil spirits of Ugandan mythology who haunt graveyards and feed on the dead.[2]

When I was in the country, the Global Fund commissioners were questioning the director of the Uganda Center for Accountability, which received $120,000 from the Global Fund to train local community-based organizations in financial management. The director, Mr. Teddy Cheeye, a gentle-looking man wearing a patterned dashiki shirt, was also an official in Uganda's main spy agency. Bank records show that two days after the Global Fund money was transferred to the Center for Accountability in March 2005, Cheeye withdrew $33,000 and bought a plane ticket to China. With a bemused, insouciant air, as if to say "Who, me?" Cheeye told the commissioners that he mixed up his accounts and the plane ticket had nothing to do with the Global Fund money. When asked for evidence that he had used the Global Fund money for management training, Cheeye produced a sheaf of gas-station chits to prove he had been traveling to workshops all over the country. In Uganda, gas-station attendants write the registration number of the vehicle on receipts. The commissioners checked with the motor-vehicle registry and discovered that the vehicle Mr. Cheeye said he used to drive to these workshops was a 1977 Caterpillar tractor.

All this was personally depressing to me, because I love Uganda. When it became the first African country to record a nationwide decline in HIV rates during the 1990s, perhaps a million lives were saved. The heated debate about whether this resulted mainly from abstinence, condom use, or (my preferred explanation) pragmatic avoidance of casual sex had obscured the fact that what really made the difference was none of these things in themselves. At a time when public health experts claimed no magic formula for fighting AIDS, Ugandans organized their own diverse and vibrant responses to the crisis. Yoweri Museveni himself was deeply concerned about AIDS, and his pragmatic statements and policies both clarified the nature of the threat and enabled community-based programs to flourish.

Now some members of Museveni's National Resistance Movement party seemed to be mistaking the Global Fund for an all-you-can-eat buffet. The commission heard that three NRM cabinet ministers working for the Ministry of Health had colluded with a local bank to fix the exchange rates for Global Fund disbursements, hired unqualified relatives for highly paid posts, issued grants to nongovernmental organizations consisting only of a post office box, and used Global Fund money for political campaigns. The ministers denied all responsibility and accused the commission of disloyalty to Uganda for even making the allegations. President Museveni himself warned that he might not accept the commission's conclusions. "Some of those commissions are not serious," he told Uganda's *New Vision* newspaper.[3]

This was the same President Museveni who had said in a speech fifteen years earlier, "Every Ugandan should ask themselves the question, 'What am I doing to make the lives of people with AIDS more livable? What assistance have I rendered to these people today? This week? This year?'"[4] Had the president and his party really forsaken the cause of fighting AIDS? If so, why? The answer, if it can ever be known, lies tangled in Uganda's recent history and contemporary patterns of foreign aid.

EVERY TIME I visit Uganda, I am amazed at how rapidly it is changing. When I left Uganda for England in 1995, the concrete buildings in downtown Kampala were still streaked with filth and riddled with bullet holes from the civil war of the 1980s. Construction cranes, immobile since the days of Idi Amin, hung over the skyline among the minarets of half-finished mosques, relics of Amin's failed program to Islamicize this deeply Christian country. There were building lots filled with rubble and piles of rotting banana peels, fed upon by giant marabou storks, scavengers with bald pink gullets shaped like the trap under a sink.

A decade later, Kampala's once-derelict streets were lined with freshly painted shops and new hotels and glass office buildings had risen in the center of town. The marabou storks were still there, but the paralyzed construction cranes were gone. Uganda is one of the few countries where Structural Adjustment, the World Bank's economic program based on economic liberalization and privatization, civil-service reform, and reduced government spending, has been moderately successful.[5] The GDP grew by about 6 percent a year throughout the 1990s, and Uganda was now exporting coffee, sesame seeds, fish, vanilla beans, tea, cotton, and other commodities to the rest of the world. According to the World Bank, the number of people living in poverty in Uganda had fallen from 56 percent in 1992 to 38 percent in 2004. Poverty remained severe in many areas, especially in the north, where a brutal civil war continued. But for many Ugandans life was better than it had been in more than a generation.

This new prosperity owed as much to foreign aid as it did to economic performance. More than half of Uganda's roughly $1.5 billion government budget was paid for by donors, including the World Bank, the U.S. and U.K. governments, and others. Nearly all health spending was donor funded, including some 90 percent of the fifty million dollars spent on AIDS in Uganda each year—amounting to nearly a third of the country's entire health budget for this one disease alone.

AIDS funding began to ramp up in the early 1990s, and by 2006, the fruits of this spending were everywhere to be seen. When I am in Kampala, I often take walks around the Mulago Hospital grounds. On the hill where I used to work, American university research teams and pharmaceutical companies have refurbished the old labs and clinical blocks and built new ones devoted to AIDS treatment and research. Inside these buildings, computers hum and nurses and doctors in white coats swish by. In one of the labs there is now a machine that can perform in seconds the experiment that took me half a day when I ran it by hand back in 1993.

Many of the exemplary AIDS organizations begun in the 1980s and early 1990s have expanded. Condoms are more widely available, and AIDS testing and treatment services have vastly improved. The AIDS Support Organization today receives $2 million annually from PEPFAR and other donors to deliver antiretroviral drugs to thousands of Ugandans with AIDS. TASO's headquarters are in a brand-new three-story office block, and when I stopped in once looking for someone I knew, I met a young man who asked me where I was from. When I told him, he said he was taking antiretrovirals paid for by PEPFAR. "We are so grateful to you Americans," he said. "I owe my life to you."

Uganda's AIDS programs are now managed by a World Bank–funded system of district AIDS committees (DACs), subcounty AIDS committees (SACs), village AIDS task forces (VATs), and even resistance AIDS task forces (RATs). Every government ministry, from Education to Labor to Defense, now has an AIDS budget. The big hotels in the capital play host to a perpetual round of AIDS-related conferences and workshops, and the streets are jammed with the vehicles of AIDS NGOs.

Although the AIDS money has been welcome, some Ugandans worried that it contributed to what they call the "Pajero culture"—a reference to the fancy four-wheel-drive aid-agency vehicles that are now ubiquitous in Kampala.[6] With so much new money, some canny people had come to see the disease less as a terrible scourge and more as a growth industry and career opportunity. It's worth noting that as the Pajero culture grew between the mid-1990s and the present day, the HIV rate in Uganda declined ever more slowly. As AIDS spending skyrocketed between 2000 and 2005, the HIV rate did not decline at all.

Many factors are responsible for this trend and it's unfair to blame it all on the aid industry. People may have grown indifferent to repeated warnings about AIDS, and new antiretroviral drug programs may have created a false sense of security. Those most able to protect themselves now probably do, while others—poor women married to abusive, unfaithful men and lonely, disaffected migrants detached from their communities—may need more than just information and education to avoid infection.

Nevertheless, the fact that Uganda's ballooning AIDS budget has not coincided with a sustained drop in new infections hints at a disturbing paradox. William Easterly, a New York University professor and former World Bank economist, argues in his 2006 book *White Man's Burden: Why the West's Efforts to Aid the Rest Have Done So Much Ill and So Little Good*[7] that some poorly administered foreign-aid programs can create perverse incentives, especially when foreign aid electrifies the power grid of traditional patronage networks that lies just beneath the surface of many African bureaucracies.[8]

It's not that all Africans are corrupt, or that corruption is unknown elsewhere. Indeed, the British director of the Global Fund himself resigned in March 2006 amid allegations of mismanagement.[9] But in Africa, corruption may be symptomatic of a "crisis of modernity" as the continent undergoes the fraught transition from a tribal society based on interpersonal ties and allegiances to a modern bureaucratic state. The very cohesiveness of African societies, the binding social force that enables survival under conditions of extreme poverty and hardship, has also contributed to a political culture in which the demands of kin, clan, and tribe too often take precedence over the good of unrelated others, however needy.

The failure of many African leaders to take AIDS seriously so worried Western aid officials that they resolved to try to break the spell with financial incentives. By the early 2000s, money for AIDS was pouring in from the World Bank, the Global Fund, PEPFAR, and other sources. Unfortunately, little is known about how much of the money was spent on what it was supposed to be spent on. We do know that a million dollars intended for Kenya's AIDS orphans "disappeared" and, in a separate case, the director of the National AIDS Control Council was jailed for forging documents and defrauding the government of some $300,000.[10]

In Zambia, a former permanent secretary for health was accused of diverting a million dollars intended for food supplements for AIDS patients to purchase a quack AIDS remedy from a Bulgarian business partner.[11] In May 2006, President Olusegun Obasanjo of Nigeria hosted an African Union summit on HIV/AIDS at which he called for increased funding for the Global Fund. As he spoke, the Global Fund was in the process of suspending Nigeria's grant for mismanagement.[12]

It is possible that as the response to AIDS became bureaucratized by foreign aid, and as informal local efforts morphed into "strategic frameworks," "operational plans," "workplace issues," and "focal points"—all with vast budgets—the crucial human element, without which no development program in Africa can possibly succeed, was lost. AIDS can't be fought without this sense of solidarity and commitment, no matter how much money is thrown at the problem. But a bad situation can be made worse.

As Easterly writes in *White Man's Burden*, the golden rule of development is . . . well, there is no golden rule. Just as ecologists have learned that you don't bulldoze complex virgin forests and plant daffodils, and just as city planners have learned that urban-renewal programs can uproot poor but functioning communities, and just as everybody knows planned economies are a no-no, we learn from Easterly that if you firehose poor countries with development dollars, you risk generating a mad scrum for money, and it's no use blaming Africans (again) when the money is misused. Truly well-designed aid programs, like those that supported Uganda's TASO, Kitovu Mobile, and other exemplary care programs, involve hard, unglamorous work and have very pragmatic goals. They involve close monitoring of simple projects, and they are run by officials who learn fast from their mistakes and recognize that aid is inevitably political, and they address the problems that arise as a result.

WHILE THE Global Fund hearings were going on, the Uganda AIDS Commission held its annual AIDS Partnership Meeting at the Speke Resort Hotel in the lush Kampala suburb of Munyonyo. The conference hall overlooks a croquet lawn, a riding ring, and a vast swimming pool. Inside, hundreds of AIDS experts from governmental and nongovernmental agencies debated policy and planned strategy for the coming year. On the agenda were several presentations by Ugandan health officials, some of whom would soon be answering questions before the Global Fund commission. They stood on a podium and read from PowerPoint slides on such topics as "Strategic Information for Policy Development and Programming," "Programme Management and Coordination," "Resource Mobilization and Review of Funding Mechanisms," and "Coordination and Management of HIV/AIDS Responses at National and District Level."

A USAID official I met at the conference muttered to me, "These people have all these plans, but they don't know how to do anything." She and the other donors were deeply concerned that all the new AIDS funding they were pouring into Uganda seemed to be having little effect on the HIV infection rate, so far. She knew that something was missing from the agenda the Ugandan health officials were proposing, but she couldn't put her finger on it. She told me she had invited a consultant from Brazil to lecture the Ugandans about Brazil's AIDS programs. "We are also looking closely at importing programs from the United States," she said. When I pointed out that the Ugandan AIDS epidemic was very different from that in either Brazil or the United States, where the epidemic was concentrated among intravenous drug users and homosexuals, and that public health programs imported from such vastly different countries might not work in Uganda, she said she didn't know what else to do.

"Why don't you speak to some of the Ugandans who worked on the AIDS program here in the late 1980s, especially the Zero Grazing campaign?" I asked. "After all, those were the most successful campaigns in Africa, and some of the people who designed them are still around." She said she hadn't thought of that. Anyway, she added, "that all happened a long time ago, and the people in the Ministry of Health don't ever talk about it."

THE FRONT LINES

CHAPTER THIRTEEN

The Lost Children of AIDS

SISTER URSULA SHARP had been running a program to help Uganda's AIDS orphans for ten years when she realized how little she knew about how these children experienced the deaths of their parents. Much was known about how European and American children experienced grief, but Ugandans are a stoic people and do not express their feelings easily. When children came to her to collect blankets or food for their families, Ursula would ask them whether they needed anything themselves, and they would look at her as though they didn't understand the question.

Over the years her organization, Kitovu Mobile, had helped thousands of Ugandan children care for their sick parents. "I never once saw a patient who wasn't properly looked after," she told me. "Never once saw a parent lying in her own excrement." When Sharp set out to interview these children, she found that even those who had lost their parents long ago could remember how they felt at every stage when their parents were dying. "I'd ask them how often they went to funerals, and they said they went all the time, just to cry there. The Baganda have a belief that after a person is buried you can't cry for them because you'll disturb the spirits, but at a funeral, it was OK, because you could cry for someone else. I'd hold their hands when we were speaking and they'd clutch onto me. I saw that they were all wondering, 'Who will care for me?'"

By 2006, some twelve million African children had lost at least one parent to AIDS. A small fraction received help from dedicated, community-based organizations like Kitovu, but there were not nearly enough of such programs to reach all needy children. For years, the vast majority were cared for by relatives, often desperately needy themselves, and had been all but forgotten by their own governments and by foreign donors.

Recently, this has begun to change. In 2007, rich governments and private donors are projected to spend roughly $2 billion on programs to help what are known in aid circles as "orphans and vulnerable children," or OVCs. These are children who lack parental care because their parents have died of AIDS or are too sick to look after them. The OVC category also includes the relatively small number of such children who are born HIV positive. About one-third of children born to HIV-positive mothers inherit the virus during childbirth or breastfeeding. Most of these children die of AIDS by age five, although a growing number are now being kept alive longer with antiretroviral drugs.

But even HIV-negative orphans need assistance. It is part of the cruel logic of the AIDS epidemic that orphans—even those born HIV negative—are especially vulnerable to infection when they become sexually active themselves. Several studies have shown that orphans are three to four times more likely to contract HIV in their teens than other young people.[1] Why this is the case is not known, but it probably has something to do with emotional and material deprivation.[2] Orphans are less likely to be enrolled in school than other children and are more likely to fall behind if they are enrolled. They have more medical and psychological problems, and they are more likely to experience discrimination and abuse within foster homes than the biological children of their guardians. Poverty, abuse, and neglect may propel these children into risky relationships, sustaining the epidemic from one generation to the next. Organizations like Kitovu that care for these young people are thus not just dealing with one tragic consequence of the epidemic; they are also on the front lines of the fight against the virus itself.

The new funding for orphan programs is welcome, but it is also cause for concern. As foreign-aid budgets rise, they can become more political and sometimes less effective. Around the time I arrived in Uganda in 1993, foreign donors were beginning to pour money into the country, but it wasn't always clear whether it was going to the right places. European and American consultants came and went from the airport, and their brand-new sport-utility vehicles were churning up the narrow lanes of slums and villages across the country. They hired servants and guards and drivers and translators and set up offices in newly renovated buildings in Kampala's genteel suburbs. Ugandans tended to greet them with outward courtesy and inward skepticism. In private discussions they wondered why the aid workers were spending so much money on offices and vehicles and staff residences that were palatial by local standards, when so many Ugandans were sick and poor and hungry.

The Ugandans were right to wonder. At least 60 percent of U.S. foreign-aid funding never leaves the United States, but is instead spent on overhead, travel, and procurement of American-made cars, computers, and other equipment, as well as salary-and-benefit packages so generous that just one of them would be enough to feed, clothe, and educate hundreds of African children for years.[3] Some of the money that arrives in Africa is well spent, but much of it is wasted on ill-conceived projects designed by foreign technocrats with little sense of African realities. In the high-stakes scramble for funding, the best projects—those that truly meet the needs of local people so that they can eventually support themselves—are often overlooked.

In June 2005, I accompanied Jonathan Cohen of Human Rights Watch on a mission to South Africa to report on discrimination against AIDS orphans in the education system.[4] Among the many organizations we visited were two OVC programs funded by George Bush's PEPFAR that made me wonder whether history might be repeating itself. Between them, these programs had received roughly ten million dollars from the U.S. government to help AIDS orphans but, like some of the foreign-aid programs I had seen in Uganda, much of this money seemed to be bypassing the people who needed it most.

It would be unfair to pass judgment on the entire PEPFAR program based on these two programs. Most PEPFAR funding is being used to support some exemplary organizations.[5] But some PEPFAR programs made me wonder whether sending money to Africa doesn't sometimes do little else than make Americans feel good about themselves.

IN DECEMBER 2002, Oprah Winfrey rented a sports complex near Soweto, the vast black township on the outskirts of Johannesburg, and gave a party for 124 AIDS orphans. There are around a million such children in South Africa. Most live in extreme poverty and many suffer from abuse, discrimination, and neglect. At the party there was food, dancing and singing, and a gift for each child—for some, it was the first they had ever received. "One little girl was so excited that she could not open her present, and instead was kissing the plastic," Oprah told South Africa's *Star* newspaper after the party.

When we were in South Africa, Jonathan and I met some of the orphans who had attended Oprah's Christmas party. We were introduced to them by Elizabeth Rapuleng, a stout, elderly African woman who lives in Meadowlands, a bleak neighborhood of tiny concrete houses on a flat, dusty plain on the edge of Soweto. At the time of Oprah's party, Elizabeth was working for Hope Worldwide, a U.S.-based Christian charity that runs medical relief programs in seventy-five countries. Hope is linked to the International Church of Christ, a fundamentalist evangelical Christian group, and receives funding from the church itself, the U.S. government, and various private donors.

In 2002, Hope was one of the largest U.S. nongovernmental organizations working on AIDS in South Africa and had been providing counseling, medical care, and HIV prevention advice to patients for some ten years. So when Oprah wanted to give a party for orphans in Soweto, her staff naturally contacted Mark Ottenweller, the director of Hope's South African office. At the time, Hope had just begun to work with orphans, but Ottenweller knew that his colleague Elizabeth ran an organization in Meadowlands called Sizanani Home-Based Caregivers that provided food, counseling, and other services to many such children, and he asked Elizabeth to invite them to the party.

As publicity for Hope, Oprah's party was a great success. Oprah's Angel Network charity produced a film in which Ottenweller introduces Oprah to some of the orphans. Hope's press release about the party was still on its Web site three years later. Around the time of the party, Hope began negotiations with PEPFAR officials, and in 2004 it received an $8 million U.S. government contract to provide services to 165,000 AIDS-affected children in South Africa and five other African countries.

Meanwhile, Sizanani—Elizabeth's organization—was struggling for funds. In 2001, Elizabeth, along with her two grown daughters, Florence and Dorothy, had established Sizanani with small grants from the South African government's Department of Social Development and a private donor. While the administration of President Thabo Mbeki has been rightly criticized for its policy on AIDS treatment, since 2001 it had been funding a small number of "Drop-In Centres" like Sizanani that offered AIDS-affected children a place to play after school and receive emotional counseling, meals, and other material necessities.

Africa has few formal orphanages. It is the policy of African governments and international agencies to keep as many children as possible out of institutions, and to encourage extended families to take in orphans. However, the South African government recognized that many families were too poor to care for extra children, and that their own government child-welfare officers and social workers—of which there were only three for all of Soweto, with a population of well over a million in 2005—could not meet the needs of the nation's rapidly growing orphan population either. Experience from other African countries, including Uganda, has shown that small, locally run and managed organizations can provide a crucial safety net for AIDS orphans.[6] So the Department of Social Development began funding a small number of organizations throughout the country—Sizanani among them—to provide basic social services to AIDS-affected children.

Just as in Uganda, many of these organizations were run by charismatic African women who had seen with their own eyes the devastation of the AIDS crisis. Elizabeth had been born and raised in Meadowlands, and during the preceding decade she had seen the epidemic unfold in her community. The willingness of African families to take in orphans has been seen as an expression of the spirit of *ubuntu*—the ancient African concept of shared humanity captured in the traditional Zulu saying "A person is a person through other people." However, Elizabeth knew that *ubuntu* had its limits. As she witnessed the horror of the AIDS crisis, she wanted to create a community-based center that would be open all the time, where orphans and children with sick parents could receive free food and other necessities, and where they could play safely and find adults who could help them if they were in distress. She wanted, as far as possible, to give these children the care they lacked. When she heard about the new government funding, she jumped at the chance.

Sizanani's headquarters were in a shipping container behind a church in Meadowlands. It employed twenty-eight staff who worked as counselors, cooks, drivers, and drama and sports coaches. After school hours and on weekends, the yard outside the shipping container is alive with children's shouts and games until the church gates close at dusk. The children receive three meals a day and snacks, as well as clothes, toothpaste, and other necessities. When the principal of a local state-run school tried to expel some Sizanani children because they could not afford tuition, Elizabeth badgered him into letting them attend for free. In South Africa, even state-run schools charge fees, but by law, principals must admit all children, even if they are too poor to pay. In practice, many schools refuse to waive the fees and many poor children—especially orphans—drop out, unless an adult is willing to advocate for them.

When Elizabeth finds a child being beaten or otherwise abused, she calls the police. When the abuse doesn't stop, she moves the children into her own tiny house. So far she has rescued eight children from particularly abusive homes, including a teenage girl whose uncle used to drag her from her bed night after night and send her out in the dark to buy beer for him at a local pub. Even now, the uncle sometimes comes around to Elizabeth's place and calls for his niece in a drunken rage. Another fifteen-year-old orphan decided she could stand her aunt's beatings no longer and fled to Johannesburg, where, she said later, she planned to kill herself. Elizabeth frantically looked for her everywhere. The aunt seemed unconcerned. Elizabeth contacted local government social workers, who got in touch with their colleagues in Johannesburg. They discovered the girl three days later, wandering the streets of the city, and brought her back to Meadowlands. She now lives with Elizabeth too.

Elizabeth pays for the care of all these children out of her own Sizanani salary of $400 per month. The government offers a foster-care grant to guardians like her, but the application process is so laborious that only some 2 percent of eligible children benefit from it.[7]

In her small office inside the shipping container, Elizabeth spent most of her time writing letters and making phone calls, trying to raise money. She worried about whether there was enough food for the children, whether they all had toothpaste and shoes, and whether they were all in school. The South African government provides Sizanani sixty thousand dollars a year, an amount that Elizabeth reckoned permitted the group to help about half the orphans in Meadowlands who need it. Moreover, the payments from the government sometimes arrived months late. She received occasional donations of food and clothing, but never enough. So, shortly after Oprah's party, Elizabeth asked her supervisors at Hope Worldwide whether they would be willing to help support Sizanani.

Elizabeth reasoned that Hope's existing programs, though valuable, could not reach most of the children who needed help. Hope runs group counseling services in health clinics for AIDS patients and their children, but the counseling sessions took place only once a week and were not open to children whose parents had already died of AIDS or were in a state of denial and refused to be tested for HIV or to enroll in antiretroviral drug programs. Hope also placed social workers in a small number of schools around the country to train teachers to run group therapy sessions for troubled children and to conduct a fifteen-step "bereavement curriculum." But Elizabeth knew that traumatized children needed more than occasional support groups and short-term counseling services; they needed stable, daily human contact—a group of people to rely on and trust, to make them feel less abandoned—something a weekly support group can't provide.

Hope officials in South Africa declined to support Sizanani, saying that Hope did not support "feeding programs"—an odd claim in view of all the help Sizanani gives aside from meals. Eventually, Elizabeth quit her job at Hope to run Sizanani full-time. She received occasional donations of food or other items from Hope but otherwise did not hear from them. Then, in 2004, officials from Hope contacted her again. They wished to offer Sizanani a "memorandum of understanding," or MOU. According to this document, Hope would promise to help Sizanani by "reviewing its current HIV/AIDS-related needs and responses," by "developing/strengthening a local working group on HIV/AIDS," by "developing HIV/OVC strategies," by "developing community competency," and by performing other similarly vague activities. Meanwhile, Sizanani would continue to pay its own staff, purchase all supplies of food and other commodities for the children, and provide space and resources for its programs. In addition, Sizanani would be required to fill out three sets of forms each month listing the number of children helped, the "kids' clubs" set up, and other data, and send these forms to Hope. Hope would provide no money.

Elizabeth declined the offer. "I'd been running this program for three years," she said. "Why would I need advice from them?"

The offer seemed odd to me too. What was Hope up to? Hope officials did not comment on the MOU,[8] but it is possible to imagine their concerns. In 2004, Hope Worldwide received an $8 million grant from PEPFAR to "support the care" of 165,000 orphans. Hope officials probably knew this was an overly ambitious target. However, like other organizations that receive PEPFAR funding, Hope was under pressure to produce statistics on the numbers of children it has helped in some way. This could explain the mysterious MOU, which was presented to Sizanani in late 2004, around the time Hope received its PEPFAR grant. Had Sizanani signed the MOU, Hope would have been able to claim that it was "supporting care" for all three hundred of the children registered with the organization at the time, even though it was doing virtually nothing for them.

Every month, PEPFAR officials were required to report to Congress the number of people helped by its programs overseas. This was important to the Bush administration because PEPFAR had political as well as humanitarian goals. President Bush announced the fifteen-billion-dollar PEPFAR program on national television one week before the start of the war against Iraq, and it was meant to send a clear signal that his foreign policy was compassionate as well as tough. Bush pledged that by the end of 2008, PEPFAR-funded programs would have supported antiretroviral drug treatment for two million people living with HIV/AIDS, prevented seven million new HIV infections, and supported care for ten million people infected with and affected by the disease, including orphans and other vulnerable children.

U.S. government–funded programs routinely set such targets because they make it easier to evaluate the success or failure of particular projects; and in attempting to meet the targets, PEPFAR had put thousands of people on antiretroviral drug treatment.[9] However, measuring the care of children affected by AIDS is much more difficult than measuring the number of patients treated with antiretroviral drugs, because there is no pill that can be given to an abused or neglected child. Thus "supporting care" can mean many things, including "mentoring" an organization like Sizanani that may not need it.

Shortly after Hope received its grant, it established the ANCHOR program—the letters stand for "African Network for Children Orphaned and at Risk." According to its Web site, ANCHOR will do the following things: "promote effective OVC policies"; "provide training and support for scaling up HIV/AIDS treatment, care and prevention"; "coordinate and facilitate capacity building in communities using tested community support and mobilization strategies and technical assistance"; and carry out "monitoring and evaluation to assess program impact."[10]

I was curious to know what these goals meant in practice. Activities such as "technical assistance" and "capacity building"—which means helping organizations to improve management—can help fledgling community-based groups become self-sustaining. But the same terms can also serve as jargon behind which public health contractors can hide when donors make impossible demands on them for political purposes. Such activities can also allow these organizations to appear to be helping far more people than they actually are.

The emphasis on "meeting targets" may well be having a detrimental effect on U.S.-funded AIDS programs. At least seven of Hope's counselors had quit in recent years, because, as one of them told Jonathan Cohen and me, the pressure from PEPFAR to produce numbers made their work all but impossible. One former counselor explained to us how she had worked for Hope for years and had been devoted to the organization, but then something changed when its officials started angling for PEPFAR's millions.

"You cannot give quality counseling anymore because PEPFAR has counseling quotas. If you have to do one thousand people by the end of the month, you end up not doing good counseling. It compromises people's dignity. And the stress on people from the paperwork! All the time we were thinking, 'I have to fill this form because PEPFAR is coming!' They're not asking, 'Are we really meeting the needs of these people?'"

In order to receive ongoing funding from PEPFAR, organizations like Hope must meet their targets—however superficial. Their predicament reminded me of Nikolai Gogol's novel *Dead Souls*, in which the main character, a minor nobleman named Chichikov, travels through the countryside, trying to purchase the names of dead serfs from local landowners, reasoning that landowners would be only too happy to hand over the names of serfs who had died between one census and another, because then they wouldn't have to pay taxes on them. Chichikov planned to mortgage the dead serfs to an unsuspecting bank, which—thinking the serfs were alive—would give Chichikov a loan with which he could build a real fortune of his own.

We wanted to do something on a huge scale," explained Greg Ash, the white South African plastic surgeon who founded NOAH—or Nurturing Orphans of AIDS for Humanity—another South African orphan program that had received approximately $1.5 million from PEPFAR. "We acted as though the responsibility for every orphan in the country was ours." I had been referred to Ash's organization by a press officer at the U.S. embassy in Pretoria. He said it was a PEPFAR success story—a truly indigenous South African organization that was helping thousands of children.

Ash hadn't thought much about AIDS before he started NOAH. Like many white South Africans, he considered leaving the country after the ANC came to power in 1994. But then he was offered a job at a private hospital in Umhlanga Rocks, an exclusive beach community of swaying palms, oceanfront high-rises, and luxurious shopping malls, and he decided to stay. Having made a commitment to raise his own children in South Africa, he began to think more seriously about the country's future, and that's when he began to worry about AIDS orphans. "Apartheid," he said, "gave us this feeling about ourselves, like we're bad people. Maybe that's why an amazing number of people want to do something for the first time. It's relatively easy to get money for kids. People are just waiting for someone to tell them what to do." In 2001, he approached officials at the U.S. embassy with a scheme that he said would help a million AIDS orphans in South Africa by 2008, and in 2003 NOAH began receiving U.S. government funding.

NOAH is a franchise organization. It funds the construction of "resource centers" in schools—separate buildings that, according to the plan, house a small library and five or ten computers, where orphans can stay after school and receive a free meal, read books, and learn how to use computers. NOAH was in the process of building twenty-two such centers—at a cost of roughly a million dollars—and the plan is to build many more.

I asked Ash why it was necessary to build new buildings and buy computers when so many of the orphans I had met in South Africa seemed to have much simpler needs. "We need to break the cycle of AIDS and poverty," he said. "Many of the schools in South Africa are, frankly, not very good, but in the future South African kids will have to compete for jobs with kids from Korea, from Shanghai. . . . They need that competitive advantage. And setting up some computers is easy, it doesn't cost anything, and the kids teach themselves how to use them." The resource centers have a staff of six people, and local volunteers are also recruited from the community to work with especially needy children.

ONE DRIZZLY Wednesday morning in June 2005, I went to visit a NOAH center in a poor black township known as Nkobongo, some thirty miles and a world away from Umhlanga Rocks. Nkobongo sprawls over the veldt behind the town of Shaka's Kraal, named for the powerful king who consolidated the Zulu tribe in the early nineteenth century.

The manager of the local NOAH program was not around when I arrived, so I waited for him at the Nkobongo community center. The community center is on a hill with a view of the whole region: the neat rows of tiny box-shaped houses spread across barren hillsides, a latrine in each front yard. Right below the community center, I noticed that a large crowd had gathered. About two hundred people, young and old, men and women, were sitting around the periphery of a rain-soaked tarmac lot. "Those people really appreciate the bones," said a woman I had met at the community center. "What bones?" I asked. Just then, a pickup truck arrived and parked in the middle of the lot. Two men got out and began off-loading stripped pork bones—refuse from a local abattoir—which they piled up in a heap on the tarmac. The crowd looked on keenly as the men began to distribute the bones—five or six to each person—until the heap disappeared.

Overseeing this extraordinary event was Charles Southwood, a retired white South African businessman who volunteers to help numerous charities in the area, including NOAH. He'd been distributing bones for a local Catholic charity for years, he said. When he started, there would be such a mob when the bones arrived that they knocked Charles over several times, and almost overturned the vehicle once or twice. "I told them they had to sit down and form an orderly queue; otherwise there would be no more bones."

According to the Ministry of Agriculture, roughly one-third of all South Africans experience "food insecurity," meaning that they live in fear of hunger.[11] At a high school in Soweto, a teacher described to Jonathan and me how many of the students, especially those who were orphans, complained that they did not get enough food at home. Sometimes they would stare through the windows of the faculty room at the teachers eating lunch. "How do you teach a hungry child?" she asked us.

South Africa is the richest country in sub-Saharan Africa. There are no wars here, no refugee camps; the country has a social-welfare system, a free press, and regular peaceful elections. But the agrarian traditions that once sustained people here—the techniques they had developed over centuries of survival on the sandy marginal soils of Africa, and that one nineteenth-century European visitor said showed such a profound understanding of nature that they closely resembled a science—have been all but lost.[12] Meanwhile, the high-tech future envisioned by Greg Ash has yet to arrive, and some three-quarters of all adults in places like Nkobongo are unemployed.[13] Although South Africa's powerhouse economy, based on gold, diamonds, commercial farming, and services, is growing rapidly, it produces very small numbers of highly skilled jobs. Most people therefore survive—sometimes barely—on government handouts or charities like those of the Catholic church.

After the bones had been passed out, Charles Southwood introduced me to some of the people who worked at the Nkobongo NOAH resource center. The new building was still under construction, and the resource center was temporarily housed in a church. There was no library, although there was a kitchen where a daily meal was prepared. I was also shown a room with nine computers. The 150 children registered with NOAH love them, but because demand is so high, each child is allowed only one hour of computer time every two weeks. It seemed unlikely that this would break the cycle of AIDS and poverty that seemed to be churning so rapidly here.

Back in Soweto, Jonathan and I asked Elizabeth what she knew about NOAH. She said that one of its representatives—a tall white South African woman—had visited Sizanani some months before. After a series of meetings the visitor announced that NOAH would begin funding Sizanani, but in order to obtain the funding, Sizanani would have to fire its meagerly paid staff and all of them, including Elizabeth, would have to reapply for their jobs. NOAH would rehire only six of the twenty-eight staff who worked there. The rest could volunteer for free, if they wished. "This is my dream!" Elizabeth said. "I wasn't going to let them kick me out!"

Unlike Sizanani, NOAH relies heavily on unpaid volunteers to provide care for needy children. Ash had hoped that these volunteers—"who are unemployed anyway," he told me—would serve out of a sense of altruism, or *ubuntu,* in African terms. However, NOAH's attempt to impose a "volunteer model" on South Africa's dangerous, hungry townships seemed to be squelching what little *ubuntu* remained. As Charles Southwood soon discovered in Nkobongo, few people in this troubled place wanted to help AIDS-affected families for free. "They come for a few days," Charles said of the volunteers. "Maybe a month. Then they realize there's no salary and then you never see them again. Sometimes you go to visit a sick person and the volunteer will just stand at the door and not go in.

"There's an old black man who lives on his own. He's blind and can't walk. Someone stole his wallet and pension book. Some volunteers were supposed to go and feed him, but then I found last week that no one had been there for three days. Sometimes I think the Zulus think I'm mad. When I blow my top, as I did last week about the old man, they fail to understand what I'm angry about. They just don't seem to care. They aren't kind to each other. I don't know why. I guess poverty disempowers people, makes them mean."

"Some families don't want my help," a NOAH outreach worker told me. "Some of them swear at me, chase me away. Sometimes they tell the children to tell me they aren't there. They embarrass me in front of the neighbors, say I am some kind of prostitute."

When Charles does find committed volunteers, he tries to raise money to pay them from local churches or businesses or simply from people he knows. The amounts required are small, some eighty dollars a month, but Charles hasn't had much luck. South African businesses may occasionally contribute food or toys that they can't sell, and they are often keen to donate funds for buildings and computers and other infrastructure projects they can put their names or business logos on, but few will support the salary of a sympathetic human being even if that is what orphans need most of all. "Most of the white people in our country are totally unaware of the situation of poor blacks," Charles said. "The other whites around here avoid me; no one wants to know what I am doing."

Home-care volunteers had been instrumental in the successful fight against AIDS in Uganda and Kagera. But these societies were very different from South Africa's. Most Ugandans live not in deracinated, crime-ridden townships, but in villages with strong traditions of voluntary mutual aid among neighbors and kin going back many generations. Volunteering was a natural way of gaining respect and status in the community.

After my visit to Nkobongo, I tried to visit two other NOAH sites in KwaZulu-Natal. According to the list I had been given by NOAH officials in Johannesburg, there should have been two NOAH community groups in a town called Mtubatuba that I happened to be visiting the following week. But when I arrived, I was told by a NOAH coordinator that they were not yet set up. There was not a single volunteer or community worker I could speak to.

THE WORK of small community-based care and support organizations like Sizanani is seldom written up in medical or public health journals or the official reports of donor agencies. Nevertheless, UNICEF, the U.S. government, the World Bank, and many AIDS experts officially recognize the importance of supporting such organizations. At present, there are far too few of them in South Africa, and most of their funding comes from local sources, often from the poor themselves.[14] In 2005, the South

African government was supporting only four such groups in all of Johannesburg, and there were none at all in many parts of the country.

When Jonathan and I visited the UNICEF officer in charge of orphans in Pretoria, she said she had not had time to visit Sizanani or any of the other community-based organizations supported by the South African government. In her view, NOAH provided a better model for orphan services, although she showed no close acquaintance with its programs.

She repeated a common criticism of community-based care and support organizations: that they were "unsustainable," meaning they start with good intentions and then collapse after a while. Maybe she had a point, but it seemed hollow to us. Of course these organizations collapse if no one supports them, or if they are uprooted by larger organizations with millions of dollars at their disposal. As Elizabeth said, referring to NOAH's takeover bid, "When the Americans come, we sing, we dance, they take our picture, and they go back and show everyone how they are helping the poor black people. But then all they do is hijack our projects and count our children."

CHAPTER FOURTEEN

Wartime

ONE OCTOBER EVENING in 2001, in an impoverished shantytown in the Northern Cape province of South Africa, David Potse entered the house of a former girlfriend and raped her nine-month-old daughter. The child was later taken to a nearby hospital, where her internal injuries were found to be so severe that she nearly died. After a series of operations, she miraculously survived, and the nurses nicknamed her "Baby Tshepang," which means "have hope." Potse was apprehended soon afterward. At his trial, he said that he was out drinking on the night of the assault. However, DNA tests showed his semen was present in the child's rectum, and his current girlfriend testified that she walked in on him during the rape. Potse was sentenced to life in prison in 2002.

News reports about Baby Tshepang, along with a small number of similar cases that came to light at around the same time, ignited moral horror across the nation. "South Africa has been shamed," declared the proceedings of a parliamentary committee on child abuse; addressing a group called the "Moral Regeneration Movement," then deputy president Jacob Zuma—himself soon to be accused (and later acquitted) of the rape of an AIDS activist—said the baby-rape cases displayed "barbarism and moral decay of the worst kind." The *Sowetan* newspaper called for a state of emergency and one columnist asked whether South African men were becoming "sex cannibals."[1]

South Africa has the highest rate of reported rape in the world. Were the nation's men really out of control? During colonial times, the Native Affairs Commission warned that the freedoms of civilization and the release from the constraints of traditional tribal life could unleash moral evil.[2] Now, for some observers, this prediction seemed to be coming true.

In early 2002, several journalists—most of them from Europe and the United States—reported that South Africa's epidemic of sexual violence was being fueled by a desperate myth: some African men believed that raping a virgin would cure them of HIV.[3] One BBC journalist described the Baby Tshepang incident as a typical example of such a "virgin-rape myth" case. This is probably not so. Before Potse was apprehended, six other men were charged with the crime but were soon released for lack of evidence. One of them said he had heard about the "virgin-rape cure" on the radio and the girlfriend of another died, probably of AIDS, shortly after the men were arrested. The BBC journalist put those loose facts together to draw his erroneous conclusion. In fact, these men were absolved of the crime, and there is no evidence that the true assailant—David Potse—raped Baby Tshepang because he thought doing so would cure him of HIV. Indeed, there is no evidence that he was himself HIV positive, or if he was, that he knew he was.

The idea that virgin-rape myths are a significant cause of either child abuse or the spread of AIDS in Africa is itself a myth, perpetuated by stigmatizing attitudes toward people with HIV and racist fears of black sexuality. A similar "myth about a myth" was prevalent in the United States during the nineteenth century, when there was widespread panic that the hordes of newly arrived southern and eastern European immigrants were raping virgins to cure themselves of syphilis.[4]

Although some surveys suggest that belief in the virgin-rape myth is common in South Africa, in only a tiny number of child-abuse cases has the accused himself claimed that it was a motivating factor in his crime. A study of child-rape cases in Johannesburg found that infection rates among the victims were far lower than would be expected if the children had been targeted by HIV-positive men. Very few South African men know their HIV status in any case. The same researchers found that most people who knew about the virgin-rape myth had read about it in newspapers or heard about it on the radio; none of the respondents in the study knew of a single case in which a child had been raped for that reason. In many traditional African belief systems, sex is held to have a ritualistic, purifying function. "So, if people hear of the myth they may think it sounds as if it could be true," Rachel Jewkes, head of the South African Medical Research Council's Gender and Health Research unit, told a reporter in 2002.[5] But this does not mean that people act on it.

Why did David Potse rape Baby Tshepang, if not to cure himself of AIDS? And why is rape so common in South Africa in general? Outsiders are inclined to see those South African men who beat and rape women and children as out-of-control brutes who heedlessly spread HIV. But anthropologists are finding that violent men may actually be enacting a cultural drama that is hundreds, perhaps thousands, of years old. These men are driven by myths, all right, but these are not myths about virgin-rape cures for HIV. They are far more powerful than that and much harder to dispel. The roots of these myths extend deep in the African past and are finding new life in the upheavals and inequalities of contemporary South African society.

The baby-rape cases came to light during a period of national soul-searching in South Africa. The euphoria that followed the end of apartheid in 1994 was giving way to the morning-after recognition of the challenge of developing a society wracked by poverty, crime, and a new deadly disease. Roughly a quarter of adults in the country were HIV positive and everyone was trying to understand why. Bizarre rumors swirled in townships and rural areas: AIDS was caused by witchcraft, germ warfare against blacks, or something in the food.[6] President Thabo Mbeki declared that Africans were prone to AIDS because of poverty and malnutrition—in other words, AIDS was one of the many legacies of past oppression by whites.[7] But other observers—including UN officials and journalists—had another theory. They attributed the AIDS epidemic to the subjugation of women in South African society, of which the nation's high rates of child abuse and rape were symptoms. The baby-rape cases bolstered their claims and came to symbolize just how dire the situation was.[8]

Until the furor over Baby Tshepang, rape was not a crime that had aroused much public concern in South Africa. The vast majority of rape victims here are not infants, but mature women or teenagers, and most incidents are treated with remarkable indifference.[9] Few cases are reported to the police; if the assault is committed by a boyfriend or husband, it is usually not even considered a crime, and a victim's screams are usually ignored.[10] A large proportion of both men and women in South Africa blame women—not men—for rape. Asked for suggestions about how to reduce the incidence of rape, respondents on one study said that women should be taught how to "dress and behave" and should not be allowed out after 7:00 p.m. One of the reasons rape is so seldom reported to the police in South Africa is that many women also internalize this logic, and fear that if the incident becomes widely known, others will wonder what they did to deserve it.[11]

When former deputy president Jacob Zuma was accused of rape, he admitted having sex with the woman in question but claimed that she had visited his house wearing a knee-length skirt. "Under normal circumstances, if a woman is dressed in a skirt, she will sit properly with her legs together." But this woman "would cross her legs and wouldn't even mind if the skirt was raised very much." This signaled that she was "ready," Zuma testified. "You cannot just leave a woman if she is ready," he said.[12] When Zuma was acquitted in May 2006, his supporters were overjoyed, but many observers around the world were stunned.

In 2000, the Johannesburg police department's sexual offenses unit had only three officers and they were saddled with two hundred new cases a month.[13] As dockets pile up in police stations around the country, many victims are advised to negotiate restitution privately with the alleged rapist's family. Sometimes the accused make their own arrangements with the police, who have been known to "lose" a docket for three U.S. dollars.[14] The conviction rate for reported rapes is about 7 percent, and most of these cases involve children. Among cases of adult rape, the conviction rate is 1 percent. "It's a logic problem," says Jewkes. "There is legislation that says rape is illegal, but it is at odds with what a great many people believe to be true."

Even child-rape cases may be treated casually. In her 2001 book *Proud of Me: Speaking Out About Sexual Violence and HIV*, the South African journalist and activist Charlene Smith describes a scene that defies comment. An eight-year-old girl had been raped in a township near Durban, a large port city on the Indian Ocean. She was taken to a hospital where she lay on a trolley in a corridor for four hours, waiting for someone to examine her. Meanwhile, the rapist, who had been beaten up by a vigilante crowd, was being treated by the district surgeon. Smith was alerted to the case, and after she screamed at the district surgeon over the phone, he agreed to go see the girl. What he did not tell Smith was that he planned to bring the rapist with him to the hospital. The rapist was placed in a wheelchair and wheeled down the same corridor where the girl was lying. When she saw him, she became so hysterical that any examination became impossible.

IN 2001, the University of Pretoria anthropologist Isak Niehaus began studying a series of rape cases that had occurred in a small area of South Africa's Limpopo province. Most of the incidents followed a typical pattern. Many of the victims were known to the rapists, and they tended to be women with an air of independence—women coming home from shops with grocery bags, teachers, nurses, shop assistants on the way to work, women in a technical college, female business owners. Some victims were single women who drank and flirted openly in bars. In one case, an unemployed, dope-smoking criminal raped a total stranger, but only after he had been rejected by several girls in a bar where he had been drinking earlier in the evening.

In contrast to their seemingly "liberated" victims, the men who committed these crimes seemed to be fighting some challenge to their sense of masculinity. Once a father raped his teenage daughter because, he said, she had disobeyed him by staying out late. Another rapist forced one of his victims to cook for him after he assaulted her.

As the feminist historian Susan Brownmiller and many others have written, rape is an assertion of male power, not sexuality.[15] Niehaus speculates that the men in his account found in acts of violence against women temporary relief from the humiliations of living in a society based on the presumption of white superiority. But these acts were not only misdirected expressions of racial anger. They were also "desperate protests against men's loss of control" over women. Over the past century, radical changes in South Africa's economy have profoundly affected gender norms and expectations and altered the balance of power between the sexes. Today, the new South Africa has provided considerable opportunities for women. Gender equality is now enshrined in the constitution, girls are more likely to be enrolled in and graduate from school than boys are, and women are finding new opportunities in the nation's expanding service sector. But as subsistence farming becomes increasingly unsustainable and as the manufacturing and mining sectors steadily collapse, many men are being left behind. The epidemic of rape may be a reaction to their perceived loss of status. In response they are reviving "scripts of male domination" with deep historical resonance.[16]

This may be why rapists often target women who seem independent, especially sexually independent single women. "Men seemed aware that these independent women were a nail in the coffin of patriarchy," wrote the anthropologist Virginia Van der Vliet in the 1970s. "They reserved a special scorn for single women and their children."[17] When a girl sleeps around, a young rapist told the anthropologist Kate Wood in 2004, "you think you should discipline her."[18] "She was my friend's girlfriend," another rapist explained to Wood. "My friend was not in love with her anymore because of her promiscuity. He called us during the day and told us at night we must streamline [gang-rape] her. Then he fetched her at her home and took her to his home. We were three, including the boyfriend. . . . My friend, her boyfriend, started, and we followed after him, and we all did one round and left."[19]

Some rapists carry out the worst punishment of all. Rather than raping the women themselves, they rape the children of the women they wish to discipline. This could be the reason David Potse raped Baby Tshepang. Potse denied that he had committed the crime, so we don't know what his reasons were, but he was a former boyfriend of the baby's mother, and he may have been angry because he suspected her of drinking and sleeping with other men. She was sixteen, and in addition to Potse, she had had an affair with the father of Baby Tshepang, and perhaps with other men. We are not told where she was when her daughter was being assaulted; some accounts say she was shopping, others that she was drinking and that she was drunk at the time. It was evening, not a usual time for shopping.

In one of Niehaus's case studies, a young man named Makandeni brought his girlfriend, Shelly, to a friend's house where a group of young men were hanging around drinking. Makandeni spiked Shelly's wine with brandy and she soon became very drunk: "Shelly wanted to go outside to urinate," said a witness, "but the boys would not let her. One boy sent the other boy to fetch a bucket. They gave the bucket to the girl and she started vomiting. They were afraid that she would flee if she got out of the room." By eight o'clock, Shelly was being gang-raped by seven men, who took turns until dawn. "Some visitors peeped through the window and laughed," said the witness.

Makandeni probably wouldn't have been aware of this, but he may have been enacting a hideous version of an ancient southern African custom. In precolonial times, chiefs of the Sotho tribe would sometimes allow other men to have sex with their wives to secure the men's loyalty. This was considered statesmanlike behavior and is celebrated in traditional myths and poems.[20] Contemporary gang rape may be a violent reprise of this male-bonding tradition. As the witness explained to Niehaus, Makandeni offered up his girlfriend to the others "because he was the youngest member of the group and wished to win their friendship."

The vast majority of HIV transmission in Africa occurs in long-term, consensual relationships and is not a result of rape. Nevertheless, a sizable number of women and children and some men do contract HIV as a result of rape, and the horror of the crime has drawn attention from the U.S. government, the World Bank, and other funding agencies. There are now many programs to "empower women" by, for example, increasing girls' school enrollment, promoting female employment, and teaching women—through media campaigns, community workshops, and school-based programs—how to assert their right to control their own sexuality and childbearing.

But as Delphine Serumaga, executive director of People Opposing Women Abuse, a South African advocacy group, told a reporter from the newspaper *The Star* in 2003, these efforts may be insufficient: "There needs to be a mind change in society as a whole," she said.[21] "We've taught women about their rights and responsibilities," explained Debbie Harrison, director of LifeLine and Rape Crisis, "but we've done nothing to teach men about theirs."

The South African government ceased publishing rape statistics after the press furor over the baby-rape cases a few years ago, so we don't know what effect these programs are having on HIV incidence or sexual violence. However, care must be taken to ensure they don't backfire. The epidemic of sexual violence in South Africa is part of a wider war between men and women that is as fierce and partisan as any other on the African continent, and it has been raging far longer. Empowering individual women without addressing the attitudes of men and society in general risks creating empowered women who antagonize men and playing right into the rapists' hands.

IN 2001, South Africa's Department of Education launched a new national AIDS-and-sex-education curriculum for secondary schools, known as "Life Orientation." In February 2004, I visited a school where the program was under way. The school was in northern KwaZulu-Natal, a rural area of tiny homesteads scattered over desolate green hills. Researchers from Columbia University in New York and the South African Medical Research Council had enhanced the curriculum, so that it emphasized gender equality. The program used skits, quizzes, and instructive games to challenge traditional patriarchal gender norms and stereotypes and explore issues such as sexual rights, domestic violence, and interpersonal communication.

On the day I visited, the teachers and students had planned a session called "Relationships." The class began with a group exercise in which the students were asked to list the characteristics of a "good relationship" and a "bad relationship." The students shouted out the answers and the teacher wrote them on the blackboard. The students got everything right. Good-relationship qualities included "cooperation, respecting each other, loving each other truly, not forcing each other, not cheating, romance, responsibility." Bad-relationship qualities included "no respect, no trust, forcing each other, abuse, rape." Two student volunteers then enacted a short play about a pregnant girl who wants her boyfriend to accompany her to the clinic. The boy wants to play football instead, but they discuss it, and eventually he agrees to go with her.

"Once you engage in a love affair, you are not a child," the teacher said sternly at the end of the skit. "You have to learn to discuss things first and change the way you talk to each other."

Just then, another teacher entered the classroom. He was tall, with very short hair, and his shirt and tie were as crisp as a soldier's uniform. In his hand he carried a sapling that had been stripped of its leaves and fashioned into a whip. Suddenly he struck it with such force against one of the students' desks that I almost fell over backward. "If you don't involve yourselves in good relationships you will end up with HIV and AIDS!" he shouted. "You must stand firm!" And he whacked the stick on the desk again.

Afterward I asked some of the students whether the teacher ever beat them. "Not me," said one girl. "But he does beat others."

The next day, I met that teacher again and asked to interview him. Now he was carrying a section of black hosepipe. As we walked together to his office for the interview, we passed some girls who were standing around in a group talking. One of them had her back to us, and the teacher casually swatted her on the behind as we passed. She laughed it off. When we sat down in his office, the teacher laid the hosepipe on the table between us. It reminded me of the instruments the apartheid police used to beat their prisoners with. Corporal punishment in schools is illegal in South Africa, the teacher explained, but many of the children were being raised by aunts and grandmothers who said they couldn't handle them. So these guardians begged the teachers to start beating the children again, even though it was against the law.

Perhaps it was true, as the teacher told me, that some of the students took drugs and cut school, but threatening children with a hosepipe seemed an odd way to teach them about the importance of negotiation and dialogue in relationships, and resolving differences without violence.

South Africa may be the most violent society on earth that is not at war. All forms of violent crime are common there; domestic violence and the beating of children are routine; even nurses in hospitals frequently assault their patients.[22] Many of South Africa's young rapists were themselves abused as children.[23] Long before AIDS created more than a million South African orphans, apartheid policies meant millions of parents were forced to leave their children behind in rural areas while they went to work in cities, factories, mines, or the houses of white families. Children remained in the care of grandmothers, aunts, or unrelated guardians, where they were vulnerable to abuse and exploitation, and some grew into the hardened adults of today.[24]

While I was at the school, I spoke to some of the students from the "Relationships" class. As an AIDS prevention measure, elders from the local Zulu tribe had recently revived the traditional custom of "virginity testing," in which older women inspect the genitalia of younger women to ensure their hymens are intact. I asked some of the girls whether they had ever been to the virginity tester.

"I would go," one fifteen-year-old told me, "but I can't. I was raped by my uncle when I was seven." Her parents were recently separated at the time, and her mother had gone off to the city, leaving her behind at her grandmother's house, where her uncle also lived. He did it twice, both times when her independent-minded mother was away. The second time, the girl contracted a sexually transmitted disease that was so painful she could not walk.

"I wasn't the first victim," she said. "He was doing it to two other kids. I told my mother and she wanted to report it to the police, but my grandmother wouldn't allow it." Eventually her mother found another husband and she and her daughter moved away.

"There is abuse," the girl sighed, "but you can't report it because it happens in the family, and everyone will be embarrassed if other people find out."

It makes you wonder what "empowerment" means in such a context. A major theme of South Africa's Life Orientation program is "negotiation skills" that help young people acquire the language to express their sexual desires, refuse unwanted sex, or insist on condom use. But how do you negotiate anything in a society where social tensions between men and women and between elders and young people are so great and so easily triggered into violence?

"When you tell a child she has sexual rights, you're just talking," an African woman who worked for a large nongovernmental organization in Zimbabwe told me once. "Then you send her back somewhere. In what way have you empowered that child? The child has all these rights, but how does the community react to this 'empowered child'? She's just an entity, lost to society. If a child goes and reports that an aunt or uncle is abusing her, and then is removed from the family, where does she go then?"

With these concerns in mind, I contacted Albertina Dano, the official in South Africa's Department of Education in charge of life orientation programs. She was a large, kind-looking woman who clearly understood the complexities of her job. She admitted that "negotiation" had its limits. "Some students are abused, and in that situation it's beyond your control; you can't negotiate about condoms or anything else," she told me.

But sometimes you can be clever. "Here's an example I like to give," she said, and she told me the following story: "There was an old pensioner, a lady. She was walking in the road. There were no minibuses in those days. It was before AIDS came, but there were young people who would lie down in the tall grass beside the road to the hospital and attack passersby. This old mama knew someone who had been raped on that road. But she had to go to the hospital for a check-up, so she set off anyway. On the way there, a man grabbed her. He had a knife. She said, 'Let's talk. I will agree to have sex with you, but please don't hurt me.' The man got excited and began to take off his trousers. What he didn't know is that the lady had taken a knife of her own from home." As the rapist was preparing to have sex with the old lady, she pulled out the knife and cut off what Ms. Dano called his "front parts." She then found a plastic packet and wrapped them up. Soon the police and an ambulance arrived and rushed them both to the hospital.

Ms. Dano insisted the story was true, but it sounded to me like one of Africa's famous "trickster tales" about a clever, wily underdog whose tribulations reflect the anxieties of an entire society.

"That was negotiation," she said with satisfaction. "It shows you that some people are skillful enough to negotiate. It all depends on how brave you can be. We are trying to convey that to the young ones."

CHAPTER FIFTEEN

The Underground Economy of AIDS

IN 2000, a group of researchers at the University of California, San Francisco, and the University of Zimbabwe came up with a scheme they hoped would protect young African women from HIV. They had been working in the slums around Zimbabwe's capital, Harare, and like most AIDS experts, had come to recognize how the spread of HIV was driven by poverty and by deeply rooted inequalities between men and women. At the time, around a quarter of all Zimbabwean adults were infected with HIV, and the virus was spreading rapidly, especially among sexually active young women.

The researchers had interviewed scores of teenage girls living in the slums around Harare and had found that, although most said they had only one sexual partner and were not prostitutes, most were involved in transactional relationships with men who had other partners, and this placed them at very high risk of HIV. Some of the girls said they used condoms, but since several of them had been pregnant, they cannot have used them all the time.

When asked why they took such risks, they said that their economic difficulties were a far greater concern for them than AIDS was. Although few of the girls were truly destitute, their bleak, impoverished lives led them to place great value on the smallest gifts of cash, jewelry, makeup, and clothes. Boys could always find odd jobs like running errands or helping out in the bus park, the girls said, but people didn't hire girls.

The researchers decided to set up a "microcredit" program to enable the girls to start their own small businesses. As part of the program, the girls would be expected to participate in a series of "life skills" seminars about AIDS and relationships, similar to the life orientation programs in South Africa. In theory, this would give the girls the knowledge, self-esteem, and financial independence to decide for themselves whether to have sex or not, and insist on condom use if they did. Since the 1970s, similar microfinance programs have helped many poor people, especially women, from Bangladesh to Brazil gain a degree of independence by setting up small businesses such as growing fruits and vegetables, raising animals, or buying and selling food, clothes, or cosmetics. Foreign-policy experts increasingly favor these programs because they recognize that gender inequality is not only an injustice in its own right, it also hinders development. In agricultural societies, women perform most of the labor—cooking, farming, and working for family businesses, for example—but most of this work is unpaid. Microfinance programs bring women into the cash economy, instill the poor with entrepreneurial skills, and sometimes help spur economic growth.[1] Although hardly a panacea for the myriad hardships faced by poor people in developing countries, microfinance programs have improved many women's lives. Women who participate in such programs tend to have fewer children than other women, and the children they do have tend to be healthier.[2] In places like Zimbabwe, these programs may also awaken a spirit of ambition and purpose in women long demoralized by lack of opportunity and by a culture of gender inequality that has numbed many of them into dependence upon men.[3] The researchers in Zimbabwe wanted to see whether microloans could reduce the spread of HIV in Chitungwiza by giving young women more personal autonomy and control over their sexual lives.[4]

Admittedly, this was not an auspicious time for anyone to start a business in Zimbabwe. The economy was in a dire state, due to a combination of disastrous leadership by the country's president, Robert Mugabe, and ruinous advice from foreign creditors such as the IMF and World Bank. The 1990s had seen the closing of numerous factories and the firing of thousands of public-sector teachers and health-care workers. The poor young women the researchers wanted to help had few skills; some could barely read. Even in better days, Zimbabwe's formal economy would have offered them few opportunities. However, the slums around Harare, like those surrounding cities and towns across Africa, were home to a bustling informal economy in which cheap food, clothes, and household products were traded at makeshift markets and among neighbors, relatives, and friends. Millions of poor, unskilled Africans, including women, earn their living in the informal economy, even in relatively wealthy countries like South Africa and Botswana. The researchers reasoned that, with a small amount of capital, girls in the slums of Zimbabwe could do so too.

During the summer of 2004, Shaping the Health of Adolescents in Zimbabwe, or SHAZ, as the program was known, recruited fifty young women aged sixteen to twenty from Chitungwiza and Epworth, two slum neighborhoods near Harare. The girls were given training in entrepreneurial skills such as making a business plan, identifying markets, and managing finances. They also attended a series of "life skills" seminars on AIDS prevention, sexual relationships, gender inequality, and the use of condoms. In September, each girl chose a business to go into and received a loan of about $150, to be repaid in monthly installments from their profits.

When I arrived in Harare six months later, only 5 percent of the girls had met their loan-repayment targets, one of the worst records of any microfinance project anywhere in the world. Zambuko Trust, the microfinance agency that administered the loans for SHAZ, had actually lost track of nearly half the girls in the program. More worrying still, SHAZ seemed to be having the opposite of its intended effect on the girls' sexual behavior. The researchers had not anticipated that their attempt to empower these poor young women was placing some of them right in the path of HIV.

SHORTLY after I arrived in Harare, I met Tafadzwa Mandipaza-Jemwa, the Zambuko Trust loan officer who was working with SHAZ. "I knew there were going to be problems from the beginning," she said. "The greatest error the researchers made was to assume that any poor person can just go out and start a business. Many of them just can't do it on their own."

Tafadzwa told me she was still in touch with many of the girls, and she offered to take me to their homes in Chitungwiza, about fifteen miles from Harare. For three days, Tafadzwa and I drove through the rain-soaked slums, searching for SHAZ participants and listening to stories of one failed business venture after another.

We met a bright twenty-year-old named Proud, who used her loan to buy a sack of used clothes from a dealer in Harare. The clothes in turn came from dealers in the United States who collected donated items and shipped them overseas. Zimbabwe once had a lively manufacturing sector of its own that produced clothing for the local market. The factories were protected by tariffs and subsidies, but in the 1990s, the World Bank and IMF, which loaned the Zimbabwean government millions of dollars a year, insisted that these barriers to free trade be eliminated. This move all but wiped out Zimbabwe's clothing factories and threw thousands of people, many of them women, out of work. Before long, the local market was flooded with cheap secondhand clothing from the United States and cheap imports from China, two countries that use trade barriers to protect their own manufacturers.[5]

The imported secondhand clothes created new opportunities for unemployed, unskilled people, who began to transport and trade them all over Africa. Proud planned to resell the used clothes she bought in Harare in the rural village where her grandmother lived. On her first business trip she found that although people in the village wanted to buy the clothes, they had no money. Instead, they offered to pay her in sacks of maize meal—the staple food of Zimbabwe, which they grew on their own plots of land.

Proud's timing seemed favorable. She knew that the maize meal would fetch a good price in Harare. In recent years there had been periodic food shortages all over the country, and people were eager to stock up. Until recently, Zimbabwe had been the breadbasket of the region. Millions of tons of maize were grown on vast commercial farms owned by whites whose pioneer ancestors had settled more than a century ago in what was then known as Southern Rhodesia. These mostly British settlers displaced thousands of African peasants and at independence, in 1980, President Robert Mugabe promised his people that this land would be returned to them. By the late 1990s, a period of deepening poverty in Zimbabwe, Mugabe declared that the process of restitution was going too slowly.

Cadres of young Mugabe loyalists claiming to be veterans of the liberation war then appropriated virtually all of the commercial farms in the country and expelled their white owners. Mugabe instructed the "war veterans" to parcel off the land into small farms for landless peasants. Unfortunately, many of these peasants lacked the seeds, fertilizers, capital, and skills to run the farms; others had no idea how to farm at all. Food production fell sharply, and in order to avert famine, the government was forced to regulate prices. This created a black market, which provided opportunities for traders like Proud.

Proud packed the maize meal into a large canvas sack and set out for Harare by bus. On the way, the vehicle was stopped by the police, who soon found Proud's contraband maize and confiscated it. When Proud protested, one of the policemen made a pass at her.

Everywhere the SHAZ girls went, it seemed, men tried to seduce them. Several feared they would be raped. A girl named Margaret told me she had hoped to use her loan to work with a friend of her mother's who was a cross-border trader. Every Saturday night, the older woman boarded a bus to Zambia, where prices were lower, and on Sunday she brought a load of goods—kitchenware, toys, and other cheap imported items—back to sell in Chitungwiza. Margaret arranged to join one of these buying trips, and set out one Saturday afternoon for Harare. She made it as far as the bus station. She stood for a while amid the noise and the dust and the leering strangers, and then she just went home.

Several girls vanished entirely after receiving their loans. When Tafadzwa went to visit them, their relatives said they had moved away. SHAZ was an experiment, and girls who did not repay their loans were not penalized. But Tafadzwa suspected many were afraid she would punish them anyway. A loan officer previously employed by SHAZ had warned some of the girls that they would go to jail if they did not make timely repayments. While Tafadzwa tried to reassure them that this was not the case, some girls remained unconvinced. Some would shout at her, and others just burst into tears when they saw her. "I don't know why they did that," Tafadzwa said. "Maybe it's a way of avoiding repayment. Maybe, when they think about the loan, they also start to think more deeply about their other problems. The other day I went to visit a girl at her house and her grandmother told me she wasn't around. She said the girl had gone up-country somewhere. But then a few hours later, I saw the same girl in the road."

At a tiny crumbling house on the edge of an alley in Chitungwiza, we met the aunt of one of the girls who had disappeared. She said her niece had become "unruly" after receiving her loan, and was now out of town with a boyfriend. "The trouble started when the first loan payments were due," the aunt explained. "She ran away because she can't repay that loan. The way girls escape from trouble is by getting a man, so that's what she's doing. She's looking for that money now."

The grandmother of another girl whom Tafadzwa had not seen in months told us, "When she got her loan she went and bought six pairs of slippers. I don't know what she did with them. Then she eloped with a man in the road. What did you teach them at that program?" she asked. "To go after men?"

At another house, the brother of a loan recipient told us that his sister was not around, and then he swore at us and told us never to come back again.

Most of the girls who disappeared were orphans, a group that is especially vulnerable to HIV. After talking to the SHAZ girls—or the people who knew them—it is easy to speculate about why. Some, lacking parents to protect them, are raped or seduced, sometimes within their own homes; others are propelled by necessity into prostitution. Others, neglected and abused, turn bitter and rebellious.

Tafadzwa's male colleagues at Zambuko were afraid of some of the SHAZ girls. "When we went to give out the loan money, some of the girls were flirting with us," a male Zambuko accountant told me. "They kept saying, 'You are very handsome!' The orphans were the toughest of all."

WHAT SOME Western researchers and aid workers don't realize when they advocate for the economic empowerment of African girls is that sex is integral to the frontier economy in which the poor live. You don't see this when you drive around the muddy lanes of places like Chitungwiza and gaze out the window of your vehicle. You see the Chitungwiza market, with its wooden stalls tented with plastic sheets; you see stout women in headscarves, long dresses, and heavy cardigans bustling over heaps of vegetables; you see women selling fly-strewn coils of raw meat, or dusty pairs of shoes displayed on tarps on the ground, or racks and racks of clothing—frilly Chinese-made party dresses, polyester men's dress shirts, shiny track suits. You see ancient minibuses heaving along with bales of goods teetering on their roofs. You get a powerful sense of interdependent, organic complexity; you see how creative the poor can be, even in the wreckage of an economy like Zimbabwe's. Poor people are ingenious at finding livelihoods. They seem to recover from the worst blows the way forests regenerate after a fire, and they often do better if no one tries to cultivate them. But the rules governing this seemingly spontaneous process are as intricate and subtle—and as tough—as those of any other system in nature.

Throughout history, poor young women have used their sexuality to cope with poverty, a trend that has almost certainly increased with economic globalization. Traditionally, most poor women in developing countries worked on family farms and their sexuality was generally supervised by their relatives. However, as the system of small-scale, family-based agriculture has become increasingly unsustainable, impoverished young women all over the world have responded by negotiating new survival strategies. Interestingly, impoverished women in Africa and Asia have tended to adapt to this situation in different ways, and this may partly explain why HIV infection rates in southern Africa are ten to one hundred times higher than they are almost anywhere in Asia.

In Asia, many impoverished women end up in the organized brothels of Bombay, Bangkok, Shanghai, and other cities, and in India there are even dedicated hereditary castes of prostitutes, known as devadasis. These women are at high risk of HIV, but because their male partners tend to have sex with them infrequently, and because condom use is increasingly the norm in encounters with prostitutes, these men, and their wives, are at relatively low risk of infection. This probably explains why in Asia, HIV rates in the general population are low and stable or declining, and mainly concentrated where the brothels and prostitutes are, or where there are large numbers of intravenous drug users.[6]

Compared to Asia, a relatively small fraction of impoverished young women in sub-Saharan Africa work exclusively in the sex trade, and the continent has few organized brothels. Instead, many poor African women work in the informal economy as traders, hairdressers, shopkeepers, and so on. Although these women are not considered prostitutes and have many fewer sexual partners than Asian prostitutes do, some of them make casual sexual arrangements with male "facilitators"—for example, the man who delivers the clothing they sell, or the police officer at the roadblock, or the man who rents them space in the market. Such relationships, though implicitly coercive, are often based on friendship and trust as well as economic expedience. Nevertheless, the risk of contracting HIV in transactional relationships can be just as great as it would be if the women were prostitutes with hundreds of partners a year, because when it comes to HIV risk, it is not only the number of sex partners that matters, but whether those partners are part of a larger sexual network involving long-term concurrent relationships.

This may be why HIV rates in Africa tend to be lowest in farming communities that are largely isolated from the cash economy, and highest wherever the informal trading economy is most active, such as in small market towns along truck routes or beside large development projects, in peri-urban slums like Chitungwiza, or in those rural areas where people have abandoned farming and rely instead on remittances from migrant workers.

In both Asia and Africa, the AIDS epidemic is driven partly by the struggles of poor young women in declining agrarian societies to find new livelihoods. Why have Asian women tended to resort to formal prostitution, while African women have tended to rely on informal sexual bartering in longer-term relationships with men they know? The Australian demographer John Caldwell has suggested there may be historical reasons for this.[7] In Asia, as in Europe, land was traditionally a family's most valuable asset, and families had to guard a daughter's virginity to ensure she did not lose her dowry to a rogue pretender from a lower social class. A clear cultural distinction emerged between "good" or "moral" women, who had sex only in marriage, and "fallen" women, who became prostitutes.

African soils tend to be far less fertile than those in Asia or Europe, and land was traditionally far less valuable. Most African Iron Age farmers practiced shifting agriculture, settling in one place for a period of time and moving on when the soil was exhausted. Their most valuable assets were labor and interpersonal alliances, not land, so the economic consequences of out-of-wedlock births were less serious. The distinction between a "moral" and an "immoral" woman was based on a range of characteristics, including her manners, generosity, and respectful demeanor.[8] A fallen woman was not necessarily one who failed to abstain until marriage and remain faithful thereafter, but rather a woman who was openly flirtatious or whose behavior otherwise disrupted the fragile web of social relationships upon which everyone's survival depended.

As demographer John Caldwell has pointed out, while in Europe and Asia cults of chastity emerged around the Virgin Mary and the Indian goddess Pattini, no such wan figures emerged in African religious cults, which exclusively celebrated fertility.

ELEANOR ROOSEVELT was among the first to recognize that human rights begin at home. "The neighborhood he lives in, the school or college he attends; the factory farm or office where he works. Such are the places where every man, woman and child seeks equal justice, equal opportunity, equal dignity without discrimination. Unless these rights have meaning there, they have little meaning anywhere."[9]

In the years since Roosevelt wrote those words, two generations of feminist scholars have demonstrated the ways in which women in developing countries have been brutalized by traditions that constrict their lives in ways that sometimes resemble slavery. According to the Global Coalition on Women and AIDS, a campaign run by a consortium of public-health and women's rights agencies based in Europe and the United States, there is no commonly accepted formula for "empowering women," and entrenched male-chauvinist gender norms will evolve only slowly. "The changes required in attitudes, behaviors, and societal structures may well take generations," the coalition concluded in 2005.[10]

But a promising study from South Africa suggests a way forward. In 2001, a group of researchers from South Africa's University of the

Witwatersrand School of Public Health and the London School of Hygiene and Tropical Medicine set out to study the impact of a microfinance program that offered small business loans to poor African women living in Limpopo, one of South Africa's poorest provinces. The program had the same goal as SHAZ did: to give women a greater sense of personal control over their lives in the hope that this would improve gender relations and reduce the spread of HIV in the community. However, unlike SHAZ, the program worked with older women, many of whom were grandmothers and thus largely immune to the predations of male strangers. Any effect on the spread of HIV would have had to occur indirectly; it was hoped that these older women would pass on their sense of confidence and empowerment to younger women by means of education or changes in social norms.

In collaboration with the Small Enterprise Foundation (SEF), a local microfinance organization, the South African researchers introduced "Sisters for Life," a series of workshop sessions addressing problems of gender and HIV to groups of about forty women who were already meeting every two weeks to repay loans and discuss business plans. The women were obliged to attend the workshops as a condition of receiving further loans. Each session was run by a woman from the local community who had been trained to lead open-ended discussions about sexuality, relationships, the different roles of men and women in daily life, and the effects of local culture on the treatment of women. The women would then act out before their peers the real-life domestic situations in which they found themselves, and discuss them frankly.

At first the women, especially the older ones, didn't like the meetings. "We don't feel comfortable talking about such issues. It is not our culture," said one. But soon they began to open up. In one session, they sang traditional wedding songs instructing new wives how to behave toward their husbands. As the words of one popular song cautioned, "The road ahead will be rocky, but no matter what happens, you must stay with it." This in turn prompted a discussion about their personal experiences of being beaten by their husbands or boyfriends and of looking away in silence when their own daughters suffered the same fate. For many, this was the first time they had shared such painful personal stories without fear of ridicule or judgment.

As in other South African communities, domestic violence in Limpopo was seen as culturally entrenched. Victims seldom called the police, neighbors rarely intervened, and even the police and courts didn't take cases seriously. But as the women talked about their lives, they began to ask themselves whether this was the way things ought to be. Were the old ways necessarily good ways? they wondered. Was this the experience they wanted for their own daughters? Who decided what constituted "culture"? Could it be that culture was not set permanently, but could change?

Perhaps it can be. Two years after the program, known as IMAGE, or Intervention with Microfinance for AIDS and Gender Equity, was initiated, participating women's risk of domestic violence was reduced by half compared to the risk of women who had not participated in the program. Rates of divorce and separation did not increase; instead, women's status, and men's perceptions of them, changed. Women reported that their partners placed greater value on their contributions to the household and treated them with more respect.

According to Kim and her coinvestigator, Paul Pronyk, the key to IMAGE's success resided less in the personal empowerment of individual women than in the collective social energy the program created, which brought the women together to solve common problems that none of them could solve on their own.[11] It sounds simple, but in the field of public health this is actually a radical idea. Most public health interventions tend to address health problems on a case-by-case basis—by, for example, delivering drugs, vaccines, contraceptives, and other items to individual people, or by supplying individuals with information on which to base personal decisions concerning their health.

IMAGE, on the other hand, seemed to give women a new language. Soon they began to speak openly about women's rights, not only in workshop meetings and among themselves but before church congregations, school assemblies, and even a football club. Before joining the loan program, most of the women had known the humiliation of having to beg for food or money from their neighbors, and this discouraged them from speaking out against abuse. As one woman put it, in the past "they'd look at us and say, 'Your grandmother came from the poorest family in this village. What could you possibly have to teach us?'" Now the income from their businesses and a shared commitment to the cause of women's rights gave them the confidence to speak out together. "Women supporting women" became their slogan.

When a girl in one village was raped and the police did nothing, the women started a rape committee and marched to the police station demanding action; then they marched to the hospital to demand better HIV/AIDS services; then they marched to commemorate the "16 Days" international campaign against gender violence, making headlines in their local newspaper.

Although the researchers were unable to measure an effect on HIV incidence, it is quite likely the program could have had some effect on this, given a few more years. Like the women's rights activists who led the fight against AIDS in Uganda in the 1980s, and like the returned prostitutes who led the fight against syphilis in Kagera in the 1950s, the IMAGE women seemed to spark a shift in attitudes. If its effect on domestic violence is confirmed by further resarch, IMAGE could become a model for women's rights programs in Africa.

The American women of the 1960s—whose ideas shaped contemporary feminism and are now helping to shape contemporary development policies—saw gender inequality as being entirely due to the arbitrary economic and social discrimination against women by men. Freedom meant striking out on your own, getting a job and an apartment, choosing for yourself when and whether to have sex or bear children. Empowerment for African women, however, has a different meaning. As their families are being torn apart by poverty, and as institutions to protect them fail to emerge, they are obliged to use whatever resources they have to negotiate a livelihood for themselves in a world wracked by forces they can barely comprehend. They can fight back, but they cannot do it alone.

THE AIM OF the SHAZ program was to give the girls of Chitungwiza more personal autonomy and independence, but some relatives, sensing the inevitable sexual risks such independence involved, tried to rein them in. One mother offered to keep her daughter's loan money for "safekeeping" but then spent it herself and never returned it. In another case, a young woman named Precious told me how she had used her loan money to buy and sell firewood. The profits came in quickly and at first she was able to make the repayments. She had already taught herself hairdressing and she planned to open a salon when she had enough money.

As her firewood business took off, Precious noticed a change in her husband's behavior. He was a factory worker and the marriage had gone well at first. But after a few years, he started drinking and coming home late and spending his money on other women. When Precious asked him where he had been, or requested money for their small child, he beat her up. When, with help from SHAZ, Precious began earning her own money, her husband started to treat her with more respect. He brought more of his own money home, and sometimes in the evening the two of them would sit and plan their future together. Then one day, another man made a casual pass at Precious when she met him on the road. She blew him off. "I am not the Scramble for Africa," she said, referring to the nineteenth-century competition among the imperial powers of Europe for sovereignty over different parts of the continent. But she made the mistake of telling her husband about the incident. A few days later, he broke the man's glasses in a barroom brawl. Precious had to spend every penny she had earned to get her husband out of jail, and now, she says, he has no intention of paying her back.

"Does he think you would leave him if you got the money back?" I asked.

"Yes, he's aware," said Precious.

"In Africa, you can't empower women and girls in isolation," a Zimbabwean woman who worked briefly for SHAZ explained to me. "African society isn't individualistic. When the Western people promote 'empowerment,' they just end up promoting the breakdown of families, which is happening anyway."

African society is like a giant web. Remove one strand and you risk destroying the entire thing. This connectedness is captured in the ancient African concept of *ubuntu*—a term that has many meanings. When the anti-apartheid hero Archbishop Desmond Tutu uses the word in his speeches, his Western listeners usually assume he is referring to a special African version of humanitarianism or solidarity. But *ubuntu* also captures the system of obligations and responsibilities that constrain behavior, restrict individualism, and limit freedom. IMAGE, by strengthening ties among women and within extended families, overturned the culture of silence around domestic violence and AIDS in a small part of Africa. SHAZ, by encouraging young women to strike out on their own without the anchor of social ties, set them adrift.[12]

EPILOGUE

Traditional Medicine

In Uganda, I once attended a musical AIDS play put on by a local community group. The central character and his wife lived in a village near Kampala with their four children. The man sang about how he wanted his wife to have another baby. She sang back that she didn't want another baby. She wanted him to use condoms. He went to a bar, where he met two girls. They thought he was rich, and behind his back they sang about how they looked forward to filling their bellies. Soon, one of them became pregnant. The man brought both girls back to his house in the village. The girls gave the man HIV, which he transmitted to his wife. In the end, the man, his wife, the two girls, and the girl's baby all died. In the finale, the man's relatives all came onstage and fought over his property.

The sparse audience consisted mainly of friends of the actors. An American woman who worked for the development agency that was supporting the theater project wanted to know what the people thought of the play. "What was the message here?" she asked. "Don't go out with bar girls," said a young man laconically. "Stick to one partner," said another. Then an older woman spoke up. She was a traditional healer and wore a voluminous green *basuti*, the traditional costume of her tribe. "AIDS has come to haunt a world that thought it was incomplete," she said. "Some wanted children, some wanted money, some wanted property, some wanted power, but all we ended up with is AIDS."

Today, in a growing number of African communities, a layman's understanding of how sexual networks put everyone at risk of infection, combined with a more compassionate attitude toward the suffering of

AIDS victims and new ideas about gender relations, is helping to reduce AIDS stigma, change sexual behavior, improve relationships between men and women, and reduce the spread of HIV.

Social mobilization is the best weapon we have against the epidemic. But what does this mean for policy? What can health officials do to mobilize people? There is no textbook strategy for motivating the broad social and normative changes in sexual behavior that occurred in Uganda, in Kagera, and for that matter, among gay men. The expertise of the international public health community lies in formulating short, medium, and long term plans; setting up national AIDS committees in African countries; and developing surveillance networks, laboratories, and procurement systems for pharmaceuticals, condoms, and other health related technologies.

Although there are no easy answers, one thing that always mobilizes people is a common enemy. In southern Africa (indeed, in much of the rest of the world), programs for "high-risk" groups and abstinence-only compaigns have sent the message that the enemy is people with AIDS. Ugandans along with gay men the world over, recognized early that the enemy was HIV itself.

The most urgent intervention may be the simplest. People must be made aware of the dangers of long-term concurrency and the risks this sexual system poses even to faithful people and those with few sexual partners. Simply explaining to people how the virus is spreading could help destigmatize the disease, open up discussions of sexuality, generate a more compassionate response to people with AIDS, and mobilize a more vibrant community-based response.

Many people are skeptical that information alone can save lives. After all, the connection between smoking and cancer was known in the 1950s, but US smoking rates remained high for decades. It's important to remember that during those some decades, people received mixed messages about how risky the habit was. Phony tobacco industry–funded research promoted the idea that the risks of smoking were "unknown" or that filters and low tar brands were not very dangerous, when they were. When respected entities such as the American Medical Association and the New England Journal of Medicine, went along with the story, this may have reinforced people's natural tendency to deny the risks they were taking. In the 1980s the US government began to realize just how much smoking related diseases were costing the Medicare program. The subsequent tobacco trials of the 1990s exposed the companies' tactics, and since then, the government has imposed new anti-smoking regulations and launched anti-smoking campaigns, some of which have been extremely effective. Similarly, behavior change in response to HIV may be more rapid when people receive clearer messages about where their risks are coming from.

For too long, people in Southern Africa have been under that impression that typical "promiscuity" is at the root of the epidemic in their communities. The truth itself, in all its complex detail, will almost certainly get people talking more openly about HIV, examining their own behavior and beliefs, and working together to change the things they can change. It is not only an urgent public health priority that they be properly informed. Access to accurate public health information is also a human right.

In southern Africa, the silence surrounding AIDS is partly due to the shadow cast by past racist discourses about black sexuality. In Uganda, where the colonial experience was more benign, where people's dignity had not been ruined by centuries of racism, discrimination, and forced displacement, discussions of sex and AIDS may have been easier. In the 1980s, these discussions helped Uganda's health officials analyze the situation more dispassionately, and this in turn enabled them to design pragmatic campaigns that informed people that everyone was at risk. As a result, most Ugandans understood that people with AIDS were just as "moral" and deserving of compassion as anyone else. As people began to recognize where their own risks were really coming from, they took measures—mainly partner reduction and condom use—to avoid them. Unfortunately, the relatively new abstinence-only programs are inhibiting this openness, and deepening divisions between "moral" and "immoral" behavior, which could thwart Uganda's success.

The failure of so many donor programs has left many with the mistaken impression that when it comes to behavior change, "nothing works". But a growing number of initiatives, including Stepping Stones, IMAGE, and Men as Partners, another South African program that uses peer education techniques to mobilize men against domestic violence and HIV are working, sometimes with words alone.

However, words alone are not enough. The billion-dollar aid agencies such as USAID, the World Bank and the Bill and Melinda Gates

Foundation must continue to make condoms and counseling and testing services as widely available as possible, and should also continue to extend the offer of AIDS treatment to all who need it. But they should be aware that these programs, though vitally important, are unlikely to bring the epidemic under control on their own. They also need to do more to support programs that promote a sense of solidarity among all those who care about the disease. Too many donor programs have divided people—rich from poor, old from young, HIV positive from HIV negative, "moral" from "immoral." Microfinance programs, home-based care and orphan programs, women's rights programs and other initiatives that are truly locally conceived and controlled need to be expanded. This must be done carefully and in good faith; episodic, self-serving efforts to boomerang funds back to donor agencies themselves can be worse than useless, as can opportunistic "projects" spontaneously generated in response to new donor funds.

The African AIDS epidemic is partly a consequence of patterns of sexual networking that have evolved in response to the insecurity of living in a rapidly globalizing world that is leaving the continent behind. Therefore, the industrialized countries should also reexamine their policies in trade and foreign investment so that African nations can compete on fairer terms in the global economy.

THE CONCLUSION that targeted technical public health programs such as condom promotion, HIV testing, and sexually transmitted disease services have played only a modest role in controlling the African AIDS epidemic will come as little surprise to historians of public health, to whom the power of new ideas and social mobilization is well known.[2] In late-nineteenth-century America, knowledge of the newly proven germ theory of disease saved millions of lives long before antibiotics, vaccines, and other technical advances based on this discovery became available decades later.[3] It was the age of long skirts and parasols, when women were believed to be incapable of abstract thought or action in the world. Nevertheless, legions of middle-class women, armed only with knowledge gained from newspaper reports about the germ theory, launched spontaneous public health campaigns. They printed pamphlets, held meetings, and went door-to-door lecturing about hygiene. Their efforts not only helped reduce infant mortality; they changed an entire culture. The social imperative to wash, an aversion to those who spit and cough in public, the elevation of the lowly estate of housekeeping to a "domestic science," modern kitchens and bathrooms with easily washable white surfaces, even the growing popularity of the clean lines of modernist architectural styles and the doing away with the dust-and-germ-laden draperies of the Victorian era—all these things were powerfully influenced by this revolutionary mobilization to prevent disease.

The adoption of birth control has similarly been driven as much by social mobilization and new ideas as by new contraceptive technology.[4] The first country to see a sustained, voluntary decline in birthrates was France, in the late eighteenth century. As the population grew, French farmers had been forced to divide their land into smaller and smaller parcels for the next generation, and this created pressure to reduce family size. At the time, the only form of contraception was a rudimentary condom fashioned from goat intestines. But revolutionary ideas were in the air. Philosophers and economists were debating whether population growth was creating a Malthusian nightmare, and ordinary French people were absorbing new ideas about personal rights and questioning church teaching about sexuality. Couples increasingly began to use withdrawal, masturbation, and other techniques to limit childbearing, while more and more women delayed marriage or avoided it altogether.

In 1978, the World Health Organization and UNICEF sponsored a vast conference on public health in developing countries in Alma-Ata, Kazakhstan. Thousands of experts, including the health ministers of more than one hundred countries, came together to launch the "Health for All" movement, a global campaign to deliver basic health care to the world's poor by the year 2000. The final declaration of the conference recognized that this would require more than increased funding for services and medical technology. Because poor health was partly an outcome of social and economic inequality, it would require greater popular participation in policy- and decision-making so that poor people could decide for themselves what services they received and could strive to change the social and economic conditions that placed them at risk of illness in the first place.

The Health for All movement was a fading gleam of 1960s communitarian thinking on development. But dusk was falling on the sometimes naïve optimism of those years. By 1980, global recession, the debt crisis, and a new cadre of neoliberal leaders in the United States and Europe all but drew the curtain on the Alma-Ata Health for All movement. It would soon be replaced with what UNICEF officials called the "Child Survival Revolution," which essentially employed a vertical, technocratic approach to delivering health commodities such as vaccines, antibiotics, and contraceptives in developing countries. The distribution was carried out by contract agencies that specialize in social marketing and other private-sector methods and have close ties to the pharmaceutical and medical-technology industries.

As a result of the Child Survival programs, the health of women and children in Africa did improve during the 1980s and into the 1990s, but the returns on this approach have begun to diminish. By the late 1990s, child- and maternal-health indicators had stagnated or deteriorated, especially in Africa—a trend that could not be explained entirely by AIDS. The reasons included decreased funding for health programs, increased corruption, flagging political will, and tensions within communities that only local people could comprehend or hope to resolve.[5] But while aid agencies often referred in their publicity documents to "community ownership" and "participation," and sometimes employed volunteers and community health workers, local people had no decision-making power and no voice in how programs were carried out.[6]

When HIV infection rates soared throughout Africa, the commodities-based approach was rapidly redeployed. Such programs as condom social marketing, the loveLife franchises, the voluntary testing and counseling services that dot the landscape throughout East and southern Africa—even the packaged "Life Skills" curricula distributed to schools throughout the continent—have tended to follow this model. But with AIDS, the commodities-based approach would be less successful than it was with childhood illnesses, because its effectiveness depends critically on a sense of commitment and will that cannot be bought and sold.

BACK IN the early 1990s, when I was still working in Kampala at the Uganda Cancer Institute and beginning to realize how hard it was going to be to make an AIDS vaccine, I became interested in traditional African medicine. The powerful antiretroviral drug cocktails had yet to been invented, but I had heard that Africa's traditional healers had their own cures for malaria, diarrhea, and other diseases that cause great suffering in Africa. These men and women, known for their exotic costumes and strange rituals, are consulted by millions of African people with physical and spiritual problems for which ordinary medicine is considered useless. Most combine trancelike drumming and dancing with herbal ointments and beverages they make themselves from local plants and other substances. I wondered if one of these healers might, perhaps, have discovered a substance that could treat the symptoms of AIDS.

Over the years, I made it a hobby to visit the markets where African traditional healers sell their goods. I learned that in Africa, illnesses fall into two categories.[7] There are "European" diseases, such as tuberculosis and the fevers of childhood, that occur naturally and can sometimes be cured with Western medicine. And there are "African" diseases—unusual afflictions or epidemics caused by supernatural forces, for which Western medicine is useless. When a jealous neighbor sends a spell that makes you sick, or when a person is felled by the anger of a neglected ancestor, or when a sudden epidemic strikes seemingly from nowhere and kills millions of otherwise healthy people, these are African diseases.

Treatments for African diseases tend to rely less on their chemical activity than on symbolism and ritual. In Zambia, the roots of the hookthorn tree, with its straight, narrow trunk and rough, thorny bark resembling an inverted sore throat, are used to cure coughing. In South Africa, roots are ground up and fed to mad people to keep them still, and plants that smell bad are used to chase away evil spirits. In Uganda, a chicken is placed upon the head to cure epilepsy. There are many treatments for sexual problems. In South Africa, an animal horn fashioned into a tube and blown between the legs functions as a sexual stimulant; to promote the growth of their testicles, Zambian boys drink a tea made from the roots of the bush orange tree, the branches of which bend under the weight of a large yellow fruit; when a Zambian girl rubs the huge flat leaves of a bush known as "the sex tree" on her face, it is said to arouse any man who looks at her. Fortunately, the African forest also produces abundant treatments for sexually transmitted diseases, such as the whitethorn, with its tiny red berries, or the ancylobotrys tree, the roots of which secrete a white gum resembling pus.

Some African medicine does have scientifically measurable chemical activity. African healers were among the first to develop the technique of smallpox inoculation, for example, and used quinine to cure malaria long before Europeans did. In Uganda, I befriended a local zoologist who was studying a plant mixture that had been used for centuries by Ethiopian peasants to cure a variety of ills. The zoologist was testing the substance experimentally, to see whether it killed any of the parasites common in Uganda—such as those that cause malaria and river blindness. He told me he had heard that in Ethiopia, peasants used this substance to cure yeast infections of the skin, such as athlete's foot and ringworm, an itchy but not very serious infection named for the circular, coin-sized rashes it causes. He suggested I try to determine whether this was true.

This was not a cure for AIDS, I thought, but since many AIDS patients suffer from yeast infections, it could be a start. Ringworm is extremely common among Ugandan children, so I asked a few neighbors in the semirural Kampala suburb where I was living whether they knew any children with ringworm.

At first, they came one by one. Mothers and fathers with feverish children, and children with oozing sores on their legs, arms, and faces; others in even graver condition. "That kid needs to go to the hospital," I'd say to their parents. "You take us," their parents replied. "The hospital people treat us badly unless we have money." I did go with one child. To others, I gave money for bribes.

Then, one morning when I was out of town, my landlord awoke to the sound of murmuring and clanking metal. A substantial crowd had gathered at his front gate. The visitors told him that they had heard there was a lady in the house who had special medicine for sick children. When I heard what had happened, I was relieved not to have been there. Now, looking back, I am sorry I wasn't. What I should have done was march the crowd to the hospital, to the Ministry of Health, to the president's office. What I should have done was write something for the international newspapers about the sorry state of health services in Uganda, a nation that was receiving substantial donor funding for Child Survival programs.

Instead, I went to England to attend graduate school in public health. I brought a vial of my friend's Ethiopian herbal mixture with me and asked several English people I knew with athlete's foot to try it. It didn't work, they said. I then sent a sample of the mixture to a lab at Kew Gardens that tests natural products for medicinal properties. The results came back a year later. The mixture had no activity against yeast, bacteria, HIV, or any other microbe.

Only later did I realize the opportunity I had missed. Back then I was still subject to magic-bullet thinking—the idea that serious public health problems could be addressed without considering their social and political causes. The Ugandans seemed to know better, but their message was lost on me.

Sometimes when I am in Africa staying in rural areas or the settled fringes of towns, I have lain awake at night listening to the sounds of drumming and the hoots and calls of dancers coming from the compound of a traditional healer. To describe these rituals, the anthropologist John Janzen uses the southern African term *ngoma*, which translates roughly as "Drums of Affliction."[8] According to Janzen, *ngoma* rituals tend to occur more frequently whenever a culture or way of life is threatened. They serve to reestablish community ties and social cohesion and often attract the marginalized, such as disabled people, or women, or as in Uganda, an entire society afflicted with a horrifying new disease. Like Africa's songs, dances, and sculpture, these healing customs offer more than mere relief from illness; they are part of a larger social code and system of ethics.

The Drums of Affliction are beating especially vigorously in Africa today, as the continent struggles to cope with so many scourges, including winner-take-all economic development, political corruption, civil conflict, and AIDS. Some of the cults that have developed are highly destructive, including the Lord's Resistance Army that terrorized northern Uganda for two decades and the angry gangs of thieves and rapists that haunt the townships of South Africa. But some cults are positive. They start with ideas that get people talking and they develop into social movements that change things for the better. Until we find the magic bullet, this is the only cure.

APPENDIX: A MAGIC BULLET AFTER ALL?

MALE CIRCUMCISION, ANTIRETROVIRAL DRUGS, HIV TESTING, VAGINAL MICROBICIDES

MALE CIRCUMCISION

For years, researchers puzzled over why most West African countries have lower HIV infection rates than many southern and East African countries. Some thought it must have something to do with the Muslim religion, widely practiced in West Africa, which imposes restrictions on women's sexual freedom. However, male circumcision, which is ritually practiced by Muslims and by many other groups, turns out to be highly protective against HIV.[1]

In African countries where male circumcision is common, such as Senegal, Mali, Ghana, Benin, and the entire region of North Africa, HIV rates tend to be much lower than in countries such as Botswana, Lesotho, and Swaziland, where circumcision has traditionally been rare. In countries with high rates of HIV, provinces and districts that have high rates of circumcision, such as Inhambane in Mozambique or Dar es Salaam in Tanzania, tend to have lower HIV rates. Two African tribes with very high HIV infection rates are the Zulu of South Africa and the Tswana of Botswana. Before colonial times, men in both tribes underwent circumcision rituals during adolescence. But when King Shaka united the Zulu tribe in the 1820s, he abolished the ritual after two of his comrades died from infections acquired during the operation. When Christian missionaries settled in Botswana in the late nineteenth century, they declared circumcision barbaric and banned it.

Circumcision removes mucosal tissue in the foreskin that contains Langerhans cells with special receptors for HIV. In 2006, researchers in South Africa, Kenya, and Uganda found that circumcision cuts a man's risk of contracting HIV by roughly 50 percent. The effect was so powerful that the trials were stopped prematurely, because it was considered unethical not to offer the procedure to men in the control groups.[2]

Although male circumcision doesn't protect women directly fewer infections among men will obviously help reduce infection rates for everyone. This is not true of female circumcision, or female genital mutilation, which offers no protection against HIV and is extremely dangerous for other reasons.[3]

Male circumcision offers more effective protection against HIV than any of the experimental vaccines currently undergoing clinical trials around the world. It is also cheaper, carries few side effects, if done safely requires no booster shots, and is available now. Evidence that male circumcision might be protective has been available since the 1980s, but it was only in 2000 that clinical trials to confirm its efficacy got under way. It is now high time that international public health agencies such as UNAIDS, WHO, and USAID develop guidelines to promote safe, hygienic male circumcision in African hospitals and clinics and fund operational research on the cheapest, safest ways to carry out the procedure.[4]

Although male circumcision offers powerful protection against HIV, it does not offer total protection. Some West African cities, such as Cotonou in Benin and Yaounde in Cameroon, have HIV infection rates of 5 to 10 percent even though virtually all men are circumcised. Therefore, efforts to change sexual behavior will still be necessary, even if male circumcision becomes routine.

ANTIRETROVIRAL DRUG TREATMENT PROGRAMS

In 1996, U.S. researchers discovered that a "cocktail" of three antiretroviral drugs taken in combination can suppress the growth of HIV in the body for years and restore the immune systems of AIDS patients. It has extended the lives of millions of patients the world over and is increasingly being made available to patients in Africa through foreign-aid programs.

While these programs are extremely important, they do have limitations. In Western countries, antiretroviral drugs may add decades to the life expectancy of an AIDS patient. In Africa, however, the prospects are more modest; the UN now estimates that antiretroviral drugs will add, on average, only an extra four or five years to the life of an African patient. This is because HIV mutates and soon becomes resistant to one or all of the cocktail drugs. Therefore, patients must eventually switch to a new cocktail and then to another one. In Western countries, patients have twenty different drugs to choose from, but patients in Africa, even with all the funding for treatment programs currently available, so far have a choice of roughly six. For now, the others are too expensive or too difficult to administer in countries without reliable health infrastructure, including health workers, electricity supplies, and refrigeration.

Antiretroviral drug programs also raise equity concerns. Distributing even relatively simple drug regimens on a large scale in Africa poses formidable obstacles. Many African health facilities lack trained and motivated staff, adequate management and administrative capacity, and sufficient supplies of medicines, vehicles, refrigerators, lab reagents, and other basic equipment. Some lack water, electricity, and even intact buildings.

Programs to treat people with syphilis and tuberculosis, or even to distribute vitamins, show how difficult it is to deliver health care in such countries, even if the drugs are simple to administer and virtually free. Half a million children—most of them African—die every year from measles, which is preventable with a five-cent vaccine. More than a million pregnant women in Africa have syphilis that is never treated and puts their newborns at risk of deformity or death. The tests and drugs to eliminate this risk cost only twenty-five cents. Hundreds of thousands of children go blind every year, and more than a million die, because they are deficient in Vitamin A. Vitamin A supplements, which need to be taken only twice a year, are virtually free.

Treating AIDS patients is far more complicated than testing for syphilis or administering Vitamin A drops or measles vaccines. AIDS patients need counseling, laboratory tests, and ongoing clinical care to treat opportunistic infections and monitor drug resistance and side effects. Even where the drugs and other necessary supplies are available—and in many places they aren't—antiretroviral treatment programs require considerable effort on the part of public-sector health workers. But the health workforce throughout sub-Saharan Africa is rapidly vanishing as salaries plummet and conditions deteriorate.

It will be important to ensure that antiretroviral drug treatment programs do not further degrade already fragile African health-care systems. The officials who run the new treatment programs sometimes hire away public-sector doctors and nurses who would otherwise be ensuring the safe delivery of babies or vaccinating children against deadly diseases. I once asked an American aid official whose organization was bidding on a U.S. government contract to deliver antiretroviral drugs in Africa how his group intended to deal with the stark inequalities between his own program for people with AIDS and the impoverished public health-care systems responsible for caring for everyone else. He said his organization was planning to ignore the issue. "When we get the contract, we're going to grab every trained health-care worker we can get our hands on," he replied.

While it is impossible to put a price tag on even one year of any human life, especially that of an HIV-positive mother whose children would otherwise be orphaned at even younger ages, it would be far better if that mother had never been infected in the first place. Antiretroviral drug programs are unlikely to turn the epidemic around unless they are accompanied by vigorous prevention efforts.[6]

HIV TESTING

Since the early 1990s, foreign donors, especially the U.S. Agency for International Development and the World Bank, have funded training programs to teach health workers how to administer HIV tests and conduct one-on-one counseling sessions for patients before and after they receive their results. Freestanding HIV testing kiosks, staffed by a counselor or a nurse, now dot the landscape in many African countries. Demand for these services is mixed. In some countries, such as Uganda, these services are in great demand. In much of southern Africa, however, fear and stigma leave many people with no desire to learn their status.

Some experts, reasoning that people who know they are negative should naturally wish to stay that way, and that people who know they are positive should naturally wish to protect others, have claimed that HIV testing is key to controlling the epidemic.[7] However, there is little evidence that widespread testing is either necessary or sufficient for HIV prevention. In the American gay community, the most dramatic declines in HIV incidence began in the early 1980s, before HIV was even identified, and long before a test for the virus became widely available.[8] Nor did many people in Uganda and Kagera know their HIV status when the epidemic began to subside in those regions in the late 1980s. While some studies show that HIV-positive people who discover their status do change their behavior, this may have more to do with the effects of the support groups they join afterward than with knowledge of the result itself. There is no evidence that HIV testing changes the behavior of those who find they are negative. A study in Uganda, for example, found that people who test HIV negative are just as likely to engage in risky behavior and contract HIV as those who don't know their status.[9]

In recent years, door-to-door testing programs—in which outreach workers offer HIV testing to people in their homes—have been launched in a number of African communities. The first such program, carried out in Uganda, was remarkably successful, in that more than 90 percent of people agreed to be tested. The effect of this on their future behavior and risk of HIV was not measured, but the program inspired similar efforts in other countries.

It is not clear that all societies are prepared for such programs, however. In countries where AIDS-related stigma is severe, such programs could make things worse. In KwaZulu-Natal, people living in the catchment area of a door-to-door testing program were seen running away as the HIV testing nurses drove up to their homesteads. In Malawi, an impoverished southern African country wracked by food shortages, the U.S. government hired Malawian researchers to go from house to house offering voluntary HIV tests. Very few people took up the offer, so the researchers—saying they worked for the

Malawian government—began warning people that if they did not give a blood sample, they would not be on the list for food rations.[10] Soon rumors began spreading throughout the area that people from the government were coercing people to have their "blood pumped" for Satanic vampire rituals, and the popularity of HIV testing services plummeted even further.

Some people probably have good reasons to flee from an HIV testing nurse—especially women. In a series of studies analyzed under the auspices of the World Health Organization, some 20 percent of African women who tested positive for HIV experienced some sort of negative outcome if their husbands or boyfriends found out.[11] Some women were blamed for bringing the infection into the relationship; others were beaten or thrown out of their houses. Some 40 percent were afraid to tell their partners at all. The women in these studies had chosen on their own to attend an HIV testing center. The frequency of adverse events in door-to-door testing programs would very likely be higher.

Even health workers can be abusive to women they know to be HIV positive. In 2004, I attended a meeting of the Mama's Club, a Ugandan support group for HIV-positive mothers. The women were discussing the treatment they received from nurses in the maternity ward at Mulago Hospital, one of the premier health centers on the continent when it comes to dealing with AIDS. "The nurses look at your chart and say, 'Yuck, this one is positive—someone else can deal with her,'" one woman said. "The doctor told me, 'If you move, I'll stab you with a knife,'" said another. All the health workers were afraid to touch her, she said. Another woman said she refused to go to the maternity ward after hearing an HIV-positive friend describe her experience there. "She was just left in a corner to deliver on her own. The baby died." The speaker decided to give birth in her village with a traditional birth attendant—a sympathetic, but untrained, old lady. The birth attendant did not have antiretrovirals and the baby was born infected. Breastfeeding such infants is generally preferable, even if they are already HIV positive. But this mother had received no counseling on the subject and her emaciated infant lay in her arms, drinking from a bottle of orange soda.[12]

In Botswana, two years after the government began offering free antiretroviral drug treatment, health officials reported that the program was reaching only some 15 percent of those who needed it. One reason for the low uptake was that people were reluctant to be tested, so the government implemented a routine HIV testing policy in all health centers. All patients would be offered an HIV test whether they were suffering from a cough, a fever, or a broken arm. According to one survey, 43 percent of respondents said that they thought people would avoid seeking health care because of the program.[13] While most respondents did not believe the testing program would increase HIV-related stigma, such stigma is already pervasive in Botswana, a country where HIV-positive pregnant women are known in some circles as "suicide bombers."

African people have a right to know their HIV status, and HIV testing services are vitally important. But they must be truly voluntary, and they must be accompanied by aggressive campaigns to destigmatize HIV and protect the human rights of infected people, especially women.

MICROBICIDES

Of growing interest to many HIV prevention experts are microbicides—soaps or gels that women can put in their vaginas before sex that may reduce their chances of becoming infected. Several U.S. and European labs are currently experimenting with such products. Experts from the UNAIDS program and other groups claim that microbicides will protect women who may not have the option to abstain from sex and whose unfaithful partners refuse to use condoms.[14]

While microbicides are promising in theory, they are as yet unavailable, and even if those currently under development turn out to work, it will take years for them to reach the market. There are reasons to question whether a microbicide would have a significant effect on the epidemic in Africa in any case.[15] Even the most promising prototypes are considerably less effective than condoms, even when tested on monkeys under ideal laboratory conditions.[16] It is unlikely that they will work even this well in the messy realities of everyday life in Africa. One danger is that couples who might otherwise have used condoms will switch to microbicides, thus increasing the risk of transmission if either partner is infected.

Although a microbicide might be less uncomfortable than a condom, and thus might be used more consistently, people using them will likely encounter many of the same problems that currently arise with condoms. Like condoms, microbicides must be made available in remote places and sold cheaply so that the poorest women can afford them. Women will also have to use them correctly and consistently—meaning every time they have sex. Like condoms, microbicides will not protect women who are coerced into sex or raped, unless they anticipate they will be.

In theory, microbicides should offer women more control than condoms do, but since most HIV transmission in Africa takes place in intimate, long-term partnerships, it is unlikely that a woman would be able to use one for an extended period without her partner's knowledge and cooperation. Introducing condoms into long-term intimate relationships is known to be extremely difficult. Microbicides—because of their association with disease prevention—may well suffer the same stigma that condoms do now. Certainly this is the case with the female condom—a plastic device that fits inside the vagina but otherwise functions like a male condom. Female condoms have been promoted as a female-controlled alternative to male condoms, but like male condoms, they are commonly associated with prostitution, misbehavior, and mistrust and have thus far proved highly unpopular.[17] When the social-marketing firm PSI began distributing free female condoms in Zimbabwe, officials discovered that people were removing the plastic rings and selling them as jewelry.[18]

NOTES

PREFACE

1. *Report on the Global AIDS Epidemic* (Geneva: UNAIDS, 2006).
2. K. French, *Report for UNAIDS Scenarios for Africa: The Future of the HIV/AIDS Epidemic in China, India, Russia and Eastern Europe* (London: Department of Infectious Disease Epidemiology, Imperial College, March 2004); Helen Epstein and Stewart Parkinson, "New Wave Big Enough, but No Tsunami," *AIDSLink* 93 (October 2005), 14–15.
3. Richard Knox, "AIDS Vaccine Remains Elusive," National Public Radio, June 5, 2006.
4. Richard Horton, "AIDS: The Elusive Vaccine," *The New York Review of Books*, September 23, 2004. The AIDS vaccines currently undergoing trials are estimated to be only partially effective. Such vaccines could even make things worse by driving the evolution of more aggressive strains of HIV, as seems to be the case for malaria. See M. Mackinnon and A. F. Read, "Immunity promotes virulence evolution in a malaria model," *PLoS Med* 2:9 (2004), E230.
5. See Anne-Christine d'Adesky, *Moving Mountains: The Race to Treat Global AIDS* (New York: Verso, 2004); Greg Behrman, *The Invisible People* (New York: Simon & Schuster, 2004); Raymond A. Smith and Patricia D. Siplon, *Drugs into Bodies: Global AIDS Treatment Activism* (Westport, Conn.: Praeger, 2006); Edwin Cameron, *Witness to AIDS* (Cape Town: Tafelberg, 2005); Stephen Lewis, *Race Against Time* (Toronto: House of Anansi Press, 2005).
6. M. J. Wawer et al., "Rates of HIV-1 transmission per coital act, by stage of HIV-1 infection, in Rakai, Uganda," *J Infect Dis* 191:9 (May 1, 2005), 1403–9.
7. "World Population Prospects" (New York: UN Population Secretariat, 2004), revision.
8. "Intensifying HIV Prevention: UNAIDS Policy Position Paper" (Geneva: UNAIDS, August 2005).

9. Bertran Auvert et al., "Randomized, controlled intervention trial of male circumcision for reduction of HIV infection risk: The ANRS 1265 trial," *PLoS Med* 2:11, e298. Other studies are under way to confirm this finding and the results should be available in mid-2007.
10. Auvert et al., "Male circumcision and HIV infection in four cities in sub-Saharan Africa: The multicentre study of factors determining the different prevalences of HIV in sub-Saharan Africa," *AIDS* 15 Suppl 4) (August 2001), S31–40.
11. For this section I have drawn on the following: John Iliffe, *Africans: The History of a Continent* (Cambridge: Cambridge University Press, 1995); Roland Oliver, *The African Experience: From Olduvai Gorge to the 21st Century* (Boulder, Colo.: Westview Press, 2000); Anthony Appiah, *In My Father's House: Africa in the Philosophy of Culture* (New York: Oxford University Press, 1999); John Reader, *Africa: A Biography of a Continent* (New York: Vintage, 1999).
12. Adam Ashforth, *Witchcraft, Violence and Democracy in South Africa* (Chicago: University of Chicago Press, 2005); Peter Geschiere, *The Modernity of Witchcraft: Politics and the Occult in Postcolonial Africa* (Charlottesville: University Press of Virginia, 1997); Stephen Ellis, *Worlds of Power: Religious Thought and Political Practice in Africa* (Oxford: Oxford University Press, 2004).
13. Basil Davidson, *The African Genius* (Athens: Ohio University Press, 2004).
14. During the mid-1980s, HIV incidence in U.S. gay men fell by about 80 percent. W. Winkelstein, Jr., et al., "The San Francisco Men's Health Study: III. Reduction in human immunodeficiency virus transmission among homosexual/bisexual men, 1982–86," *Am J Public Health* 77:6 (June 1987), 685–9; Martina Morris and Laura Dean, "Effect of sexual behavior change on long-term human immunodeficiency virus prevalence among homosexual men," *Am J Epidemiol* 140:3 (August 1, 1994), 217–32.
15. Wellings, K.; Collumbien, M.; Slaymaker, E.; Singh, S.; Hodges, Z.; Patel, D.; Bajos, N.; "Sexual behaviour in context: a global perspective." *Lancet* (2006) 368(9548):1706–28.
16. Epstein, H. "Why is AIDS worse in Africa?" *Discover Magazine* (February 2004) Southern African Development Community. Expert Think Tank Meeting on HIV Prevention in High-Prevalence Countries in Southern Africa (Report), Maseru, Lesotho (May 10-12, 2006); Daniel T. Halperin and Helen Epstein. "Why is HIV prevalence so severe in southern Africa? The role of multiple concurrent partnerships and lack of male circumcision." *Southern African Journal of HIV Medicine* (2007) 26: 19–25.

A NOTE ON THE STATISTICS CITED IN THIS BOOK

1. Drumright L.N., Gorbach P.M., Holmes K.K. Do people really know their sex partners? Concurrency, knowledge of partner behavior, and sexually transmitted infections within partnerships. Sex Transm Dis. 2004 Jul; 31(7):437–42.
2. "Reconciling antenatal clinic-based surveillance and population-based survey estimates of HIV prevalence in sub-Saharan Africa" (World Health Organization and UNAIDS, August 2003).
3. See the UNAIDS/WHO Global HIV/AIDS Online Database (http://www.who.int/globalatlas/default.asp).
4. K. Dzekedzeke and K. M. Fylkesnes, "Reducing uncertainties in global HIV prevalence estimates: The case of Zambia," *BMC Public Health* 6:1 (April 2, 2006), 83.
5. See, for example, Nicholas Eberstadt, "The Future of AIDS," *Foreign Affairs*, November/December 2002; Susan Hunter, *AIDS in Asia: A Continent in Peril* (Basingstoke: Palgrave Macmillan, 2004).
6. French, *Report for UNAIDS* (London: Department of Infectious Disease Epidemiology, Imperial College, March 2004); Epstein and Parkinson, "New Wave Big Enough, but No Tsunami," *AIDSLink* 93 (October 2005).
7. See, for example, Hallett T.B., Aberle-Grasse J., Bello G., Boulos L.M., Cayemittes M.P., Cheluget B., Chipeta J., Dorrington R., Dube S., Ekra A.K., Garcia-Calleja J.M., Garnett G.P., Greby S., Gregson S., Grove J.T., Hader S., Hanson J., Hladik W., Ismail S., Kassim S., Kirungi W., Kouassi L., Mahomva A., Marum L., Maurice C., Nolan M., Rehle T., Stover J., Walker N. "Declines in HIV prevalence can be associated with changing sexual behaviour in Uganda, urban Kenya, Zimbabwe, and urban Haiti. *Sex Transm Infect.* (2006 Apr.) 22 Suppl 1:i1–8.
8. Ahmed S., Lutalo T., Wawer M., Serwadda D., Sewankambo N.K., Nalugoda F., Makumbi F., Wabwire-Mangen F., Kiwanuka N., Kigozi G., Kiddugavu M., Gray R. "HIV incidence and sexually transmitted disease prevalence associated with condom use: a population study in Rakai, Uganda." AIDS. 2001 Nov; 15(16):2171–9.

CHAPTER ONE: THE OUTSIDERS—APRIL 1993

1. Yoweri Museveni, *What Is Africa's Problem?* (Minneapolis: University of Minnesota Press, 2000); Henry Kyemba, *A State of Blood: The Inside Story of Idi Amin* (Kampala: Fountain Publishers, 1997).
2. V. Simon and D. D. Ho, "HIV-1 dynamics in vivo: Implications for therapy," *Nature Reviews Microbiology* 1:3 (December 2003), 181–90.

3. J. D. Smith et al., "Reactions of Ugandan antisera with peptides encoded by V3 loop epitopes of human immunodeficiency virus type 1," *AIDS Res Hum Retrov* 10:5 (May 1994), 577–83; M. A. Rayfield et al., "A molecular epidemiologic survey of HIV in Uganda, HIV variant working group," *AIDS* 12:5 (March 26, 1998): 521–7.
4. Quoted in Michael Tuck, "Syphilis, Sexuality, and Social Control: A History of Venereal Disease in Colonial Uganda," Ph.D. diss., Northwestern University, 1997.
5. Ibid.
6. Ibid.
7. Richard Horton, "AIDS: The Elusive Vaccine," *New York Review of Books*, September 23, 2004.
8. M. J. Wawer et al., "Control of sexually transmitted diseases for AIDS prevention in Uganda: A randomised community trial, Rakai Project Study Group," *Lancet* 353:9152 (February 13, 1999), 525–35; A. Kamali et al., "A community-based randomized controlled trial to investigate impact of improved STD management and behavioural interventions on HIV incidence in rural Masaka, Uganda: Trial design, methods and baseline findings," *Trop Med Int Health* 7:12 (December 2002), 1053–63; H. Grosskurth et al., "Impact of improved treatment of sexually transmitted diseases on HIV infection in rural Tanzania: Randomised controlled trial," *Lancet* 346:8974 (August 26, 1995), 530–6; R. Kaul et al., "Monthly antibiotic chemoprophylaxis and incidence of sexually transmitted infections and HIV-1 infection in Kenyan sex workers: A randomized controlled trial," *JAMA* 291:21 (June 2, 2004), 2555–62. Michael Carter "IAS: Daily aciclovir doesn't reduce HIV risk in HSV-2 infected women—was poor adherence the reason? AIDSMap News Monday, July 23, 2007.
9. Grosskurth et al., "Control of sexually transmitted diseases for HIV-1 prevention: Understanding the implications of the Mwanza and Rakai trials," *Lancet* 355:9219 (June 3, 2000), 1981–7. For a different view, see Christopher Hudson, "Community-based trials of sexually transmitted disease treatment: Repercussions for epidemiology and HIV prevention," *B World Health Organ* 79:1 (2001), 48–58.

CHAPTER TWO: THE MYSTERIOUS ORIGINS OF HIV

1. T. Zhu et al., "An African HIV-1 sequence from 1959 and implications for the origin of the epidemic," *Nature* 391:6667 (February 5, 1998), 594–7.
2. Tom Curtis, "The Origin of AIDS: A Startling New Theory Attempts to Answer the Question: Was It an Act of God or an Act of Man?" *Rolling Stone*, March 19, 1992, 54–61, 106–8.

3. J. Mokili and B. Korber, "The spread of HIV in Africa," *J Neurovirol* 11 Suppl 1 (2005), 66–75.
4. E. Hooper, *Slim: A Reporter's Own Story of AIDS in East Africa* (London: Bodley Head, 1990).
5. Dale Peterson and Karl Amman, *Eating Apes* (Berkeley: University of California Press, 2003).
6. Megan Vaughan, *Curing Their Ills: Colonial Power and African Illness* (Cambridge: Polity Press, 1991).
7. Boston: Little, Brown, 1999.
8. Nathan Wolfe et al., "Naturally acquired simian retrovirus infections in central African hunters," *Lancet* 363:9413 (March 20, 2004), 932–7; P. A. Marx, C. Apetrei, and E. Drucker, "AIDS as a zoonosis? Confusion over the origin of the virus and the origin of the epidemics," *J Med Primatol* 33:5–6 (October 2004), 220–6.
9. Marx, Apetrei, and Drucker, "AIDS as a zoonosis?"
10. See *Philosophical Transactions of the Royal Society: Biological Sciences* 356:1410 (June 29, 2001). This entire issue was devoted to the question of the origin of HIV, with special reference to the "polio hypothesis."
11. See Hooper, *The River*, chap. 49, "Preston Marx and the Alternative Hypothesis." Also see Zhu et al., "African HIV-1 sequence." This article contains the following aside: "The factors that propelled the initial spread of HIV-1 in central Africa remain unknown: the role of large-scale vaccination campaigns, perhaps with multiple uses of non-sterilized needles, should be carefully examined, although social changes such as easier access to transportation, increasing population density, and more frequent sexual contacts may have been more important."
12. See S. V. Joag et al., "Chimeric simian/human immunodeficiency virus that causes progressive loss of CD4+ T cells and AIDS in pig-tailed macaques," *J Virol* 70 (1996), 3189–97; and K. A. Reimann et al., "A chimeric simian/human immunodeficiency virus expressing a primary patient human immunodeficiency virus type 1 isolate *env* causes an AIDS-like disease after in vivo passage in Rhesus monkeys," *J Virol* 70 (1996), 6922–8.
13. A. Chitnis, D. Rawls, and J. Moore, "Origin of HIV type 1 in colonial French Equatorial Africa?" *AIDS Res Hum Retrov* 16:1 (January 1, 2000), 5–8.
14. Jim Moore, "The Puzzling Origins of AIDS," *American Scientist*, November–December 2004.
15. Hooper, *The River*, p. 673.
16. Helen Epstein, "Bugs Without Borders," *New York Review of Books*, January 16, 2003; Mike Davis, *The Monster at Our Door: The Global Threat of Avian Flu* (New York: New Press, 2005); Laurie Garrett, *The Coming Plague: Newly Emerging Diseases in a World out of Balance* (New York: Penguin, 1995).

CHAPTER THREE: WHY ARE HIV RATES SO HIGH IN AFRICA?

1. *Report on the Global AIDS Epidemic* (Geneva: UNAIDS, 2006).
2. Ibid.
3. K. French, *Report for UNAIDS Scenarios for Africa: The Future of the HIV/AIDS Epidemic in China, India, Russia and Eastern Europe* (London: Department of Infectious Disease Epidemiology, Imperial College, March 2004); John Cleland and Benoit Ferry, eds., *Sexual Behavior and AIDS in the Developing World: Findings from a Multisite Study* (London: Taylor and Francis, 1995); and Kaye Wellings et al., "Sexual behavior in context: A global perspective," *Lancet* (November 1, 2006), 24–46.
4. Renee Sabatier, *Blaming Others: Prejudice, Race and Worldwide AIDS* (London: Panos Institute, 1989).
5. Hooper, *Slim*.
6. Ibid.
7. Alan Cochrane, *Daily Telegraph*, September 20, 1986, referred to in Sabatier, *Blaming Others*.
8. See Sabatier, *Blaming Others*.
9. Hooper, *Slim*; Karen Booth, *Local Women, Global Science: Fighting AIDS in Kenya* (Bloomington: Indiana University Press, 2004).
10. Jonathan Mann and Daniel Tarantola, eds., *AIDS in the World II* (Oxford: Oxford University Press, 1996); M. H. Merson, "Slowing the spread of HIV: Agenda for the 1990s," *Science* 260:5112 (May 28, 1993), 1266–8. The historian John Iliffe still maintains that that is the case—that HIV rates are higher in Africa because the virus appeared there first. However, most epidemiologists now maintain that the epidemic has had plenty of time to catch up in other countries. See John Iliffe, *The African AIDS Epidemic: A History* (Oxford: Oxford University Press, 2006).
11. See John C. Caldwell, Pat Caldwell, and Pat Quiggin, "The Social Context of AIDS in sub-Saharan Africa," *Popul Dev Rev* 15:2 (June 1989), 185–234. But also see Marie-Nathalie LeBlanc, Deidre Meintel, and Victor Piche, "The African sexual system: Comment on Caldwell et al.," *Popul Dev Rev* 17:3 (September 1991), 497–505; and Caldwell, Caldwell, and Quiggin, "The African sexual system: Reply to LeBlanc et al.," *Popul Dev Rev* 17:3 (September 1991), 506–15.
12. See Michel Carael, "Sexual Behavior," in *Sexual Behavior and AIDS in the Developing World*, ed. Cleland and Ferry.
13. See, for example, Carael, "Sexual Behavior"; A. Buve et al., "The multicentre study of factors determining the different prevalences of HIV in sub-Saharan Africa," *AIDS* 15 Suppl 4 (August 2001); Denise Gilgen et al., "The Natural History of HIV/AIDS in South Africa: A Biomedical and Social Survey in Carletonville" (Johannesburg: CSIR, 2000); Martina Morris,

"The Thailand and Ugandan Sexual Network Studies," in *Network Epidemiology: A Handbook for Survey Design and Data Collection*, ed. M. Morris (Oxford: Oxford University Press, 2004).

14. Adele Baleta, "Concern voiced over 'dry sex' practices in South Africa," *Lancet* 352:9136 (October 17, 1998), 1292.
15. Hooper, *Slim*; Hillary Standing and M. Kisekka, *Sexual Behaviour in Sub-Saharan Africa: A Review and Annotated Bibliography* (London: Overseas Development Administration, 1989).
16. Q. Gausset, "AIDS and cultural practices in Africa: The case of the Tonga (Zambia)," *Soc Sci Med* 52 (2001), 509–18; M. E. Beksinska et al., "The practice and prevalence of dry sex among men and women in South Africa: A risk factor for sexually transmitted infections?" *Sex Transm Infect* 75:3 (1999), 178–80; and R. S. McClelland et al., "Vaginal washing and increased risk of HIV-1 acquisition among African women: A 10-year prospective study," *AIDS* 20:2 (January 9, 2006), 269–73. But also see J. Van de Wiggert et al., "Is vaginal washing associated with increased risk of HIV-1 acquisition?" *AIDS* 20:9 (2006), 1347–48, and McClelland et al.'s reply, ibid., 1348–49.
17. M. Essex, "Human immunodeficiency viruses in the developing world," *Adv Virus Res* 53 (1999), 71–88.
18. Eileen Stillwagon, "AIDS and Poverty in Africa," *Nation*, May 21, 2001.
19. J. D. Shelton, M. M. Cassell, and J. Adetunji, "Is poverty or wealth at the root of HIV?" *Lancet* 366:9491 (September 24, 2005), 1057–8.
20. In her book *AIDS and the Ecology of Poverty* (Oxford: Oxford University Press, 2005), Eileen Stillwagon also argues that helminth infections predispose African people to HIV infection. This appears not to be the case in Uganda; see Michael Brown et al., "Helminth infection is not associated with faster progression of HIV disease in coinfected adults in Uganda," *J Infect Dis* 190:10 (November 15, 2004), 1869–79, although there may be some evidence for it in Zimbabwe; see E. F. Kjetland, "Association between genital schistosomiasis and HIV in rural Zimbabwean women," *AIDS* 20:4 (February 28, 2006), 593–600.
21. S. S. Bloom et al., "Community effects on the risk of HIV infection in rural Tanzania," *Sex Transm Infect* 78:4 (August 2002), 261–6.
22. See R. M. Anderson et al., "The spread of HIV-1 in Africa: Sexual contact patterns and the predicted demographic impact of AIDS," *Nature* 352:6336 (August 15, 1991), 581–9; and Anderson et al., "The Spread of HIV and Sexual Mixing Patterns," in Mann and Tarantola, eds., *AIDS in the World II*. During the 1990s, there was a shift in nomenclature. Reference to "high-risk groups" was seen as stigmatizing, so public health agencies increasingly referred instead to "high-risk behaviors," but the policy of "targeting" programs to those who practiced such behaviors remained the same.

23. Among many references, see Isaac Shapera, *Married Life in an African Tribe* (New York: Sheridan House, 1941), and *Migrant Labour and Tribal Life* (London: Oxford University Press, 1945); Ruth First, *Black Gold: The Mozambican Miner, Proletarian and Peasant* (London: Palgrave Macmillan, 1983); and Benedict Carton, *Blood from Your Children: The Colonial Origins of Generational Conflict in South Africa* (Charlottesville: University Press of Virginia, 2000).
24. S. L. Kark, "The social pathology of syphilis in Africans, 1949." *Int J Epidemiol* 32:2 (April 2003), 181–6.
25. Peter Piot and Michel Carael, "Epidemiological and sociological aspects of HIV infection in developing countries," *Brit Med Bull* 44:1 (January 1988), 68–88; J. O. Ndinya-Achola et al., "Acquired immunodeficiency syndrome: Epidemiology in Africa and its implications for health services," *Afr J Sex Transm Dis* 2:2 (October 1986), 77–80; Piot et al., "Acquired immunodeficiency syndrome in a heterosexual population in Zaire," *Lancet* 2:8394 (July 14, 1984), 65–9.
26. See J. W. Carswell, G. Lloyd, and J. Howells, "Prevalence of HIV-1 in East African lorry drivers," *AIDS* 3:11 (November 1989), 759–61.
27. M. Potts and W. Carswell, "AIDS: Losing the battle and the war?" *Lancet* 341:8858 (June 5, 1993), 1442–3; G. P. Garnett and R. M. Anderson, "Strategies for limiting the spread of HIV in developing countries: Conclusions based on studies of the transmission dynamics of the virus," *J Acq Immun Def Synd Hum Retrovirol* 9:5 (August 15, 1995), 500–13.
28. See, for example, Martha Ainsworth and Meade Over, *Confronting AIDS: Public Priorities in a Global Epidemic* (Washington, D.C.: The World Bank, 1999); Project Support Group of Zimbabwe, "Corridors of Hope in Southern Africa: HIV Prevention, Needs and Opportunities in Four Border Towns," monograph prepared for Family Health International, Research Triangle Park, North Carolina, 2006.
29. Gilgen et al., "Natural History"; Antonio Mussa, "Seroprevalence of HIV Among Miners in Mozambique," Ph.D. diss., University of Washington, Seattle, 2001; M. P. Coffee et al., "Patterns of movement and risk of HIV infection in rural Zimbabwe," *J Infect Dis* 191 Suppl 1 (February 1, 2005), S159–67.
30. AIDSMark, "HIV prevalence and condom sales in Africa," Population Services International, presentation at USAID, Washington, D.C., 2002; Gilgen et al., "Natural History."
31. Wawer et al., "Control of sexually transmitted diseases"; Kamali et al., "A community-based randomized controlled trial"; Grosskurth et al., "Impact of improved treatment"; and Kaul et al., "Monthly antibiotic chemoprophylaxis."
32. S. Ray et al., "Sexual behaviour and risk assessment of HIV seroconvertors

among urban male factory workers in Zimbabwe," *Soc Sci Med* 47:10 (November 1998), 1431–43; Gilgen et al., "Natural History"; Carael, "Sexual Behavior"; Buve et al., "The multicentre study of factors"; French, *Report for UNAIDS*; Cleland and Ferry, *Sexual Behavior*; and Wellings et al., "Sexual Behavior."

33. C. H. Watts and R. M. May, "The influence of concurrent partnerships on the dynamics of HIV/AIDS," *Math Biosci* 108:1 (February 1992), 89–104. Christopher Hudson would later expand upon their theory; see "AIDS in rural Africa: A paradigm for HIV-1 prevention," *Int J STD & AIDS* 7 (1996), 236–43.
34. M. L. Plummer et al., "'A bit more truthful': The validity of adolescent sexual behaviour data collected in rural northern Tanzania using five methods," *Sex Transm Infect* 80 Suppl 2 (December 2004), ii49–56; S. Nnko et al., "Secretive females or swaggering males? An assessment of the quality of sexual partnership reporting in rural Tanzania," *Soc Sci Med* 59:2 (July 2004), 299–310.
35. M. Morris and Mirjam Kretzschmar, "A microsimulation study of the effect of concurrent partnerships on the spread of HIV in Uganda," Population Research Institute, Pennsylvania State University, 2000.
36. Henry Kyemba, *A State of Blood: The Inside Story of Idi Amin* (Kampala: Fountain Publishers, 1977). See also Maxine Ankrah et al., "AIDS in Uganda: Analysis of the Social Dimensions of the Epidemic," National Survey, September–December 1989 (Kampala: Makerere University, May 1993).
37. Speech given at the Fifteenth International Conference on AIDS, Bangkok, Thailand, July 21, 2004.
38. Carael, "Sexual Behavior."
39. See Garnett and Johnson, "Coining a new term in epidemiology: Concurrency and HIV," *AIDS* 11:5 (April 1997), 681–3.
40. See E. Lagarde et al., "Concurrent sexual partnerships and HIV prevalence in five urban communities of sub-Saharan Africa," *AIDS* 15:7 (May 4, 2001), 877–84.
41. See P. M. Gorbach, L. N. Drumright, and K. K. Holmes, "Discord, discordance & concurrency: Comparing individual and partnership level analyses of new partnerships of young adults at risk of STI," *Sex Transm Dis*, 32:1 (January 2005), 7–12.
42. M. Morris, and M. Kretzschmar "Concurrent partnerships and the spread of HIV." *AIDS* 11: 641–8.
43. H. Chakraborty et al., "Viral burden in genital secretions determines male-to-female sexual transmission of HIV-1: A probabilistic empiric model," *AIDS* 15:5 (March 30, 2001), 621–7.

44. Christopher Pilcher et al., "Quest study; Duke-UNC Emory Acute HIV Consortium: Brief but efficient: Acute HIV infection and the sexual transmission of HIV," *J Infect Dis* 189:10 (2004), 1785–92.
45. George Kawule, "Lutaaya Meets Students," *New Vision*, April 22, 1989.
46. Mahmood Mamdani, *Politics and Class Formation in Uganda* (New York: Monthly Review Press, 1976).
47. Gardner Thompson, *Governing Uganda* (Kampala: Fountain, 2003).
48. Paul Theroux, "Rajat Neogy Remembered," *Transition* 69 (1996), 4–7.
49. See, for example, Reginald Austin, *Racism and Apartheid in Southern Africa: Rhodesia* (Paris: UNESCO Press, 1975), and *Racism and Apartheid in Southern Africa: Namibia and South Africa* (Paris: UNESCO Press, 1974).

CHAPTER FOUR: THE AFRICAN EARTHQUAKE

1. See also Aud Talle, "Desiring Difference: Risk Behavior Among Young Maasai Men," in *Young People at Risk: Fighting AIDS in Northern Tanzania*, ed. Knut-Inge Klepp, Paul M. Biswalo, and Aud Talle (Copenhagen: Scandinavian University Press, 1995).
2. Dorothy Hodgson, *Once Intrepid Warriors: Gender, Ethnicity, and the Cultural Politics of Maasai Development* (Bloomington: Indiana University Press, 2004), 224.
3. Patrick Cull, "There Were Successes in EC Over Past Year," *The Herald Online*, February 24, 2003.
4. Carol Kaufman and Stavros Stavrou, "'Bus fare please': The economics of sex and gifts among adolescents in urban South Africa," Population Council Issue Brief No. 116 (New York: Population Council, 2002); Nancy Luke, "Cross-generational and transactional sexual relations in sub-Saharan Africa: A review of the evidence on prevalence and implications for negotiation of safe sexual practices for adolescent girls" (Washington, D.C.: International Center for Research on Women, 2001), mimeo.
5. Susan Cotts Watkins and Ann Sandler, "Ties of dependence: AIDS and transactional sex in rural Malawi," unpublished manuscript, August 2006.
6. K. L. Dunkle et al., "Transactional sex among women in Soweto, South Africa: prevalence, risk factors and association with HIV infection," *Soc Sci Med* 59:8 (October 2004), 1581–92; Dunkle et al., "Gender-based violence, relationship power, and risk of HIV infection in women attending antenatal clinics in South Africa," *Lancet* 363:9419 (May 1, 2004), 1415–21.
7. M. Hunter, "The materiality of everyday sex: Thinking beyond 'prostitution,'" *Afr Stud* 61:1 (July 1, 2002), 99–120.
8. "South Africa: Population Census 2001" (available through Statistics South Africa—www.statssa.gov.za—accessed May 13, 2004).

9. *The World Factbook* (Washington, D.C.: CIA, 2006).
10. J. D. Shelton and M. M. Cassell, "Is poverty or wealth at the root of HIV?" *Lancet* 366:9491 (September 24, 2005), 1057–8.
11. S. Mathews et al., "Every six hours a woman is killed by her intimate partner: A national study of female homicide in South Africa," *MRC Policy Brief* 5 (June 2004).
12. Claudia Garcia-Moreno et al., "Violence against women," *Science* 310 (November 25, 2005), 1282–3.
13. Rachel Jewkes, "Non-consensual sex among South African youth: Prevalence of coerced sex and discourses of control and desire," unpublished manuscript, 2005.
14. "Gender Oppression in Southern Africa's Precapitalist Societies," in *Women and Gender in Southern Africa to 1945*, ed. C. Walker (London: James Currey, 1990), 33–47, cited in Jewkes, "Non-consensual sex."
15. Iona Mayer, "Wives of Migrant Workers," in P. Mayer, ed., "Migrant Labour: Some Perspectives from Anthropology," typescript, Rhodes University, Grahamstown, 1978, cited in Virginia Van der Vliet, "Traditional Husbands, Modern Wives? Constructing Marriages in a South African Township," in *Tradition and Transition in Southern Africa: Festschrift for Philip and Iona Mayer*, ed. A. D. Spiegel and P. A. McAllister, African Studies Series, 50th Anniversary Volume, vol. 51, nos. 1 and 2.
16. "Moral renewal and African experience(s)," in *African Renaissance*, ed. Malegapuru William Makgoba (Cape Town: Mafube Publishing, 1999).
17. Van der Vliet, "Traditional Husbands."
18. Mark Hunter, "Cultural politics and masculinities: Multiple partners in historical perspective in KwaZulu-Natal," *Cult Health Sex* 7:3 (May 2005), 209–23.
19. Monde Makiwane, "The demise of marriage," *Children First* 58 (November/December 2004).
20. Cullinan, "Amorous Materialism in the Age of AIDS," *Sunday Independent* (South Africa), April 15, 2001.
21. Posel, "Getting the Nation Talking About Sex: Reflections on the Politics of Sexuality and 'Nation-Building' in Post-Apartheid South Africa," Witwatersrand Institute of Social and Economic Research, working paper, presented at Sex and Secrecy: A Conference of the International Association for the Study of Sexuality, Culture and Society, July 12, 2003.
22. Chicago: University of Chicago Press, 2003.
23. This point was originally made by Susan Watkins in "Navigating the AIDS epidemic in rural Malawi," *Popul Dev Rev* 30:4 (2004), 603–705.
24. R. Jewkes et al., "Relationship dynamics and teenage pregnancy in South Africa," *Soc Sci Med* 52:5 (March 2001), 733–44.

25. Dunkle et al., "Gender-based violence"; Audrey Pettifor et al., "HIV and Sexual Behavior Among Young South Africans: A National Survey of 15-24 year olds" (Johannesburg: Reproductive Health Research Unit, University of the Witwatersrand, 2004); Joyce Abma, Anne Driscoll, and Kristin Moore, "Young women's degree of control over first intercourse: An exploratory analysis," *Fam Plann Perspect* 30:1 (January/February 1998).
26. "Bemba marriage and present economic conditions," *The Rhodes-Livingstone Papers* No. 4 (Manchester: Manchester University Press, 1940).

CHAPTER FIVE: GOLD RUSH

1. "AIDS Epidemic Update, December 2005" (Geneva: UNAIDS, 2005).
2. See, for example, First, *Black Gold*; and Karen Jochelson, "Sexually Transmitted Diseases in Nineteenth- and Twentieth-Century South Africa," in *Histories of Sexually Transmitted Diseases and HIV/AIDS in Sub-Saharan Africa*, ed. Philip W. Setel, Milton Lewis, and Maryinez Lyons (Westport, Conn.: Greenwood Press, 1999).
3. Mark Schoofs, "African Gold Giant Finds History Impedes a Fight Against AIDS," *The Wall Street Journal*, June 26, 2001; and Dr. M. LaGrange, personal communication.
4. Antonio Mussa, "Seroprevalence of HIV Among Miners in Mozambique," MS. diss., University of Washington, Seattle, 2001.
5. Mozambique consists of three regions: southern, central, and northern. The central region has the most severe epidemic of HIV. Mozambique was at war in the 1980s, and refugees from the central region fled to neighboring countries, including Malawi and Zimbabwe, where infection rates were already very high by 1990. According to the health ministry, the virus came to the central region with the approximately 1.5 million refugees who returned home in the early 1990s. It is also likely that high HIV rates among Zimbabwean soldiers guarding transport corridors in the central region contributed to high infection rates in the local population. While the HIV situation in the central region of the country became dire almost overnight in the early 1990s, infection rates in the northern and southern regions seemed to be much lower, at least until recently, when infection rates soared in the southern region, but not in the northern region, where rates have remained relatively low. HIV could have spread into the southern region from the central region, but this is unlikely, because there is little migration between the central and southern regions of the country. A far more likely possibility is that the epidemic in southern Mozambique spread from South Africa, with returning miners and other migrant workers.
6. See Catherine Campbell, "Selling Sex in the Time of AIDS: The psycho-

social context of condom use by sex workers on a South African mine," *Soc Sci Med* 50 (2000), 479–94.

7. See, for example, "HIV/AIDS at a Glance," on the World Bank's Web site (www.worldbank.org), and The World Bank, *Confronting AIDS: Public Priorities in a Global Epidemic* (Oxford: Oxford University Press, 1997).
8. The figure for miners might have been an underestimate. At the time, miners were given a physical exam at the beginning of every contract, or about once a year. Although they were not tested for HIV, those who were too sick to work, perhaps because they were in the early stages of AIDS, might have been rejected, and thus excluded from HIV surveys of working miners.
9. Gilgen et al., "Natural History."
10. Ibid. See also Norman Hearst and Sammy Chen, "Condom promotion for AIDS prevention in the developing world: Is it working?" *Stud Fam Plann* 35:1 (March 2004), 39–47.
11. At the time, a USAID survey found only two AIDS-prevention groups working in Gaza province: Population Services International, which markets condoms, and an umbrella group that was trying to mobilize the NGO community by holding workshops and conferences. See David Wilson, Claudia Werman Connor, and the Project Support Group, "An AIDS Assessment of the Maputo Corridor: Ressano Garcia to Chokwe and Vilankulo" (USAID, 2001).
12. M. N. Lurie et al., "Who infects whom? HIV-1 concordance and discordance among migrant and non-migrant couples in South Africa," *AIDS* 17:15 (October 17, 2003), 2245–52. A study in Uganda came to similar conclusions: R. H. Gray et al., "Probability of HIV-1 transmission per coital act in monogamous, heterosexual, HIV-1-discordant couples in Rakai, Uganda," *Lancet* 357 (April 14, 2001), 1149–53.
13. Judith Glynn et al., "HIV risk in relation to marriage in areas with high prevalence of HIV infection," *J Acq Immun Def Synd* 33:4 (August 1, 2003), 526–35.
14. "Sex in Geneva, sex in Lilongwe, sex in Balaka," *Soc Sci Med* (forthcoming).
15. See Mozambique National Human Development Report (UNDP, 2000); "MOZAL Responsible for 60 Percent of Exports," *AIM Reports* No. 217 (October 15, 2001); and "Growth Lower than Expected in 2000," *AIM Reports* No. 205 (April 20, 2001).
16. See "Drug Trafficking Is Big Business in Mozambique," *AIM Reports* No. 210 (June 29, 2001).
17. Joseph Hanlon, *Peace Without Profit: How the IMF Blocks Rebuilding in Mozambique* (Portsmouth, N.H.: Heinemann, 1996). Industries in other countries have been adversely affected by such policies as well. See, for example, Pádraig Carmody, *Tearing the Social Fabric: Neoliberalism, Deindustrialization, and the Crisis of Governance in Zimbabwe* (Portsmouth, N.H.:

Heinemann, 2001). For a critique of World Bank/IMF development policies in general, see Joseph E. Stiglitz, *Globalization and Its Discontents* (New York: W. W. Norton, 2002).

18. Hanlon, "Banking in the transition from socialism to capitalism in Mozambique, and the struggle to maintain a developmental focus," *Rev Afri Poli Econ* 29:91 (March 2002), 41–60. Views about how liberal economic reforms have unintentionally contributed to government corruption can also be found in Jean-François Bayart, Stephen Ellis, and Béatrice Hibou, *The Criminalization of the State in Africa*, trans. Stephen Ellis (Bloomington: Indiana University Press, 1999).
19. See Merle L. Bowen, *The State Against the Peasantry: Rural Struggles in Colonial and Postcolonial Mozambique* (Charlottesville: University Press of Virginia, 2000).
20. In 2001, it was common for Mozambican doctors not to tell patients found to be HIV positive their diagnosis.
21. See Wilson and Connor, "AIDS Assessment."
22. See Joseph Collins and Bill Rau, "AIDS in the Context of Development," UNRISD Program on Social Policy and Development Paper No. 4 (UNRISD/UNAIDS, December 2000); and Paul Farmer, *Infections and Inequalities: The Modern Plagues* (Berkeley: University of California Press, 1999).
23. "Former Mine Workers Yet to Claim Compensation," report by *AIM*, September 11, 2001.
24. Neil White, "Dust-Related Diseases in Former Miners—the ODMWA Legacy," *Occupational Health Southern Africa*, July/August 1997, 20–24.
25. *World Development Report 2002: Building Institutions for Markets/The World Bank* (New York: Oxford University Press, 2002).
26. Peter R. Lamptey, "Reducing heterosexual transmission of HIV in poor countries," *BMJ* 324:7331 (January 26, 2002), 207–11.

CHAPTER SIX: A PRESIDENT, A CRISIS, A TRAGEDY

1. Mary Robertson, "An overview of rape in South Africa," *Continuing Medical Education Journal* 16 (February 1998), 139–42.
2. See, for example, numerous articles at www.virusmyth.com (accessed July 12, 2006); Peter Duesberg, *Inventing the AIDS Virus* (Washington, D.C.: Regnery Publishing, 1997); Gary Null, *AIDS: A Second Opinion* (New York: Seven Stories Press, 2001).
3. For a discussion of the evidence that HIV is the sole cause of AIDS on the Web site of the National Institutes of Health (www.niaid.nih.gov/factsheets/evidhiv.htm). See also Richard Horton, "Truth and Heresy About AIDS," *New York Review of Books*, May 23, 1996.

4. See Howard Barrell and Stuart Hess, "Zuma Defends AZT Policy," *Mail & Guardian* (Johannesburg), October 16, 1998.
5. See "AIDS Exists. Let's Fight It Together," *Mail & Guardian* (Johannesburg), February 11, 2000. AZT and other antiretroviral drugs are unlikely to be toxic to unborn children in the doses needed to prevent HIV transmission. The Centers for Disease Control and Prevention has followed the cases of more than twenty thousand children born to women in the United States who took AZT during pregnancy, and found no evidence of long-term toxic effects. In France, two children died from what seemed to be toxic exposure to AZT and another antiretroviral drug, 3TC. These children were exposed to higher doses of the drugs than would be administered in South Africa. See "Timeline of events related to follow-up of children exposed to anti-retrovirals perinatally," Centers for Disease Control and Prevention, 2000.
6. "Buying Anti-AIDS Drugs Benefits the Rich," *Business Day*, March 20, 2000.
7. Laura Guay et al., "Intrapartum and neonatal single-dose nevirapine compared with zidovudine for prevention of mother-to-child transmission of HIV-1 in Kampala, Uganda: HIVNET 012 randomised trial," *Lancet* 354:9181 (September 4, 1999), 795–802.
8. See "Ministry Refuses Anti-HIV Drug Discount," *Mail & Guardian*, May 7, 1999.
9. "Triangle Pharmaceuticals Announces Clinical Hold on Study FTC-302," *PR Newswire*, April 7, 2000.
10. See "AIDS Trial Woman Dies," *Citizen*, April 24, 2000.
11. "A Duty of Care Means Good Money Shouldn't Lie Idle," *Financial Mail*, March 17, 2000; Ivor Powell, "Uproar over AIDS Council," *Mail & Guardian*, January 28, 2000; Judith Soal, "HIV Patient Was Denied Treatment," *Cape Times*, May 11, 2000; N. Lamati, testimony given at the Health Portfolio Committee, May 10, 2000.
12. The names of the trial participants and Dr. Steenkamp have been changed.
13. "Privacy, confidentiality and stigma: The case of NM, SM and LH v Patricia De Lille, Charlene Smith and New Africa Books Publishers," AIDS Law Project, www.alp.org.za (accessed July 12, 2006).
14. William Mervin Gumede, *Thabo Mbeki and the Battle for the Soul of the ANC* (Cape Town: Zebra Press, 2005).
15. Cape Town: Mafube/Tafelberg, 1999.
16. Gumede, *Thabo Mbeki.*
17. See James Myburgh, "The Virodene Trials" and "Who Owns Virodene?" ever-fasternews.com, September 5, 2005; and "Anti-retrovirals vs Virodene," ever-fasternews.com, September 8, 2005.
18. James Myburgh, "The Virodene affair parts I-V" *Politicsweb* 17–21

September 2007. (www.politicsweb.co.za) and Fiona Forde "Mbeki link to toxic 'cure.'" *The Independent* (South Africa) September 15, 2007.

19. "New Technology to Fight HIV/Aids Investigated," South African Press Association (Johannesburg), April 3, 2003; "Companies Struck 'Secret Deal' to Distribute Unregistered Herbal AIDS Treatment in 12 African Countries," *Kaiser Network Daily HIV/AIDS Report*, December 19, 2001.
20. Nawaal Deane, David Macfarlane, and Mungo Soggot, "SA Tests Coal-Fired AIDS Muti on Tanzanian Soldiers," *Mail & Guardian*, September 28, 2001; Mariette Botes et al., "Phase trial with oral oxyhumate in HIV-1 infected patients," *Drug Development Research* 57 (2002), 34–39.
21. William Finnegan, "The Poison Keeper: Biowarrior, Brilliant Cardiologist, War Criminal, Spy—Can a Landmark Trial in South Africa Reveal Who Wouter Basson Really Was?" *New Yorker*, January 15, 2001, p. 58.
22. "Politicisation of debate on HIV care in South Africa," *Lancet* 355:9214 (April 29, 2000), 1473.
23. Smuts Ngonyama (head of the ANC Presidency), "Democratic Alliance's hypocrisy," ANC press statement, October 19, 2000, cited in Myburgh, "Anti-retrovirals vs Virodene."

    After Medicines Control Council officials were fired for blocking Olga Visser's Virodene trials in South Africa, the MCC's new leadership also declined to approve the trials. Then, in 2001, health authorities in Tanzania discovered Visser testing Virodene on Tanzanian soldiers and expelled her from the country. In a subsequent court battle over the ownership of Virodene, it emerged that millions of dollars had been invested in Visser's Tanzanian experiments. Although it is not known for certain where the money came from, much of it passed through the hands of various ANC heavyweights, including the husband of Health Minister Tshabalala-Msimang and other close associates of Mbeki. See Myburgh, "Virodene Trials," "Who Owns Virodene?" and "Anti-retrovirals vs Virodene."
24. Gumede, *Thabo Mbeki*.
25. "South African Health Minister Tshabalala-Msimang Defends Group Claiming Vitamins Can Prevent AIDS-Related Death," *Kaiser Network Daily HIV/AIDS Report*, April 15, 2005 (http://www.kaisernetwork.org/daily_reports/rep_index.cfm?DR_ID=29367).

CHAPTER SEVEN: AIDS, INC.

1. Helen Schneider, "On the fault-line: The politics of AIDS policy in contemporary South Africa," *Afr Stud* 61:1 (July 1, 2002), 145–67; Samantha Power, "The AIDS Rebel," *New Yorker*, May 19, 2003, pp. 54–67.
2. Rob Dorrington et al., "The Impact of HIV/AIDS on Adult Mortality

in South Africa" (Cape Town: Burden of Disease Research Unit, Medical Research Council of South Africa, September 2001); "Mortality and causes of death in South Africa, 2003 and 2004," Statistics South Africa, May 2006.

3. Richard Delate, "The Struggle for Meaning: A Semiotic Analysis of Interpretations of the loveLife His&Hers Billboard Campaign," November 2001, http://www.comminit.com/stlovelife/sld-4389.html.
4. Personal communication, February 2003.
5. For more about this, see Malcolm Gladwell, *The Tipping Point* (Boston: Little, Brown, 2000), and Everett Rogers, *Diffusion of Innovations* (New York: Free Press, 1983).
6. Delate, "Struggle for Meaning."
7. See Prishani Naidoo, "Youth Divided: A Review of loveLife's Y-Centre in Orange Farm" (Johannesburg: CADRE Report, 2003).
8. Nancy Luke and Kathleen M. Kurtz, "Cross-Generational and Transactional Sexual Relations in Sub-Saharan Africa: Prevalence of Behavior and Implications for Negotiating Safer Sexual Practices," International Center for Research on Women, 2002, http://www.icrw.org/docs/CrossGenSex_Report_902.pdf; J. Swart-Kruger and L. M. Richter, "AIDS-related knowledge, attitudes and behaviour among South African street youth: Reflections on power, sexuality and the autonomous self," *Soc Sci Med* 45:6 (1997), 957–66; Editorial, "Reassessing priorities: Identifying the determinants of HIV transmission," *Soc Sci Med* 36:5 (1993), iii–viii.
9. Daniel Low-Beer and Rand Stoneburner, "Uganda and the Challenge of AIDS," in *The Political Economy of AIDS in Africa*, ed. Nana Poku and Alan Whiteside (London: Ashgate, 2004).
10. See Helen Epstein, "Fat," *Granta* 49 (1995). Low-Beer and Stoneburner make this observation, too, as do Janice Hogle et al. in *What Happened in Uganda? Declining HIV Prevalence, Behavior Change and the National Response* (USAID, 2002).
11. In 2006, *The Washington Post* reported that the HIV infection rate in Rwanda, once estimated to be 15 percent, was now estimated to be 3 percent. See Craig Timberg, "How AIDS in Africa Was Overstated: Reliance on Data from Urban Prenatal Clinics Skewed Early Projections," *Washington Post*, April 6, 2006, p. A1. Timberg attributed the downward revision to a new U.S. government survey and suggested that the earlier estimate, issued by the UNAIDS program, had been inflated, perhaps to raise money or appease AIDS activists. Although the old UNAIDS statistics were in need of correction, there clearly had been a decline in the true infection rate. A population-based survey carried out in Rwanda in 1986 found that prevalence was 17.8 percent in urban areas and 1.3 percent in rural areas. (Rwandan HIV Seroprevalence Study Group, "Nationwide community-based

serological survey of HIV-1 and other human retrovirus infections in a country," *Lancet* 1 (ii) (1989), 941–943.

12. A. E. Pettifor et al. "Young people's sexual health in South Africa: HIV prevalence and sexual behaviors from a nationally representative household survey," *AIDS* 19:14 (September 23, 2005), 1525–34; but see R. Jewkes, "Response to Pettifor et al., *AIDS* 20:6 (April 4, 2006), 952–3; author reply, 956–8; and W. M. Parker and M. Colvin, "Response to Pettifor et al.," *AIDS* 20:6 (April 4, 2006), 954–5.
13. In 2005, an article in the prestigious medical journal *AIDS* reported that young people who had attended at least one loveLife program were slightly, but significantly, less likely to be HIV positive than those who had not. The author argued that this was consistent with the possibility that loveLife reduced risky sexual behavior. However, there could well be another explanation. From what I saw, loveLife attracted young people who would have been at lower risk of infection in the first place, either because they were wealthier or better educated or less vulnerable to abuse. (While the loveLife study attempted to control for education and wealth, it did not do so rigorously.) Indeed, the tendency to avoid the subject of AIDS would seem to discourage HIV-positive young people from attending loveLife's programs, and this could make it look as though loveLife protected young people when in fact it merely alienated those most at risk. Most loveLife materials were in English, and thus accessible only to young people with higher social status. This would have sent a clear signal to those—often marginalized and vulnerable young people—who could not speak English well that loveLife was not for them. The main author of the article reporting lower HIV rates among young people exposed to loveLife admitted to me in an interview that an anthropologist hired by loveLife itself had come to these same conclusions, but her results remain unpublished. See Pettifor et al., "A community-based study to examine the effect of a youth HIV prevention intervention on young people aged 15–24 in South Africa: results of the baseline survey," *Trop Med Int Health* 10:10 (October 2005), 971–80; but see also Jewkes, "Response to Pettifor et al.," author reply, and Parker and Colvin, "Response to Pettifor." Information re the loveLife anthropologist from Pettifor, personal communication, April 2006.

CHAPTER EIGHT: WHY DON'T THEY LISTEN?

1. Africa Centre for Health and Population Studies, Mtubatuba, South Africa, unpublished report, 2005.
2. Between 2000 and 2004, nurses from the Africa Centre for Health and Population Studies interviewed thousands of relatives of deceased AIDS

victims in the area. However, only one in fifty admitted that AIDS was, in fact, the cause of death. Adam Ashforth, "Will anti-retrovirals cure AIDS stigma in South Africa?" *Passages* ns2 (June 2005).

3. Africa Centre for Health and Population Studies, unpublished report, 2005.
4. J. C. Caldwell, "Rethinking the African AIDS epidemic," *Popul Dev Rev* 26:1 (March 26, 2000), 117–35.
5. When I contacted the Treatment Action Campaign and The National Association of People Living with AIDS in 2005, they could not put me in touch with a single activist in northern KwaZulu-Natal.
6. A. Castro and P. Farmer, "Understanding and addressing AIDS-related stigma: From anthropological theory to clinical practice in Haiti," *Am J Public Health* 95:1 (January 2005), 53–9.
7. Andrew Furber et al., "Barriers to better care for people with AIDS in developing countries," *BMJ* 329:7477 (November 2004), 1281–3. In 2006, Sheila Tlou, Botswana's minister of health, told me that prominent Batswana remained unwilling to "go public" about their HIV status, even though antiretrovirals became available through the public sector in 2003. See also Seth Mydans, "In Thailand, More Survive AIDS, Only to Face Rejection," *International Herald Tribune*, October 6, 2006.
8. Deborah Posel, "Sex, Death and Embodiment: Reflections on the Stigma of AIDS in Agincourt, South Africa," paper presented at the symposium on Life and Death in a Time of AIDS: The Southern African Experience, Witwatersrand Institute for Social and Economic Research, October 14–16, 2004.
9. Edward C. Green and Allison Herling, "Paradigm shift and controversy in AIDS prevention," *Journal of Medicine and the Person* 4:1 (2006), 23–33.
10. Betsy Hartmann, *Reproductive Rights and Wrongs: The Global Politics of Population Control and Contraceptive Choice* (New York: Harper and Row, 1987).
11. J. C. Ling et al., "Social Marketing," *Annu Rev Publ Health* 13 (May 1992), 341–62.
12. "Condoms Fight for Space on Shelves," *Daily Nation* (Kenya), May 2, 2006.
13. James Pfeiffer, "Condom social marketing, pentecostalism, and structural adjustment in Mozambique: A clash of AIDS prevention messages," *Med Anthropol Q* 18:1 (March 18, 2004), 77–103.
14. Norman Hearst and Sammy Chen, "Condom promotion for AIDS prevention in the developing world: Is it working?" *Stud Family Plann* 35:1 (March 2004), 39–47.
15. See Suzette Heald, "It's never as easy as ABC: Understandings of AIDS in Botswana," *Afr AIDS Research* 1:1 (2002), 1–10.
16. Sunanda Ray et al., "Sexual behavior and risk assessment of HIV serocovertors among urban male factory workers in Zimbabwe," *Soc Sci Med* 47:10 (1998), 1431–43.

17. This section draws heavily on John Iliffe's *Honour in African History* (Cambridge: Cambridge University Press, 2004).
18. Athens: Ohio University Press, 2004.
19. New York: Farrar, Straus and Giroux, 1977.
20. Isak Niehaus and G. Jonsson, "Dr. Wouter Basson, Americans, and wild beasts: Men's conspiracy theories of HIV/AIDS in the South African lowveld," *Med Anthropol Q* 24:2 (April–June, 2005), 179–208.
21. Pfeiffer, "Condom social marketing."
22. A. Nicoll et al., "Lay health beliefs concerning HIV and AIDS—A barrier for control programmes," *AIDS Care* 5:2 (1993), 231–41; Seth Kalichman and L. Simbayi, "Traditional beliefs about the causes of AIDS and AIDS-related stigma in South Africa," *AIDS Care* 16:5 (July 16, 2004), 572–80; Alexander Rodlach, *Witches, Westerners and HIV: AIDS and Cultures of Blame in Africa* (Walnut Creek, Calif.: Left Coast Press, 2006).
23. See especially Deborah Posel, "Sex, death and the fate of the nation: Reflections on the politicisation of sexuality in post-apartheid South Africa." *Africa* 75:2 (2005), 125–53. For other insightful speculations, see Allister Sparks, *Beyond the Miracle: Inside the New South Africa* (Chicago: University of Chicago Press, 2003); Iliffe, *Honour in African History*; Virginia Van der Vliet, "AIDS: Losing 'The New Struggle'?" *Daedalus* 130 (Winter 2001), 151–84; Gumede, *Thabo Mbeki*.
24. http://www.virusmyth.net/aids/data/ancdoc.htm.
25. Gumede, *Thabo Mbeki*.
26. Quoted in Dial Ndima, *The Law of Commoners and Kings: Narratives of a Rural Transkei Magistrate* (Pretoria: University of South Africa Press, 2004).
27. Chicago: University of Chicago Press, 1990.
28. Sampie Terreblanche, *A History of Inequality in South Africa, 1652–2002* (Durban: University of Natal Press, 2002), cited in Adam Ashforth, *Witchcraft, Violence and Democracy in South Africa* (Chicago: University of Chicago Press, 2005), p. 90.

CHAPTER NINE: THE INVISIBLE CURE

1. Birgitta Larsson, *Conversion to Greater Freedom? Women, Church and Social Change in North-Western Tanzania Under Colonial Rule* (Stockholm: Almqvist and Wiksell International, 1991), 106; see also, Bengt Sundkler, *Bara Bukoba, Church and Community in Tanzania* (London: C. Hurst, 1980); Marja-Liisa Swantz, *Women in Development: A Creative Role Denied? The Case of Tanzania* (London: C. Hurst, 1985).
2. Luise White, *The Comforts of Home: Prostitution in Colonial Nairobi* (Chicago: University of Chicago Press, 1990).

3. Barbo Johansson, "The position of women in Hayaland," *Book of the Jubilee of the Church of Sweden Mission, 75th Anniversary* (Uppsala, 1949). Referred to in Larsson, *Conversion*, 153. Many thanks to Aili Marie Tripp, Marja-Liisa Swartz, and Sister Deborah Bryck for discussions concerning Bukoba.
4. G. Kwesigabo et al., "HIV-1 infection prevalence and incidence trends in areas of contrasting levels of infection in the Kagera region, Tanzania, 1987–2000," *J Acq Immun Def Synd* 40:5 (December 15, 2005), 585–91.
5. G. Asiimwe-Okiror et al., "Declining trends in HIV infection in urban areas in Uganda," paper presented at the 9th International Conference on AIDS and Sexually Transmitted Diseases in Africa, Kampala, Uganda, 1995; Alex Opro et al., "Declining Trends of HIV Transmission in Uganda," 12th International Conference on AIDS, Vancouver, July 7–12, 1996.
6. U.S. Census Bureau, HIV/AIDS Surveillance Database, 2000.
7. John Stover et al., "Can we reverse the HIV/AIDS pandemic with an expanded response?" *Lancet* 360:9326 (July 6, 2002), 73–7.
8. R. L. Stoneburner and D. Low-Beer, "Population-level HIV declines and behavioral risk avoidance in Uganda," *Science* 304:5671 (April 30, 2004), 714–8; Gary Slutkin et al., "How Uganda reversed its HIV epidemic," *AIDS Behav* 10:4 (July 2006).
9. "What Happened in Uganda?", a short film produced by Jeffrey Rosenberg for the Gerard Health Foundation, 2003; Maria Wawer et al., "HIV Prevalence Decline in Uganda: Evidence from Rakai, Uganda," presentation at the 12th Annual Conference on Retroviruses and Opportunistic Infections, Boston, February 22–25, 2005; Edward C. Green, *Rethinking AIDS Prevention* (Westport, Conn.: Praeger, 2003); Slutkin et al., "How Uganda reversed"; Ronald Gray et al., "Uganda's HIV prevention success: The role of sexual behavior change and the national response. Commentary on Green et al," *AIDS Behav* 10:4 (July 2006), 347–50; E. C. Green et al., "Uganda's HIV prevention success: The role of sexual behavior change and the national response," *AIDS Behav* 10:4 (July 2006), 335–46, discussion on 347–50.
10. For more about "social cohesion" and the public good, see Peter Kropotkin, *Mutual Aid* (London: Heinemann, 1902); Felton Earls and M. Carlson, "The social ecology of child health and well-being," *Annu Rev Public Health* 22 (2001), 143–66; Robert D. Putnam, *Bowling Alone: The Collapse and Revival of American Community* (New York: Simon & Schuster, 2000); Tony Barnett and Alan Whiteside, *AIDS in the Twenty-first Century: Disease and Globalization* (New York: Macmillan, 2002).
11. R. J. Sampson, S. W. Raudenbush, and F. Earls, "Neighborhoods and violent crime: A multilevel study of collective efficacy," *Science* 277:5328 (August 15, 1997), 918–24.
12. During the mid-1980s, HIV incidence in U.S. gay men fell by about 80

percent. W. Winkelstein, Jr., et al., "The San Francisco Men's Health Study: III. Reduction in human immunodeficiency virus transmission among homosexual/bisexual men, 1982–86," *Am J Public Health* 77:6 (June 1987), 685–9; Martina Morris and Laura Dean, "Effect of sexual behavior change on long-term human immunodeficiency virus prevalence among homosexual men," *Am J Epidemiol* 140:3 (August 1, 1994), 217–32.

13. For more on the discovery of the first cases of AIDS in Uganda, see Hooper, *Slim*.
14. Noerine Kaleeba, *We Miss You All* (Harare, Zimbabwe: SAFAIDS, 2002).
15. "AIDS War Begins," *New Vision*, October 3, 1986.
16. Samuel I. Okware, "Towards a national AIDS program in Uganda," *Western J Med* 147 (1987), 726–9; Paul Kaagwa, head, Health Education Section, Ministry of Health, Kampala, Uganda, interview, September 21, 2004; Gary Slutkin, former WHO/GPA representative for East Africa, interview, August 13, 2004; Green et al., "Uganda's HIV Prevention Success"; Slutkin et al., "How Uganda reversed."
17. Eckhard Breitinger, "Popular urban theatre in Uganda: Between self-help and self-enrichment," *New Theat Q* 8:31 (1992), 270–90.
18. See Maryinez Lyons, "The Point of View: Perspectives on AIDS in Uganda," in *AIDS in Africa and the Caribbean*, ed. George Bond et al. (Boulder, Colo.: Westview Press, 1997).
19. See *Keeping the Promise: An Agenda for Action on Women and AIDS* (Geneva: UNAIDS, 2004).
20. Miria Matembe, *Gender, Politics and Constitution Making in Uganda* (Kampala: Fountain Publishers, 2002); Aili Marie Tripp, *Women and Politics in Uganda* (Oxford: James Curry, 2000); Sylvia Tamale, *When Hens Begin to Crow: Gender and Parliamentary Politics in Uganda* (Kampala: Fountain Publishers, 1999); Tripp and Joy Kwesiga, eds., *The Women's Movement in Uganda: History, Challenges and Prospects* (Kampala: Fountain Publishers, 2002); and Maxine Ankrah, interview, February 6, 2006, Kampala, Uganda.
21. Tripp, *Women and Politics*.
22. Matembe, *Gender, Politics*; Tamale, *When Hens Begin to Crow*.
23. Harare: SAFAIDS, 2000.
24. Kaleeba et al., "Participatory evaluation of counselling, medical and social services of The AIDS Support Organization (TASO) in Uganda," *AIDS CARE* 9:1 (February 1997), 13–26.
25. Beatrice Were, "The Destructive Strings of U.S. Aid," *International Herald Tribune*, December 15, 2005.
26. Slutkin, personal communication, July 2006.
27. However, Botswana's businesses and other institutions were well aware of the threat the disease posed. In the early 1990s, a negative HIV test was

required of those seeking bank loans or certain civil-service jobs. For background on one such case, see *Sarah Diau v Botswana Building Society*, Case No. IC 50/2003, Industrial Court of Botswana, Gaborone, 2003.

28. Low-Beer, "Going Face to Face with AIDS," *Financial Times*, November 28, 2003.
29. Busisiwe Ncama, Ph.D. thesis, University of KwaZulu-Natal School of Nursing, 2005.

CHAPTER TEN: FORENSIC SCIENCE

1. *Sexual Behavior Change in Response to HIV: Where Have the Theories Taken US?* (Geneva: UNAIDS, 1999).
2. See John P. Elder, *Behavior Change and Public Health in the Developing World* (Thousand Oaks, Calif.: Sage Publications, 2001), and references therein.
3. See, for example, Ruth Bessinger, Priscilla Akwara, and Daniel T. Halperin, *Sexual Behavior, HIV, and Fertility Trends: A Comparative Analysis of Six Countries; Phase I of the ABC Study* (Measure Evaluation, 2003), at http://www.cpc.unc.edu/measure/publications/special/abc.pdf (accessed June 22, 2004); Joint United Nations Programme on HIV/AIDS (UNAIDS), "A measure of success in Uganda: The value of monitoring both HIV prevalence and sexual behaviour" (Geneva: UNAIDS, May 1998) (UNAIDS Case Study, UNAIDS Best Practice Collection—UNAIDS, August 1998); G. Asiimwe-Okiror et al., "Change in sexual behaviour and decline in HIV infection among young pregnant women in urban Uganda," *AIDS* 11:14 (November 15, 1997), 1757–63; Slutkin et al., "How Uganda reversed," 351–60.
4. "HIV/AIDS Surveillance Report; March 1995," STD/AIDS Control Programme, Ministry of Health, Entebbe, Uganda; referred to in Joshua Musinguzi et al., "Results of population-based KAPBP surveys on HIV/AIDS and STDs in four districts in Uganda," STD/AIDS Control Programme, Ministry of Health, Uganda, October 1996.
5. Asiimwe-Okiror et al., "Change in sexual behaviour."
6. Martha Ainsworth and Mead Over, *Confronting AIDS: Public Priorities in a Global Epidemic* (Washington, D.C.: World Bank, 1997); "HIV/AIDS: Observations on USAID and UN Prevention Efforts," statement for the record by Benjamin F. Nelson, director, International Relations and Trade Issues, National Security and International Affairs Division (Washington, D.C.: U.S. General Accounting Office), September 16, 1998; Norman Hearst and Sammy Chen, "Condom promotion for AIDS prevention in the developing world: Is it working?" *Stud Family Plann* 35:1 (March 2004), 39–47.

7. "HIV prevalence and condom sales in Kenya, Botswana, and Cameroon," PSI/AIDSMark presentation at USAID, 2002.
8. Gilgen et al., "Natural History"; Hearst and Chen, "Condom promotion."
9. S. J. Forster and K. E. Furley, "1988 public awareness survey on AIDS and condoms in Uganda," *AIDS* 3:3 (March 1989), 147–54; Tom Barton, "Epidemics and Behaviours: A Review of Changes in Ugandan Sexual Behavior in the Early 1990s," unpublished report for UNAIDS, Geneva, 1997; Joshua Musinguzi et al., "Results of population-based KAPBP surveys on HIV/AIDS and STDs in four districts in Uganda," STD/AIDS Control Programme, Ministry of Health, Uganda, October 1996; Uganda Demographic and Health Survey 1995. Uganda Ministry of Health. Kampala, Uganda: Ministry of Health. Calverton, MD: Macro International Inc; Edward C. Green, unpublished trip report for World Learning Inc. Washington DC, April 18–25, 1993 and "Report on the situation of AIDS and the role of IEC in Uganda" unpublished report for the World Bank December 15, 1998.
10. Bessinger, Akwara, and Halperin, *Sexual Behavior*.
11. Barbara de Zalduondo, UNAIDS, interview March 16, 2006.
12. S. J. Forster and K. E. Furley, "1988 public awareness survey on AIDS and condoms in Uganda," *AIDS* 3:3 (March 1989), 147–54; Maryinez Lyons, "The Point of View."
13. For a review of these studies, see Daniel Low-Beer and Rand Stoneburner, "AIDS communications through social networks: Catalyst for behavior changes in Uganda," *Afr AIDS Research* 3:1 (2004), 1–13; and Tom Barton, "Epidemics and Behaviours: A Review of Changes in Ugandan Sexual Behavior in the Early 1990s," unpublished report for UNAIDS, Geneva, 1997.
14. Saifuddin Ahmed et al., "HIV incidence and sexually transmitted disease prevalence associated with condom use: a population study in Rakai, Uganda," *AIDS* 15:16 (November 9, 2001), 2171–9.
15. See for example, Janice Hogle et al., "What happened in Uganda? Declining HIV prevalance, behavior change, and the national response," Synergy Project, USAID, 2002; Low-Beer and Stoneburner, "Behaviour and communication change in reducing HIV: Is Uganda unique?" *Afr AIDS Research* 2:1 (May 2003), 9–21 (13); S. Gregson et al., "HIV decline associated with behavior change in eastern Zimbabwe," *Science* 311:5761 (February 3, 2006), 664–6; B. Cheluget et al., "Evidence for population level declines in adult HIV prevalence in Kenya," *Sex Transm Infect* 82 Suppl 1 (April 2006), i21–6; Warren Winkelstein, Jr., et al., "The San Francisco Men's Health Study: Continued decline in HIV seroconversion rates among homosexual/bisexual men," *Am J Public Health* 78 (November 1988), 1472–4.
16. M. H. Becker and J. G. Joseph, "AIDS and behavioral change to reduce risk:

A review," *Am J Public Health* 78:4 (April 1988), 394–410. For San Francisco, see Warren Winkelstein, Jr., et al., "The San Francisco Men's Health Study: Continued decline in HIV seroconversion rates among homosexual/ bisexual men," *Am J Public Health* 78:11 (November 1988), 1472–4; for New York, see Martina Morris and Laura Dean, "Effect of sexual behavior change on long-term human immunodeficiency virus prevalence among homosexual men," *Am J Epidemiol* 140:3 (August 1, 1994), 217–32. For other U.S. cities, see Raoul Coutinho et al., "Effects of preventative efforts among homosexual men," *AIDS* 3 Suppl 1 (1989), S53–S56, and references therein.

17. In 2005, various U.S. newspapers suggested that increased condom use and the death of AIDS patients were the main reasons for the decline in HIV infection rates in Uganda. See Lawrence K. Altman, "Study Challenges Abstinence as Crucial to AIDS Strategy," *New York Times*, February 24, 2005; and David Brown, "Uganda's AIDS Decline Attributed to Deaths," *Washington Post*, February 24, 2005.

These news reports were based on a study from the Rakai district of southern Uganda that had been under way for more than a decade. The reports on the study were misleading for several reasons. First, although AIDS certainly increased death rates in Uganda, it has done so throughout eastern and southern Africa. However, HIV rates in Uganda fell by 75 percent in the 1990s but rose or stabilized everywhere else. The HIV epidemic in Zimbabwe, Zambia, and Malawi began only a year or two after Uganda's. If deaths from AIDS were the main reason for Uganda's decline, huge declines in HIV infection rates similar to Uganda's should have occurred in these countries by the late 1990s. However, in 2004, HIV rates in these countries were three to five times higher than they were in Uganda, and had fallen very little, if at all, in the previous decade.

Because HIV infection has no cure, deaths need to occur for HIV prevalence to decline. What happened in Uganda (but not elsewhere) is that sexual behavior changed, so that when people died of AIDS, they were not replaced by an equal number of newly infected people. In other countries, there has been very little prevalence decline, despite a great many deaths. See also Albert H. D. Kilian et al., "Reductions in risk behaviour provide the most consistent explanation for declining HIV-1 prevalence in Uganda," *AIDS* 13:3 (1999), 391–8.

Although increased condom use probably did contribute to the decline of HIV infection rates in Uganda, it is unlikely to have been the main reason for this success. The survey of sexual behavior in Rakai district referred to in Brown's and Altman's articles was conducted between 1994 and 2003. However, there appears to have been significant behavior change in Rakai and throughout southern Uganda before 1994, which the study described in the news articles did not measure. According to scientific reports on the Rakai project (see references below), HIV rates in Rakai fell rapidly between 1990 and 1996, and much more slowly, if at all, thereafter. In 1990, the HIV prevalence rate in Rakai trading centers was around 23 percent. In 1996, it was around 16 percent. In 2004, after a decade of steeply rising condom use, it was around 14 percent. In 1996, when the decline in HIV prevalence was well under way, only 12 percent of people surveyed in Rakai had used a condom in the six months preceding the survey. Thus it is unclear how it is possible to claim that condoms were the main reason for the decline in infection rates that occurred before 1996. Nor was death, or abstinence, for that matter. See Maria J. Wawer et al., "Dynamics of spread of HIV-1 infection in a rural district of Uganda," *BMJ* 305 (November 23, 1991), 1303–6; and Wawer et al., "Control of sexually transmitted diseases for AIDS prevention in Uganda: A randomised community trial, Rakai Project Study Group," *Lancet* 353:9152 (February 13, 1999), 525–35.

Consistent with the findings of Low-Beer and Stoneburner, focus groups conducted in Rakai itself during the 1980s and early 1990s found that Zero Grazing and "sticking to one" were the most commonly reported responses to the question "What are you doing to protect yourself from HIV?" See, for example, Joseph K. Konde-Lule et al., "Focus group interviews about AIDS in Rakai district of Uganda," *Soc Sci Med* 37:5 (September 1993), 679–84; Forster and Furley, "1988 public awareness survey."

18. See, for example, Global HIV Prevention Working Group, "New Approaches to HIV Prevention Accelerating Research and Ensuring Future Access," August 2006, and "HIV Prevention in the Era of Expanded Treatment Access," June 2004; "Global Mobilization for HIV Prevention: A Blueprint for Action" (Seattle: Bill and Melinda Gates Foundation, July 2002); Department of Health, South Africa, "HIV/AIDS Strategic Plan for South Africa, 2000–2005," Cape Town, May 2000; Eliott Marseille et al., "The Cost-Effectiveness of HIV Prevention in Developing Countries," Leadership Forum on HIV Prevention, June 22, 2001, Henry J. Kaiser Family Foundation; UNAIDS, "Learning and teaching about AIDS in school," technical update, October 1997; "Guide to the strategic planning process for a national response to HIV/AIDS," UNAIDS, Geneva 1998; Ainsworth and Over, *Confronting AIDS: The World Health Report 2004: Changing History* (Geneva: The World Health Organization, 2004); U.S. Bureau of the Census, Health Studies Branch, "The Status and Trends of the HIV/AIDS Epidemic in the World (2002)" (Washington, D.C.: U.S. Department of Commerce, 2002), http://www.mapnetwork.org.
19. J. D. Shelton et al., "Partner reduction is crucial for balanced 'ABC' approach to HIV prevention," *BMJ* 328:7444 (April 10, 2004), 891–3.

20. The following reports were commissioned by UNAIDS but never made public: Barton, "Epidemics and Behaviours"; "Making condoms work for HIV prevention," unpublished Best Practice Collection report, UNAIDS Geneva, 2004; Hearst and Chen, "Condom promotion" (original report commissioned by UNAIDS, but published independently by the authors). The following reports were commissioned by the World Health Organization's Global Program on AIDS but never made public: Maxine Ankrah et al., "AIDS in Uganda: Analysis of the Social Dimensions of the Epidemic," National Survey, September–December 1989 (Kampala: Makerere University, May 1993); Stoneburner and Manuel Carballo, "Emerging Patterns of HIV Incidence in Uganda and Other East African Countries," International Centre for Migration and Health, May 1997; Joshua Musinguzi et al., "Results of population-based KAPBP surveys on HIV/AIDS and STDs in four districts in Uganda," STD/AIDS Control Programme, Ministry of Health, Uganda, October 1996.
21. Slutkin et al., "How Uganda reversed"; "SADC Expert Think Tank Meeting on HIV Prevention in High-Prevalence Countries in Southern Africa," Maseru, Lesotho, May 10–12, 2006.
22. Lori Heise and Christopher Elias, "Transforming AIDS prevention to meet women's needs: A focus on developing countries," *Soc Sci Med* 40:7 (April 1995), 931–43; Janet Fleischman, "Beyond 'ABC' Helping Women Fight AIDS," *Washington Post*, June 29, 2004.
23. K. L. Dunkle et al., "Prevalence and patterns of gender-based violence and revictimization among women attending antenatal clinics in Soweto, South Africa," *Am J Epidemiol* 160:3 (August 1, 2004), 230–9; Dunkle et al., "Gender-based violence, relationship power, and risk of HIV infection in women attending antenatal clinics in South Africa," *Lancet* 363:9419 (May 1, 2004), 1415–21; M. A. Koenig et al., "Domestic violence in rural Uganda: Evidence from a community-based study," *Bulletin of World Health Organ* 81:1 (2003), 53–60; Barton, "Epidemics and Behaviours"; J. Lugalla et al., "Social, cultural and sexual behavioral determinants of observed decline in HIV infection trends: Lessons from the Kagera Region, Tanzania," *Soc Sci Med* 59:1 (July 2004), 185–98.
24. Stoneburner and Low-Beer, "Population-Level HIV declines and behavioral risk avoidance in Uganda," *Science* 304:5671 (April 30, 2004), 714–18; Anne Case and Helen Epstein, unpublished; see also Musinguzi et al., "Results."
25. E-mail exchange between myself and Michel Carael, October 12–15, 2005.
26. Westport, Conn.: Praeger.
27. S. J. Forster and K. E. Furley, "1988 public awareness survey on AIDS and condoms in Uganda," *AIDS* 3:3 (March 1989), 147–54; Tom Barton,

"Epidemics and Behaviours: A Review of Changes in Ugandan Sexual Behavior in the Early 1990s," unpublished report for UNAIDS, Geneva, 1997; Joshua Musinguzi et al., "Results of population-based KAPBP surveys on HIV/AIDS and STDs in four districts in Uganda," STD/AIDS Control Programme, Ministry of Health, Uganda, October 1996; Uganda Demographic and Health Survey 1995. Uganda Ministry of Health. Kampala, Uganda: Ministry of Health. Calverton, MD: Macro International Inc; Edward C Green, unpublished trip report for World Learning Inc. Washington DC, April 18–25, 1993 and "Report on the situation of AIDS and the role of IEC in Uganda" unpublished report for the World Bank December 15, 1998.

28. PBS, *NOW*, transcript of November 4, 2005, broadcast, presented by David Brancaccio.
29. A 2002 U.S. Bureau of the Census report endorsed by UNAIDS stated that condoms had been responsible for Uganda's HIV decline, and warned against the introduction "of the language of 'fidelity' and 'faithfulness,'" which the authors considered moralizing. In its 2005 AIDS Epidemic Update, UNAIDS again attributed Uganda's decline to condom use, citing a study of sexual-behavior change between 1994 and 2003—years after the decline in infection rates actually began. Finally, in 2006, UNAIDS documents began to recommend that the reduction of multiple sexual partnerships should be a key goal for AIDS prevention programs in southern Africa. See U.S. Bureau of the Census, Health Studies Branch, "Status and Trends"; UNAIDS/WHO, "AIDS Epidemic Update: December 2005 Special Section on HIV Prevention," Geneva, December 2005; "SADC Expert Think Tank."
30. T. Allen, "AIDS and evidence: Interrogating some Ugandan myths," *J Biosoc Sci* 38:1 (January 2006), 7–28; J. O. Parkhurst, "The Ugandan success story? Evidence and claims of HIV-1 prevention," *Lancet* 360:9326 (July 6, 2002), 78–80; "A measure of success in Uganda: The value of monitoring both HIV prevalence and sexual behaviour" (Geneva: UNAIDS, May 1998) (UNAIDS Case Study, UNAIDS Best Practice Collection—UNAIDS, August 1998).
31. Bessinger, Akwara, and Halperin, *Sexual Behavior*; W. L. Kirungi et al., "Trends in antenatal HIV prevalence in urban Uganda associated with uptake of preventive sexual behaviour," *Sex Transm Infect* 82 Suppl 1 (April 2006), i36–41.
32. E. L. Korenromp et al., "HIV dynamics and behaviour change as determinants of the impact of sexually transmitted disease treatment on HIV transmission in the context of the Rakai trial," *AIDS* 16:16 (November 8, 2002), 2209–18; Ronald Gray et al., "Uganda's HIV prevention success."
33. C. Mulanga et al., "Political and socioeconomic instability: How does it affect HIV? A case study in the Democratic Republic of Congo," *AIDS* 18:5

(March 26, 2004), 832–4. In any case, after 1979, the Ugandan civil war mainly affected Luweero district, north of Kampala, whereas the epidemic started, and remained most severe, in the southern districts of Rakai, Masaka, and Kampala.

34. Adriana Petryna, *Life Exposed: Biological Citizens After Chernobyl* (Princeton: Princeton University Press, 2002).

CHAPTER ELEVEN: GOD AND THE FIGHT AGAINST AIDS

1. See Greg Behrman, *The Invisible People: How the US Has Slept Through the Global AIDS Pandemic, the Greatest Humanitarian Catastrophe of Our Time* (New York: Free Press, 2004).
2. T. Yamamori, D. Dageforde, and T. Bruner, eds., *The Hope Factor: Engaging the Church in the HIV/AIDS Crisis* (Waynesboro, Ga.: Authentic Media, 2003), 250.
3. Ibid., 194.
4. Debra Hauser, "Five Years of Abstinence-Only-Until-Marriage Education: Assessing the Impact" (Washington, D.C.: Advocates for Youth, 2004).
5. See Health and Development Networks, "Condom U-Turn Puts Many Young Ugandans at Risk," May 26, 2004; Human Rights Watch, "The Less They Know, the Better: Abstinence Only HIV/AIDS Programs in Uganda," March 2005; Center for Health and Gender Equity, "Where Is the 'C' in ABC: Implications of U.S. Global AIDS Policy and Funding for HIV Prevention in PEPFAR Focus Countries," March 2005; Thomas J. Coates, "Science vs. Assumption in Public Health Policy: Abstinence Alone Not the Answer," *San Francisco Chronicle*, May 25, 2004; and Esther Kaplan, *With God on Their Side: How Christian Fundamentalists Trampled Science, Policy, and Democracy in George W. Bush's White House* (New York: New Press, 2004).
6. Janice Hogle et al., in "What Happened in Uganda? Declining HIV Prevalence, Behavior Change and the National Response" (USAID, 2002).
7. "RE: Global AIDS Senate Bill," memo from Janet Museveni, First Lady of Uganda, to Richard Lugar, chair of the U.S. Senate Foreign Relations Committee, April 2, 2003.
8. Edward C. Green, "Trip report for World Learning Inc., Subcontractor for USAID; Kampala, Uganda, April 18–25, 1993," unpublished; Edward C. Green, "Report on the Situation of AIDS and the Role of IEC In Uganda," trip report for World Bank, December 15, 1998. See also Barton, "Epidemics and Behaviours"; UNAIDS, "Making Condoms Work for HIV Prevention," unpublished best practice collection report for UNAIDS, 2004; Stoneburner and Carballo, "Emerging Patterns"; Musinguzi et al., "Results of population-based KAPBP."

9. Bessinger, Akwara, and Halperin, *Sexual Behavior.*
10. Even by year. Virtually the same number of fifteen- , sixteen- , seventeen- , eighteen- , and nineteen-year-olds became pregnant in 1988 as in 1995, a period when HIV rates in the same group of pregnant girls fell by nearly half. Teenage pregnancy rates did fall significantly between 1995 and 2001, but the use of modern contraceptives, including condoms, nearly tripled during this time, so it is difficult to attribute this to abstinence alone.
11. P. A. Mardh et al., "Correlation between an early sexual debut, and reproductive health and behavioral factors: A multinational European study," *Eur J Contracept Reprod Health Care* 5:3 (September 5, 2000), 177–82.
12. Sam Okware et al., "Revisiting the ABC strategy: HIV prevention in Uganda in the era of anti-retroviral therapy." *Postgradu Med J* 81 (2005), 625–8.
13. Speech given at "AIDS Care in Africa: The Way Forward," meeting sponsored by the Rockefeller Foundation, Kampala, Uganda, April 19–21, 2001.
14. Michael Tuck, "Syphilis, Sexuality, and Social Control: A History of Venereal Disease in Colonial Uganda," Ph.D. diss., Northwestern University, 1997.
15. On Museveni's undemocratic tendencies, see Will Ross, "Museveni: Uganda's Fallen Angel," *BBC News Online*, November 30, 2005.
16. Tamale, *When Hens Begin to Crow.*
17. M. Gysels et al., "The adventures of the Randy Professor and Angela the Sugar Mummy: Sex in fictional serials in Ugandan popular magazines, *AIDS Care* 17:8 (2005), 967–77.
18. Martin Ssempa, "From vaginal monologue to intellectual dialogue," *New Vision* online bulletin board, February 24, 2005, http://www.allergodil.dk/B/detail.php?limit=28&bulletinId=395&bulletinCategoryId=5, accessed March 2, 2005. See also Andrew Rice, "Evangelicals vs. Muslims in Africa: Enemy's Enemy," *New Republic*, August 9, 2004; and Human Rights Watch, "The Less They Know."
19. Maria Wawer et al., "HIV prevalence decline in Uganda: Evidence from Rakai, Uganda," presentation at the 12th annual conference on Retroviruses and Opportunistic Infections, Boston, February 22–25, 2005; Ruth Bessinger, personal communication, August 12, 2005.
20. Emily Bass, "Fighting to close the condom gap in Uganda," *Lancet* 365:9465 (March 26–April 1, 2005), 1127–8.
21. See Priya Abraham, "Hooked on Failure," *World*, November 6, 2004; and Candi Cushman, "Burying the Truth," *Citizen*, March 2005.
22. S. J. Forster and K. K. Furley, "1988 public awareness survey on AIDS and condoms in Uganda," *AIDS* 3 (March 1989), 147–54; Gary Slutkin et al., "How Uganda reversed"; Okware, "Towards a national AIDS program in Uganda," *Western Med* 147 (1987), 726–9; Maryinez Lyons, "The Point of View."

23. Some of the money for Mrs. Museveni's program was channeled through the Children's AIDS Fund, or CAF, a U.S. organization run by friends of President Bush. In November 2004, CAF was awarded U.S. government funding, even though the grant proposal it submitted to USAID was deemed "unfit" by a review panel. USAID administrator Andrew Natsios argued that CAF had ties with Janet Museveni's Uganda Youth Forum, "a pioneer in abstinence and be faithful messages," and should therefore be given special consideration. Randall Tobias, the U.S. global AIDS coordinator, apparently agreed. CAF was formerly known as Americans for a Sound AIDS Policy. In the 1990s, it lobbied to increase federal funding for abstinence-only-until-marriage programs, and against extending Americans with Disabilities Act protection for people with HIV. The disbursement of funds under PEPFAR is disturbingly opaque. According to the Center for Health and Gender Equity, an organization that tracks U.S. government spending on reproductive health, millions of dollars disbursed so far have not been publicly accounted for, in addition to that promised to CAF. See David Brown, "Group Awarded AIDS Grant Despite Negative Appraisal," *Washington Post*, February 16, 2005, A17.
24. Human Rights Watch, "The Less They Know."
25. In 2005, USAID began funding pilot "faithfulness" campaigns in Africa, such as Swaziland's "I choose to be faithful to my family" and Uganda's "Be a Man." It remains to be seen whether this will have more success.
26. Suzanne Leclerc-Madlala, "Potecting Girlhood? Virginity Revivals in the Era of AIDS," *Agenda* 56 (2003), 16–25.
27. Thanks to Alex Coutinho of the AIDS Support Organization in Uganda for discussions on this point.
28. On April 13, 2005, Pastor Martin Ssempa of Uganda addressed a hearing before the House Committee on International Relations on PEPFAR. He urged lawmakers to reduce funds for condom social marketing in favor of faith-based organizations, such as his own, that promote abstinence-only sex education. I would like to correct, for the record, some statements he made in response to questions posed by Representative Betty McCollum that concerned a version of this chapter that appeared in the April 28, 2005, issue of *The New York Review of Books.*

    My article (and this chapter) describes how Pastor Ssempa set fire to a box of condoms belonging to some students at Makerere University in Uganda, and suggests he did so to discourage young people from using condoms.

    When Representative McCollum asked Pastor Ssempa whether he had in fact burned the students' condoms, he admitted that he had. But he also said that my article was "full of misrepresentation." He then claimed that the government of Uganda had banned that particular brand of condoms—known as Engabu—a few days before and had ordered their destruction because they were defective and posed a significant risk to the public.

This is not the case. In August 2004, the government of Uganda had received complaints that some lots of Engabu condoms smelled bad, and by early September an investigation was under way. The condom-burning incident took place during freshman orientation week, in mid-September 2004. On October 4, some three weeks later, the government issued a statement reassuring the public that Engabu condoms were safe. Then, on October 19, the government announced that tests carried out in Sweden showed that some lots of Engabu contained too much sulfur, hence the smell, and all Engabu condoms were recalled.

At the time of the condom-burning incident, the government had not issued any warning about Engabu condoms, thus it is hard to believe that this was Ssempa's sole motivation for burning them, as he contended in the congressional hearing. Nor did Ssempa advise the students to use one of the two other condom brands available in Uganda at the time, about which there had been no complaints.

Further details of the incident may help clarify Pastor Ssempa's intentions when he burned the condoms. I was not present during the incident itself, but Pastor Ssempa referred to it in his sermon the following Sunday, and I discussed it afterward with some of the students who witnessed it. In an interview with me some days earlier, Pastor Ssempa had already made clear his loathing for condoms, condom social marketing, and, in particular, the condom social-marketing activities of the organization Population Services International. I therefore assumed his motivation for burning the condoms was part of a general antipathy toward that method of HIV prevention. This seemed to be the impression of the students as well.

One student from Ssempa's congregation explained to me that the condoms Ssempa burned had been placed in front of a scrap-metal statue called Gongom, built many years ago to honor the memory of a student who had been killed by the soldiers of the former dictator, Idi Amin. Gongom had since become the official mascot of Lumumba Hall, a men's dormitory. Lumumba men were known to be rowdy and liked to carry on affairs with girls in the dorm next door. The girls' dorm also has a statue, known as Gongomez, and at parties Gongom and Gongomez would be brought together. Gongom would be dressed in a condom, and a box of free condoms would be placed at its feet for the students. Some students saw this as a form of safe-sex education, but born-again Christians saw Gongom as a "spirit who brings death," I was told. "Every year, except the last two, someone has died in Lumumba," the student I spoke to explained. "Blood has to be shed because a demon has entered the statue."

The student explained that the new dorm representative of Lumumba Hall was a born-again Christian. He had given a Bible to Gongom, indicating that the statue had been "saved from the demon."

When Pastor Ssempa and the born-again Christian students found Gongom wearing a condom, it came as a shock: "Pastor Ssempa started shouting about the condoms." In retort, the non-Christian students started singing their anthem, "KaliKayai!" a song about street urchins, mischief, and crime. But then Ssempa started singing too: "Now I am *saved*! I used to steal!" The born-again Christian students sang along with him, and urged him to burn the condoms.

Lumumba Hall has a "culture committee" that guards Gongom, and some of its members soon arrived. "They were very drunk. 'How can you burn that! This is our culture!'" they said. They tried to prevent Ssempa from burning the condoms, but because most of them were freshmen and there were relatively few of them, they were unable to do so.

The condom-burning incident seems to have erupted during a struggle between born-again and non-born-again students over the soul of Gongom, not as a measure to prevent the circulation of defective condoms.

CHAPTER TWELVE: WHEN FOREIGN AID IS AN ATM

1. Jude Luggya and Peter Nyanzi, "VP's NGO Cited in Global Fund Scam," *Monitor* (Kampala), March 28, 2006; James Ogoola et al., "The Report of the Judicial Commission of Inquiry into the Mismanagement of the Global Fund," report submitted to the President of Uganda, May 30, 2006; Bernard Rivers, "Ugandan Official Inquiry Condemns Minister," *Global Fund Observer* 60 (June 29, 2006).
2. See also Joseph Tumushabe, "The Politics of HIV/AIDS in Uganda" (draft) (Geneva: UNRISD, 2005).
3. Nyanzi and Luggya, "Will Muhwezi Survive Again?" *Monitor Weekly* (Kampala), March 26–April 1, 2006.
4. "AIDS Awareness Is Growing," *New Vision*, December 11, 1991.
5. Ritva Reinikka and Paul Collier, *Uganda's Recovery: The Role of Farms, Firms, and Government* (Washington, D.C.: The World Bank, 2001).
6. See, for example, Ndyakira Amooti, "Is AIDS Commission Future in Balance?" *New Vision*, March 2, 1993.
7. New York: Penguin Press, 2006.
8. Patrick Chabal and Jean-Pascal Daloz, *Africa Works: Disorder As Political Instrument* (Bloomington: Indiana University Press, 1999); Stephen Ellis, *The Criminalization of the State in Africa* (Bloomington: Indiana University Press, 1999).

9. It should also be noted that in Uganda, it was local activists who blew the whistle when they discovered that Global Fund money was being misused. They are part of a growing indigenous social movement across the continent, from Kenya to South Africa, that is deeply concerned with the threat corruption poses to the future of the continent. See, for example, Michela Wrong, "NS Profile—John Githongo," *New Statesman*, February 6, 2006.
10. Editorial, "How Aids Money Is 'Eaten,'" *Daily Nation* (Nairobi), August 3, 2005.
11. Noel Sichalwe, "Bulaya Put On His Defence," *Post* (Lusaka), April 19, 2006.
12. "Global Fund Suspends HIV/AIDS Grants to Nigeria," *Kaiser Network Daily HIV/AIDS Report*, May 2, 2006.

CHAPTER THIRTEEN: THE LOST CHILDREN OF AIDS

1. S. Gregson et al., "HIV infection and reproductive health in teenage women orphaned and made vulnerable by AIDS in Zimbabwe," *AIDS Care* 17:7 (October 2005), 785–94; Megan Dunbar et al., unpublished study; Frances Cowan et al., unpublished study.
2. See "Africa's Orphaned Generations" (New York: UNICEF, 2003); Jonathan Cohen, "Letting Them Fail: Government Neglect and the Right to Education for Children Affected by AIDS," *Human Rights Watch* 17:13(A) (October 2005); Takashi Yamano and T. S. Jayne, "Working-age adult mortality and primary school attendance in rural Kenya," *Econ Dev Cult Change* 53:3 (2005), 619–54; Anne Case and Cally Ardington, "The impact of parental death on school enrollment and achievement: Longitudinal evidence from South Africa," *Demography* 43:3 (August 2006), 401–20; David Evans and Edward A. Miguel, "Orphans and Schooling in Africa: A Longitudinal Analysis," unpublished manuscript, March 1, 2005; and Martha Ainsworth, Kathleen Beegle, and Godlike Koda, "The impact of adult mortality and parental deaths on primary schooling in North-Western Tanzania," *J Dev Stud* 41:3 (April 2005), 413–15.
3. Curt Tarnoff and Larry Nowels, "Foreign Aid: An Introductory Overview of U.S. Programs and Policy," Congressional Research Service, Library of Congress, updated January 19, 2005.
4. See Cohen, "Letting Them Fail."
5. Some treatment programs are reaching fewer people than was originally hoped. The dire state of African clinics and hospitals is part of the problem, but the greed of U.S.-based contractors is also a factor. For example, the Maryland-based Institute of Human Virology proposed to spend $600,000 to hire three consultants to "mentor" South African health workers—an amount that could have been spent on antiretroviral drug treatment for some five hun-

dred poor South Africans. In another example, the North Carolina–based Family Health International proposed to hand over $1 million of a $3 million PEPFAR grant to Northrop Grumman, a military contractor, which would conduct "monitoring and evaluation" of Family Health's orphan programs. Under the terms of the original contract, which was fortunately changed, Family Health International and Northrop Grumman would have each received more than twice as much money as all the orphans combined.

6. See Geoff Foster, "Supporting community efforts to assist orphans in Africa," *NEJM* 346:24 (June 13, 2002), 1907–10.
7. See Case and Ardington, "Parental Death."
8. See Mark Ottenweller, Marion Bunch, and Helen Epstein, "'The Lost Children of AIDS': An Exchange," *New York Review of Books*, December 15, 2005.
9. Although perhaps not as many as the United States claims. See Craig Timberg, "Botswana's Gains Against AIDS Put U.S. Claims to Test," *Washington Post Foreign Service*, July 1, 2005.
10. Ottenweller, "ANCHOR Program in Africa," *Hope Worldwide Newsletter* 2 (2004).
11. See http://land.pwv.gov.za/publications/news/speeches/didiza_telefood_concert_2march02.htm.
12. Colin Bundy, *The Rise and Fall of the South African Peasantry* (Berkeley: University of California Press, 1979).
13. See the Department of Agriculture and Environmental Affairs: KwaZulu-Natal Province, http://agriculture.kzntl.gov.za/dae/index.aspx?ID=4.
14. See Foster, "Bottlenecks and Drip-feeds: Channeling Resources to Communities Responding to Orphans and Vulnerable Children in Southern Africa" (London: Save the Children, June 2005).

CHAPTER FOURTEEN: WARTIME

1. Deborah Posel, "The scandal of manhood: 'Baby rape' and the politicization of sexual violence in post-apartheid South Africa," *Cult Health Sex* 7:3 (May 2005), 239–52(14).
2. South African Native Affairs Commission, 1903, referred to in Karen Jochelson, *The Colour of Disease: Syphilis and Racism in South Africa: 1880–1950* (New York: Palgrave Macmillan, 2001).
3. Rachel Swarns, "Grappling With South Africa's Alarming Increase in the Rapes of Children," *New York Times*, January 29, 2002; Roger Cohen, "Globalist: South Africa's Ghosts Haunt Thinking on HIV," *International Herald Tribune*, November 17, 2004; Allan Little, "AIDS: A South African Horror Story," BBC News, October 14, 2002.

4. Allen Brandt, *No Magic Bullet: A Social History of Venereal Disease in the United States Since 1880* (Oxford: Oxford University Press, 1987).
5. "In a country long sickened by the level of sexual violence, a shocking series of child rapes has stunned South Africa and left people grasping for answers," Integrated Regional Information Network, April 25, 2002; see also R. Jewkes, L. Martin, and L. Penn-Kekana, "The virgin cleansing myth: Cases of child rape are not exotic," *Lancet* 359:711 (February 23, 2002); Linda Richter, Andrew Dawes, and Craig Higson-Smith, eds., *The Sexual Abuse of Young Children in Southern Africa* (Cape Town: HSRC Press, 2004).
6. Niehaus and Jonsson, "Dr. Wouter Basson."
7. Speech of the president of South Africa at the opening session of the 13th International AIDS Conference, Durban, Office of the Presidency, Pretoria, South Africa, July 9, 2000.
8. Carolyn Dempster, "Rape—Silent War on SA Women," BBC News, April 9, 2002; Charlene Smith, "South Africa: A Sexual Lottery of Death," *Le Monde Diplomatique*, October 2005; Lewis, *Race Against Time* (Toronto: House of Anansi Press, 2005).
9. Smith, *Proud of Me*.
10. Adam Ashforth, "Sex and Violence, Soweto Style," paper presented to the CODESRIA L'Histoire Culturelle du Present Workshop on Sexualties, Zanzibar, July 3–5, 1999; Kate Wood, Helen Lambert, and Rachel Jewkes, "'Location love': An ethnography of young people's talk about sexual coercion in a South African township," *Med Anthropol Q*, in press; Catherine MacPhail and Catherine Campbell, "'I think condoms are good but, aai—I hate those things': Condom use among adolescents and young people in a Southern African township," *Soc Sci Med* 52:11 (June 2001), 1613–27.
11. Wood, "Contextualising group rape in post-apartheid South Africa," unpublished manuscript, 2006; Megan Power, "Why Men Rape—The Shocking Truth," *Saturday Star* (South Africa), February 8, 2003.
12. Michael Wines, "Highly Charged Rape Trial Tests South Africa's Ideals," *The New York Times*, April 10, 2006.
13. Smith, *Proud of Me*.
14. Wood, "Contextualising group rape."
15. Susan Brownmiller, *Against Our Will: Men, Women and Rape* (New York: Ballantine Books, 1993).
16. Niehaus, "'Now Everyone Is Doing It': Towards a Social History of Rape in the South African Lowveld," research working paper presented at Sex and Secrecy, a conference of the International Association for the Study of Sexuality, Culture and Society, July 12, 2003.
17. Virginia Van der Vliet, "Traditional Husbands, Modern Wives? Constructing Marriages in a South African Township," in *Tradition and Transition in*

Southern Africa: Festschrift for Philip and Iona Mayer, ed. A. D. Spiegel and P. A. McAllister, African Studies Series, 50th Anniversary Volume, vol. 51, nos. 1 and 2.

18. Wood, "Contextualising group rape."
19. R. Jewkes et al., "Rape perpetration by young, rural South African men: Prevalence, patterns and risk factors," *Soc Sci Med* 63:11 (December 2006), 2949–61.
20. Spiegel, "Polygyny as Myth: Towards Understanding Extramarital Relations in Lesotho," in Spiegel and P.A. McAllister, eds., *Tradition and Transition.*
21. Power, "Why Men Rape."
22. Jewkes, Naeemah Abrahams, and Zodumo Mvo, "Why do nurses abuse patients? Reflections from South African obstetric services," *Soc Sci Med* 47:11 (December 1998), 1781–95.
23. Jewkes, "Non-consensual sex among South African youth: Prevalence of coerced sex and discourses of control and desire," unpublished manuscript.
24. Abrahams and Jewkes, "Effects of South African men's having witnessed abuse of their mothers during childhood on their levels of violence in adulthood," *Am J Public Health* 95:10 (October 2005), 1811–16; J. Stadler, T. Collins, and S. Ngwenya, "Adolescent Sexuality and Reproductive Health in the Northern Province: A Summary of Findings of the Adolescent Health Program" (Acornhoek: Health Systems Trust, 1997).

CHAPTER FIFTEEN: THE UNDERGROUND ECONOMY OF AIDS

1. Linda Mayoux, *Beyond Rhetoric: Women's Empowerment and Micro-enterprise Development* (London and New York: Zed Press, 2001).
2. Mayoux, "Microfinance and women's empowerment: Rethinking 'best practice,'" *Development Bulletin* 57 (February 2002), 76–80.
3. Naila Kabeer, *Reversed Realities: Gender Hierarchies in Development Thought* (New York: Verso, 1994); Helen Epstein and Julia Kim, "Sisters in Health," *New York Review of Books*, January 2007.
4. Nicole Brown, "Promoting Adolescent Livelihoods," a discussion paper prepared for the Commonwealth Youth Forum and UNICEF, 2001.
5. Pádraig Carmody, *Tearing the Social Fabric.*
6. There is some debate about the outlook for India's epidemic. However, most surveys suggest the virus is not widespread in the general population, although it is common among prostitutes and intravenous drug users. R. Kumar et al., "Trends in HIV-1 in young adults in south India from 2000 to 2004: A prevalence study," *Lancet* 367:9517 (April 8, 2006), 1164–72; B. G. Williams et al., "The impact of HIV/AIDS on the control of tuberculosis in India," *P Natl Acad Sci USA* 102:27 (July 5, 2005), 9619–24.

7. "The Social Context of AIDS in Sub-Saharan Africa," *Popul Dev Rev* 15:2 (June 1989), 185–234.
8. Jessica Ogden, "'Producing' Respect: The 'Proper' Woman in Postcolonial Kampala," in *Postcolonial Identities in Africa*, ed. Richard P. Werbner and Terence Ranger (New Jersey: Zed Books, 1996), 165–92.
9. Quoted in Ellen Chesler's introduction to *Where Human Rights Begin: Health, Sexuality and Women in the New Millennium*, ed. Wendy Chavkin and Ellen Chesler (New Brunswick, N.J.: Rutgers University Press, 2005). I thank Julie Kim for help with the following section of this chapter.
10. "The Global Coalition on Women and AIDS, 2005 Progress Report" (Geneva: UNAIDS, 2005); "AIDS in Africa: Three Scenarios to 2025" (Geneva: UNAIDS, 2005).
11. P. M. Pronyk, J. R. Hargreaves, J. C. Kim, et al., "Effect of a social intervention for the prevention of intimate partner violence and HIV in rural South Africa: Results of a cluster randomized trial," *Lancet* 368 (December 1, 2006), 1973–83. For further details of the program implementation, see Paul Pronyk et al., "Integrating microfinance and HIV preventive—perspectives and emerging lessons from rural South Africa, *Small Enterprise Development* 16:3 (Septembe 2005), 26–28; see also www.wits.ac.za/radar/.
12. One of SHAZ's few successful participants was a young woman who used her loan money to help expand her mother's long-established tailoring business. In her case, the loan money helped strengthen family solidarity, but most of the SHAZ participants had been encouraged to start their own businesses, which tended to be far less successful. See "Adolescent Girls' Social Support and Livelihood Program Design Workshop Summary of Notes," Population Council/University of California, San Francisco (Nairobi, March 22–23, 2006). Available online at www.Microlinks.org.

EPILOGUE: TRADITIONAL MEDICINE

1. Craig Timberg, "In Swaziland, 'Secret Lovers' Confronted in Fight Against AIDS," *Washington Post*, October 29, 2006.
2. For more on this, see, for example, Simon Szreter, *Health and Wealth* (Rochester, N.Y.: University of Rochester Press, 2005); Thomas Scalway and James Deane, "Missing the Message: 20 Years of Learning from HIV/ AIDS," Panos Institute briefing document, November 28, 2003; Josef Decosas, "The Social Ecology of AIDS in Africa," UNRISD briefing paper, draft, 2002.
3. Martha Tomes, *The Gospel of Germs: Men, Women, and the Microbe in American Life* (Cambridge, Mass.: Harvard University Press, 1999).
4. John C. Caldwell, "Paths to lower fertility," *BMJ* 319 (October 9, 1999), 985–7; John Cleland and Christopher Wilson, "Demand theories of fertility

and causation: An iconoclastic view," *Population Studies* 41:1 (March 1987), 5–30.

5. J. Bryce, N. Terreri, C. G. Victora et al., "Countdown to 2015: Tracking intervention coverage for child survival," *Lancet* 368:9541 (2006), 1067–68; Richard Horton, "A new discipline is born: Comparative health-systems studies," ibid., 1949–50; N. Walker et al., "Meeting international goals in child survival and HIV/AIDS," *Lancet* 360:9329 (2002), 284–89.
6. David Werner and David Sanders, *Questioning the Solution: The Politics of Primary Health Care and Child Survival* (Palo Alto, Calif.: Healthwrights, 1997).
7. See, for example, Harriet Ngubane, *Body and Mind in Zulu Medicine: An Ethnography of Health and Disease in Nyuswa-Zulu Thought and Practice* (London and New York: Academic Press, 1977).
8. *Ngoma: Discourses of Health and Healing in Central and Southern Africa* (Berkeley: University of California Press, 1992).

APPENDIX: A MAGIC BULLET AFTER ALL?

1. B. G. Williams et al., "The potential impact of male circumcision on HIV in sub-Saharan Africa," *PLoS Med* 3:7 (July 11, 2006), e262; B. Auvert et al., "Randomized, controlled intervention trial of male circumcision for reduction of HIV infection risk: The ANRS 1265 Trial," *PLoS Med* 2:11 (November 2, 2005), e298.
2. Auvert et al., "Randomized, controlled intervention trial"; Donald McNeil, Jr., "Circumcision Halves HIV Risk, U.S. Agency Finds," *New York Times*, December 14, 2006.
3. E. Banks et al., "Female genital mutilation and obstetric outcome: WHO collaborative prospective study in six African countries," *Lancet* 367:9525 (June 3, 2006), 1835–41; L. Almroth et al., "Urogenital complications among girls with genital mutilation: A hospital-based study in Khartoum," *Afr J Reprod Health* 9:2 (August 2005), 118–24; L. Wallis, "When rites are wrong," *Nurs Stand* 20:4 (October 5–11, 2005), 24–6.
4. Sharon Lafraniere, "Circumcision Studied in Africa as AIDS Preventive," *New York Times*, April 28, 2006.
5. Joint Learning Initiative, "Human Resources for Health: Overcoming the Crisis," Global Energy Initiative, Harvard University, 2004.
6. R. F. Baggaley, G. P. Garnett, and N. M. Ferguson, "Modelling the impact of antiretroviral use in resource-poor settings," *PLoS Med* 3:4 (April 2006), e124.
7. Richard Holbrooke, "Sorry, but AIDS Testing Is Critical," *Washington Post*, January 4, 2006, p. A17.
8. G. Slutkin, "Global AIDS 1981–1999: The response," *Int J Tuber Lung Dis*

4:2 Suppl 1 (February 2000), S24–33; D. Low-Beer and R. L. Stoneburner, "Behaviour and communication change in reducing HIV: Is Uganda unique?" *Afr AIDS Research* 2:1 (May 1, 2003), 9–21; G. Kwesigabo et al., "HIV-1 infection prevalence and incidence trends in areas of contrasting levels of infection in the Kagera region, Tanzania, 1987–2000," *J Acq Immun Def Synd* 40:5 (December 15, 2005), 585–91.

9. J. K. Matovu et al., "Voluntary HIV counseling and testing acceptance, sexual risk behavior and HIV incidence in Rakai, Uganda," *AIDS* 19:5 (March 25, 2005), 503–11.
10. Prof. Susan Cotts Watkins, personal communication, January 2005.
11. A. Medley et al., "Rates, barriers and outcomes of HIV serostatus disclosure among women in developing countries: Implications for prevention of mother-to-child transmission programmes," *Bulletin of World Health Organ* 82:4 (April 2004), 299–307; Suzanne Maman and Anne Medley, "Gender Dimensions of HIV Status Disclosure to Sexual Partners: Rates, Barriers and Outcomes," Department of Gender and Women's Health, World Health Organization, Geneva, 2004.
12. Thomas M. Painter et al., "Women's reasons for not participating in follow up visits before starting short course antiretroviral prophylaxis for prevention of mother to child transmission of HIV: Qualitative interview study," *BMJ* 329 (September 2004), 543.
13. Sheri D. Weiser, "Routine HIV testing in Botswana: A population-based study on attitudes, practices, and human rights concerns," *PLoS Med* 3:7 (July 2006), e261.
14. Dr. Purnima Mane, director of UNAIDS for Social Mobilization and Information Department, interviewed by Jackie Judd at the 15th Annual International AIDS Conference, Bangkok, July 16, 2004, http://www.kaisernetwork.org/health_cast/uploaded_files/071604_nm_mane.pdf.
15. Dr. Ward Cates, CEO of Family Health International, PowerPoint presentation, International AIDS Society Conference, Rio de Janeiro, July 2005.
16. R. S. Veazey et al., "Protection of macaques from vaginal SHIV challenge by vaginally delivered inhibitors of virus-cell fusion," *Nature* 438:7064 (November 3, 2005), 99–102.
17. A. Kaler, "'It's some kind of women's empowerment': The ambiguity of the female condom as a marker of female empowerment," *Soc Sci Med* 52:5 (March 2001), 783–96; S. T. Murphy, L. C. Miller, J. Moore, and L. F. Clark, "Preaching to the choir: Preference for female-controlled methods of HIV and sexually transmitted disease prevention," *Am J Public Health* 90:7 (July 2000), 1135–7.
18. Steve Vickers, "Zimbabweans Make Condom Bangles," BBC News, February 10, 2005.

ACKNOWLEDGMENTS

In writing this book, I have relied heavily on the generosity, intellectual and otherwise, of large numbers of people. I am particularly grateful to Daniel Halperin. Until November 2006, Daniel was HIV/AIDS prevention advisor for USAID, where he helped change institutional thinking on AIDS in Africa while negotiating the Bush administration's troubling policies on contraception. He and I have discussed many of the ideas expressed herein, and even our arguments have been an inspiration to me.

A small number of people recognized early on various unique aspects of the African AIDS epidemic. Among them were Martina Morris, Tom Barton, Maxine Ankrah, Rand Stoneburner, Daniel Low-Beer, Ted Green, and Christopher Hudson. I thank them for sharing their insights with me.

I also thank Doug Kirby for many discussions about Uganda; Susan Watkins for her fascinating interpretations of the response to AIDS in Malawi; Rachel Jewkes for unraveling the links between gender violence and HIV; Julia Kim for her help with the description of the IMAGE project in chapter 15; Christopher Obbo for his friendship; Sam Okuonzi for wide-ranging discussions on Africa, public health, and life in general; Stewart Parkinson for his drawings on pages 57–95 and for helpful discussions about concurrency; Bob Grant for looking after me on my first trip to Uganda; Brian G. Williams and Catherine Campbell for their insights into the AIDS crisis in South Africa's mining communities; Cathy Watson of Straight Talk Uganda, Johan Viljoen of the South African Catholic Bishops Conference, and Deborah Posel of the Witwatersrand Institute for Social and Economic Research for their wisdom about the AIDS epidemic; Angus Deaton and Anne Case of Princeton University for many lively conversations; and Jonathan Cohen of the Open Society Institute, Joanne Csete of the Canadian HIV/AIDS Legal Network, and Joe Amon and

Rebecca Schlieffer of Human Rights Watch for their pioneering work on the relationship between AIDS and human rights.

For introducing me to their remarkable work with orphans, I thank Sister Deborah Brycke and Pastor Jonas Balami of the Huyawa orphan program in Bukoba, Tanzania, and Charles Matovu and Gertrude "Bob" Nabbosa of the Kitovu Mobile AIDS and Home Care Project in Masaka, Uganda.

Others who have helped me over the years are too numerous to list, but let me make a start: Martha Ainsworth, Phil Alcabes, Adam Ashforth, Bertran Auvert, Tony Barnett, Bilge Bassani, Michael and Christine Bennish, Joao Biehl, Albina du Boisrouvray, Holly Burkhalter, Wilson Carswell, Lincoln Chein, Ellen Chesler, Ernest Drucker, Siddharth Dube, Megan Dunbar, William Easterly, Lindiwe Farlane, Geoff Garnett, Mary Hallaway, Keith Hansen, Mai Harper, Jacques Holmsey, Rachel King, the late and much-missed Victoria Kipendi, Gideon Kwesigabo, Evan Lieberman, Tafadzwa Mandipaza-Jemwa, Purnima Mane, Preston Marx, Catherine Maternowska, Edward Mbidde, Nicolette Moodie, Gerry Mshana, Aldin Mutembei, Busisiwe Ncama, Sixolile Ngcobo, Peter Nsubuga (both of them), Nancy Padian, Warren Parker, Adriana Petryna, Elizabeth Rapuleng, Bernard Rivers, Alastair Robb, David Ross, the late Joseph Serunjogi, Lindah Sibanda, Gary Slutkin, John Stover, Ann Swidler, Aili Marie Tripp, Leanna Uys, Johannes van Dam, Janneke van de Wijgert, Maria Wawer, Alan Whiteside, David Wilson, Paul Wilson, and countless others cited anonymously and by name in this book.

This book is based on a series of articles written between 1995 and 2006, mostly for *The New York Review of Books*. In 1998, the *Review*'s editor, Bob Silvers, suggested I write a piece for him about the AIDS epidemic in Africa. By then, I had been working on the epidemic for five years and had grown deeply discouraged. The disease had been spreading across the continent for more than a decade, and I had no idea what I could say that was new. However, new energy, new money, and, most important, new ideas were soon to be brought to bear on the crisis, and the timing of Bob's request was highly fortuitous. His editing, legendary in literary circles, not only made me a better writer, but perhaps in some respects a better person too.

This book is dedicated to the memory of my mother, Barbara, who died in 2006. She was Bob Silvers's co-editor at *The New York Review of Books*, and they had worked together since the magazine was founded in 1963. When she was alive, I showed her everything I wrote, and she listened with the patience of a saint to every thought, however foolish or dull, that came into my head. Her influence is everywhere in this book.

The wisdom of my father, Jason, has also been crucial. Right from the start, he suspected that the response to the AIDS epidemic in Africa was at risk of being undermined by the very bureaucracies that had been erected to fight it. After traveling to the continent countless times, reading everything I could about the epidemic, and interviewing hundreds of people, I arrived at the same conclusion.

Darryl Pinckney and James Fenton provided crucial moral support for this project early on; Bill Buford, formerly of *Granta* magazine, introduced me to the rough-and-tumble world of literary quarterlies; and Sarah Richardson of *Discover* magazine, Katherine Bouton, Jerry Marzaroti and Vera Titunik of *The New York Times Magazine*; Ted Genoways of *The Virginia Quarterly Review*; and Nick Goldberg of the *Los Angeles Times* provided helpful advice on articles that formed the early drafts of chapters of this book.

I am also grateful to Jonathan Galassi and Paul Elie of Farrar, Straus and Giroux and Mary Mount of Penguin UK for their editorial comments, and likewise to Sarah Chalfant of the Wylie Agency.

For immensely appreciated financial assistance I thank the John Simon Guggenheim Memorial Foundation; the Center for Health and Wellbeing of the Woodrow Wilson School of Public and International Affairs, Princeton University; and the Open Society Institute.

Finally, I thank Jake, Susie, Sam, Natalie, and Thomas for their good humor and for reminding me that there is more to life than the AIDS epidemic. And extra *matooke* and love for my husband, Peter; if not for him, I would never have had the guts to write this book.

INDEX